WORLD HEALTH STATISTICS 2014

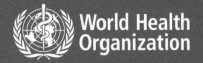

World Health Organization

WHO Library Cataloguing-in-Publication Data

World health statistics 2014.

1.Health status indicators. 2.World health. 3.Health services – statistics. 4.Mortality. 5.Morbidity. 6.Life expectancy. 7.Demography. 9.Statistics. I.World Health Organization.

ISBN 978 92 4 156471 7   (NLM classification: WA 900.1)
ISBN 978 92 4 069267 1 (PDF)

Original cover by WHO Graphics
Layout by designisgood.info
Printed in Italy.

Table of Contents

Abbreviations   7

Introduction   8

Part I. Health-related Millennium Development Goals   11

Summary of status and trends   13

Regional and country charts   20

   1. AARD (%) in under-five mortality rate, 1990–2012   22
   2. Measles immunization coverage among 1-year-olds (%)   23
   3. AARD (%) in maternal mortality ratio, 1990–2013   24
   4. Births attended by skilled health personnel (%)   25
   5. Antenatal care coverage (%): at least one visit and at least four visits   26
   6. Unmet need for family planning (%)   27
   7. AARD (%) in HIV prevalence, 2001–2012   28
   8. Antiretroviral therapy coverage among people eligible for treatment (%)   29
   9. Children aged <5 years sleeping under insecticide-treated nets (%)   30
  10. Children aged <5 years with fever who received treatment with any antimalarial (%)   31
  11. AARD (%) in tuberculosis mortality rate, 1990–2012   32
  12. AARD (%) in proportion of population without access to improved drinking-water sources 33
  13. AARD (%) in proportion of population without access to improved sanitation   34

Part II. Highlighted topics   35

Putting an ending to preventable maternal mortality – the next steps   37

Rising childhood obesity – time to act   40

Life expectancy in the world in 2012   42

Years of life lost due to premature mortality – trends and causes   45

Civil registration and vital statistics –
the key to national and global advancement   50

Part III. Global health indicators   55

General notes   57

1. Life expectancy and mortality   59
Life expectancy at birth (years)
Life expectancy at age 60 (years)
Healthy life expectancy at birth (years)
Neonatal mortality rate (per 1000 live births)
Infant mortality rate (probability of dying by age 1 per 1000 live births)
Under-five mortality rate (probability of dying by age 5 per 1000 live births)
Adult mortality rate (probability of dying between 15 and 60 years of age per 1000 population)

2. Cause-specific mortality and morbidity 71
Mortality
Age-standardized mortality rates by cause (per 100 000 population)
Years of life lost (per 100 000 population)
Number of deaths among children aged < 5 years (000s)
Distribution of causes of death among children aged < 5 years (%)
Maternal mortality ratio (per 100 000 live births)
Cause-specific mortality rate (per 100 000 population)
Morbidity
Incidence rate (per 100 000 population)
Prevalence (per 100 000 population)

3. Selected infectious diseases 93
Cholera
Diphtheria
Human African trypanosomiasis
Japanese encephalitis
Leishmaniasis
Leprosy
Malaria
Measles
Meningitis
Mumps
Pertussis
Poliomyelitis
Congenital rubella syndrome
Rubella
Neonatal tetanus
Total tetanus
Tuberculosis
Yellow fever

4. Health service coverage 104
Unmet need for family planning (%)
Contraceptive prevalence (%)
Antenatal care coverage (%)
Births attended by skilled health personnel (%)
Births by caesarean section (%)
Postnatal care visit within two days of childbirth (%)
Neonates protected at birth against neonatal tetanus (%)
Immunization coverage among 1-year-olds (%)
Children aged 6–59 months who received vitamin A supplementation (%)
Children aged < 5 years with ARI symptoms taken to a health facility (%)
Children aged < 5 years with suspected pneumonia receiving antibiotics (%)
Children aged < 5 years with diarrhoea receiving ORT (ORS and/or RHF) (%)
Children aged < 5 years sleeping under insecticide-treated nets (%)
Children aged < 5 years with fever who received treatment with any antimalarial (%)
Pregnant women with HIV receiving antiretrovirals to prevent MTCT (%)
Antiretroviral therapy coverage among people eligible for treatment (%)
Case-detection rate for all forms of tuberculosis (%)
Treatment-success rate for smear-positive tuberculosis (%)

5. Risk factors

116

Population using improved drinking-water sources (%)
Population using improved sanitation (%)
Population using solid fuels (%)
Preterm birth rate (per 100 live births)
Infants exclusively breastfed for the first 6 months of life (%)
Children aged < 5 years who are wasted (%)
Children aged < 5 years who are stunted (%)
Children aged < 5 years who are underweight (%)
Children aged < 5 years who are overweight (%)
Prevalence of raised fasting blood glucose among adults aged ≥ 25 years (%)
Prevalence of raised blood pressure among adults aged ≥ 25 years (%)
Adults aged ≥ 20 years who are obese (%)
Alcohol consumption among adults aged ≥ 15 years (litres of pure alcohol per person per year)
Prevalence of smoking any tobacco product among adults aged ≥ 15 years (%)
Prevalence of current tobacco use among adolescents aged 13–15 years (%)
Prevalence of condom use by adults aged 15–49 years during higher-risk sex (%)
Population aged 15–24 years with comprehensive correct knowledge of HIV/AIDS (%)

6. Health systems

128

Health workforce
Density of physicians per 10 000 population
Density of nursing and midwifery personnel per 10 000 population
Density of dentistry personnel per 10 000 population
Density of pharmaceutical personnel per 10 000 population
Density of psychiatrists per 10 000 population
Infrastructure and technologies
Hospitals (per 10 000 population)
Hospital beds (per 10 000 population)
Psychiatric beds (per 10 000 population)
Computed tomography units (per million population)
Radiotherapy units (per million population)
Mammography units (per million females aged 50–69 years)
Essential medicines
Median availability of selected generic medicines in public and private sectors (%)
Median consumer price ratio of selected generic medicines in public and private sectors

7. Health expenditure

141

Health expenditure ratios
Total expenditure on health as a percentage of gross domestic product
General government expenditure on health as a percentage of total expenditure on health
Private expenditure on health as a percentage of total expenditure on health
General government expenditure on health as a percentage of total government expenditure
External resources for health as a percentage of total expenditure on health
Social security expenditure on health as a percentage of general government expenditure on health
Out-of-pocket expenditure as a percentage of private expenditure on health
Private prepaid plans as a percentage of private expenditure on health
Per capita health expenditures
Per capita total expenditure on health at average exchange rate (US$)
Per capita total expenditure on health (PPP int. $)
Per capita government expenditure on health at average exchange rate (US$)
Per capita government expenditure on health (PPP int. $)

8. Health inequities   153
Contraceptive prevalence: modern methods (%)
Antenatal care coverage: at least four visits (%)
Births attended by skilled health personnel (%)
DTP3 immunization coverage among 1-year-olds (%)
Children aged < 5 years who are stunted (%)
Under-five mortality rate (probability of dying by age 5 per 1000 live births)

9. Demographic and socioeconomic statistics   165
Total population (000s)
Median age of population (years)
Population aged < 15 years (%)
Population aged > 60 years (%)
Annual population growth rate (%)
Population living in urban areas (%)
Civil registration coverage (%) of births and causes of death
Crude birth rate (per 1000 population)
Crude death rate (per 1000 population)
Total fertility rate (per woman)
Adolescent fertility rate (per 1000 girls aged 15–19 years)
Literacy rate among adults aged ≥ 15 years (%)
Net primary school enrolment rate (%)
Gross national income per capita (PPP int. $)
Population living on < $1 (PPP int. $) a day (%)
Cellular phone subscribers (per 100 population)

Annex 1. Regional and income groupings   176
WHO regional groupings   176
Income groupings   177

Abbreviations

AARD	average annual rate of decline
AFR	WHO African Region
AIDS	acquired immunodeficiency syndrome
AMR	WHO Region of the Americas
ARI	acute respiratory infection
ART	antiretroviral therapy
CRS	Creditor Reporting System
CRVS	civil registration and vital statistics
DAC	Development Assistance Committee, OECD
DHS	Demographic and Health Survey
DTP3	3 doses of diphtheria-tetanus-pertussis vaccine
EML	essential medicines list
EMR	WHO Eastern Mediterranean Region
EUR	WHO European Region
GDP	gross domestic product
GHO	Global Health Observatory
HAI	Health Action International
HALE	healthy life expectancy
HepB3	3 doses of hepatitis B vaccine
Hib3	3 doses of Haemophilus influenzae type B vaccine
HIV	human immunodeficiency virus
ICD	International Classification of Diseases
ICPD+5	International Conference on Population and Development, five-year follow-up
IGME	Inter-agency Group for Child Mortality Estimation
ITU	United Nations International Telecommunication Union
MCV	measles-containing vaccine
MDG	Millennium Development Goal
MDR-TB	multi-drug resistant tuberculosis
MICS	Multiple Indicator Cluster Survey
MSH	Management Sciences for Health
MTCT	mother-to-child transmission

NCD	noncommunicable disease
NGO	nongovernmental organization
NHA	national health account
NTD	neglected tropical disease
OECD	Organisation for Economic Cooperation and Development
ORS	oral rehydration salts
ORT	oral rehydration therapy
PPP	Purchasing Power Parity
RHF	recommended home fluids
SAVVY	Sample Registration with Verbal Autopsy
SD	standard deviation
SEAR	WHO South-East Asia Region
UNAIDS	Joint United Nations Programme on HIV/AIDS
UNDESA	United Nations Department of Economic and Social Affairs
UNESCAP	United Nations Economic and Social Commission for Asia and the Pacific
UNESCO	United Nations Educational, Scientific and Cultural Organization
UNICEF	United Nations Children's Fund
WPR	WHO Western Pacific Region
YLL	years of life lost

Introduction

The World Health Statistics series is WHO's annual compilation of health-related data for its 194 Member States, and includes a summary of the progress made towards achieving the health-related Millennium Development Goals (MDGs) and associated targets. This year, it also includes highlight summaries on the ongoing commitment to end preventable maternal deaths; on the need to act now to combat rising levels of childhood obesity; on recent trends in both life expectancy and premature deaths; and on the crucial role of civil registration and vital statistics systems in national and global advancement.

The series is produced by the WHO Department of Health Statistics and Information Systems of the Health Systems and Innovation Cluster. As in previous years, World Health Statistics 2014 has been compiled using publications and databases produced and maintained by WHO technical programmes and regional offices. A number of demographic and socioeconomic statistics have also been derived from databases maintained by a range of other organizations. These include the United Nations Population Division, United Nations International Telecommunication Union (ITU), the United Nations Department of Economic and Social Affairs (UNDESA), the United Nations Educational, Scientific and Cultural Organization (UNESCO), the United Nations Children's Fund (UNICEF) and the World Bank.

Indicators have been included on the basis of their relevance to global public health; the availability and quality of the data; and the reliability and comparability of the resulting estimates. Taken together, these indicators provide a comprehensive summary of the current status of national health and health systems in the following nine areas:

- life expectancy and mortality
- cause-specific mortality and morbidity
- selected infectious diseases
- health service coverage
- risk factors
- health systems
- health expenditure
- health inequities
- demographic and socioeconomic statistics.

The estimates given in this report are derived from multiple sources, depending on each indicator and on the availability and quality of data. In many countries, statistical and health information systems are weak and the underlying empirical data may not be available or may be of poor quality. Every effort has been made to ensure the best use of country-reported data – adjusted where necessary to deal with missing values, to correct for known biases, and to maximize the comparability of the statistics across countries and over time. In addition, statistical modelling and other techniques have been used to fill data gaps.

Because of the weakness of the underlying empirical data in many countries, a number of the indicators presented here are associated with significant uncertainty. It is WHO policy to ensure statistical transparency, and to make available to users the methods of estimation and the margins of uncertainty for relevant indicators. However, to ensure readability while covering such a comprehensive range of health topics, printed versions of the World Health Statistics series do not include the margins of uncertainty which are instead made available through online WHO databases such as the Global Health Observatory.[1]

While every effort has been made to maximize the comparability of the statistics across countries and over time, users are advised that country data may differ in terms of the definitions, data-collection methods,

---

[1] The Global Health Observatory (GHO) is WHO's portal providing access to data and analyses for monitoring the global health situation. See: http://www.who.int/gho/en/, accessed 22 March 2014.

population coverage and estimation methods used. More-detailed information on indicator metadata is available in the WHO Indicator and Measurement Registry.[1]

WHO presents *World Health Statistics 2014* as an integral part of its ongoing efforts to provide enhanced access to comparable high-quality statistics on core measures of population health and national health systems. Unless otherwise stated, all estimates have been cleared following consultation with Member States and are published here as official WHO figures. However, these best estimates have been derived using standard categories and methods to enhance their cross-national comparability. As a result, they should not be regarded as the nationally endorsed statistics of Member States which may have been derived using alternative methodologies.

---

[1] See: http://www.who.int/gho/indicator_registry/en/, accessed 22 March 2014.

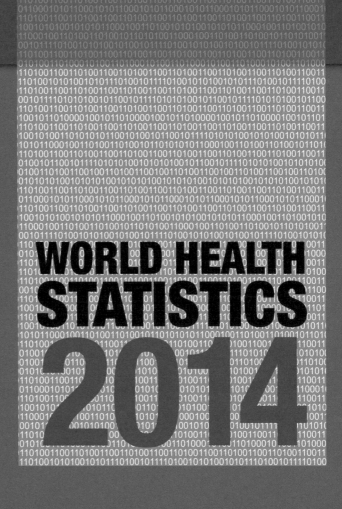

WORLD HEALTH STATISTICS 2014

Part I

Health-related Millennium Development Goals

Summary of status and trends

With one year to go until the 2015 target date for achieving the MDGs, substantial progress can be reported on many health-related goals. The global target of halving the proportion of people without access to improved sources of drinking water was met in 2010, with remarkable progress also having been made in reducing child mortality, improving nutrition, and combating HIV, tuberculosis and malaria.

Between 1990 and 2012, mortality in children under 5 years of age declined by 47%, from an estimated rate of 90 deaths per 1000 live births to 48 deaths per 1000 live births. This translates into 17 000 fewer children dying every day in 2012 than in 1990. The risk of a child dying before their fifth birthday is still highest in the WHO African Region (95 per 1000 live births) – eight times higher than that in the WHO European Region (12 per 1000 live births). There are, however, signs of progress in the region as the pace of decline in the under-five mortality rate has accelerated over time; increasing from 0.6% per year between 1990 and 1995 to 4.2% per year between 2005 and 2012. The global rate of decline during the same two periods was 1.2% per year and 3.8% per year, respectively.

Nevertheless, nearly 18 000 children worldwide died every day in 2012, and the global speed of decline in mortality rate remains insufficient to reach the target of a two-thirds reduction in the 1990 levels of mortality by the year 2015. **Table 1** shows the number of countries that have achieved this target; those that are on track to meet the target by 2015 if the current rate of progress is maintained; those that are at least halfway to achieving a two-thirds reduction in the 1990 level of mortality but are unlikely to achieve it by 2015 at the current rate of progress; and those that are less than halfway to meeting the target. Less than one-third of all countries have achieved or are on track to meet the MDG target by 2015.

Inequities in child mortality between high-income and low-income countries remain large. In 2012, the under-five mortality rate in low-income countries was 82 deaths per 1000 live births – more than 13 times the average rate in high-income countries (**Fig. 1**). Reducing these inequities across countries and saving the lives of more children by ending preventable child deaths are key priorities.

Table 1. Number of countries according to MDG Target 4.A achievement status, by WHO region, 2012

WHO region	MDG Target 4.A – achievement status				
	Achieved	On track	Halfway or more	Less than halfway	Total
African Region (AFR)	3	6	21	16	46
Region of the Americas (AMR)	5	3	22	5	35
South-East Asia Region (SEAR)	4	3	4	0	11
European Region (EUR)	17	8	28	0	53
Eastern Mediterranean Region (EMR)	6	2	11	3	22
Western Pacific Region (WPR)	2	1	18	6	27
Global	**37** (19%)	**23** (12%)	**104** (54%)	**30** (15%)	**194** (100%)

Calculated using unrounded under-five mortality rates, 1990 and 2012.

Figure 1. Neonatal and under-five mortality rates – globally and by country income group, 1990 and 2012

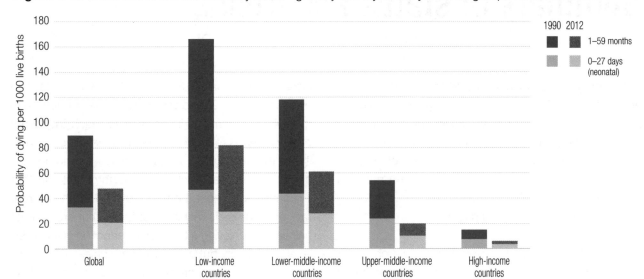

Each bar indicates the total under-five mortality rate as the sum of the neonatal mortality rate (0–27 days; lighter-shaded bars) plus the combined mortality rate for infants aged 1–11 months and children aged 1-4 years (darker-shaded bars).

The first 28 days of life – the neonatal period – represent the most vulnerable time for a child's survival. In 2012, around 44% of under-five deaths occurred during this period, up from 37% in 1990 (**Fig. 1**). As overall under-five mortality rates decline the proportion of such deaths occurring during the neonatal period is increasing. This highlights the crucial need for health interventions that specifically address the major causes of neonatal deaths, particularly as these typically differ from the interventions needed to address other under-five deaths.

Current evidence indicates that undernutrition[1] is the underlying cause of death in an estimated 45% of all deaths among children under 5 years of age.[2] The number of underweight children globally declined from 160 million in 1990 to 99 million in 2012, representing a decline in the proportion of underweight children from 25% to 15%. This rate of progress is close to that required to meet the

relevant MDG target, but varies between regions (**Fig. 2**). Beyond the MDGs, a new global target was recently set for a 40% reduction in the number of stunted children by 2025 against the 2010 baseline, along with five other targets on maternal, infant and young-child nutrition.[3] Between 1990 and 2012, the number of children affected by stunting declined from 257 million to 162 million, representing a global decrease of 37%.

In 2012, global measles immunization coverage reached 84% among children aged 12–23 months. More countries are now achieving high levels of vaccination coverage, with 66% of WHO Member States reaching at least 90% coverage in 2012, up from only 43% in 2000. Between 2000 and 2012, the estimated number of total measles deaths worldwide decreased by 78% from 562 000 to 122 000.

MDG 5 – Improve maternal health – sets out the targets of reducing the maternal mortality ratio from its 1990 level by three quarters and achieving universal access to reproductive-health services by the year 2015. The

---

[1] Including fetal growth restriction, stunting, wasting, and deficiencies of vitamin A and zinc, along with suboptimal breastfeeding.

[2] Black RE, Victora CG, Walker SP, Bhutta ZA Christian P, de Onis M et al. Maternal and child undernutrition and overweight in low-income and middle-income countries. *Lancet*. 3 August 2013;382(9890):427–51. doi:10.1016/S0140-6736(13)60937-X (http://www.thelancet.com/journals/lancet/article/PIIS0140-6736%2813%2960937-X/abstract, accessed 12 March 2014).

[3] Comprehensive implementation plan on maternal, infant and young child nutrition. Sixty-fifth World Health Assembly, WHA resolution 65.6 and Annex 2. Geneva: World Health Organization; 2012. (WHA65/2012/REC/1; http://apps.who.int/gb/ebwha/pdf_files/WHA65-REC1/A65_REC1-en.pdf, accessed 7 April 2014).

Figure 2. Prevalence of underweight children under 5 years of age – globally and by WHO region, 1990–2012

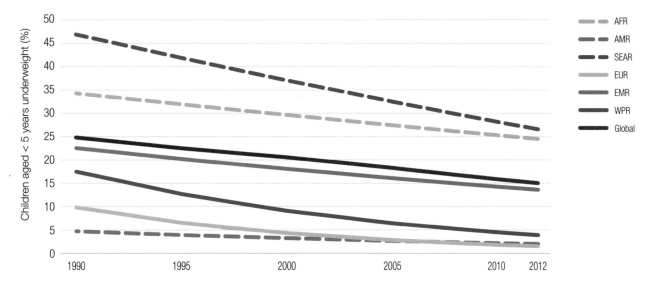

number of women dying due to complications during pregnancy and childbirth decreased by nearly 50% from an estimated 523 000 in 1990 to 289 000 in 2013. While such progress is notable, the average annual rate of decline (AARD) is far below that needed to achieve the MDG target (5.5%), and the number of deaths remains unacceptably high. In 2013, nearly 800 women died every day from maternal causes. Almost all of these deaths (99%) occur in developing countries, and most can be avoided as the necessary medical interventions exist and are well known. The key obstacle is the lack of access to quality care by pregnant women before, during and after childbirth.

In many countries, programmes have been implemented to eliminate or reduce the barriers that prevent access to effective reproductive-health interventions. Despite increasing overall levels of contraceptive use, there still remain significant gaps between the desire of women to delay or avoid having children and their actual use of contraception. Globally in 2011, around one in every eight women aged 15–49 years who were married or in a union had an unmet need for family planning. In the WHO African Region, the figure was around one in four. Although the proportion of women receiving antenatal care at least once during pregnancy was 81% globally for the period 2006–2013, the figure dropped to around 56% for the recommended minimum of four visits or more. Around seven in every 10 births globally are attended by skilled health personnel. However, coverage varies sharply across country-income level from almost all births (99%) in high-income countries to less than half of births (46%) in low-income countries.

Despite progress in reducing the birth rate among adolescents, more than 15 million of the estimated 135 million live births worldwide are to girls aged 15–19 years. Pregnant adolescents are more likely than adults to have unsafe abortions, and early childbearing increases risks for both mothers and their newborns. Complications from pregnancy and childbirth are a major cause of death among girls aged 15–19 in low- and middle-income countries.

Globally, an estimated 2.3 million people were newly infected with HIV in 2012 – representing a 33% decline compared with the 3.4 million new infections estimated for 2001. People living in sub-Saharan Africa accounted for 70% of all new infections. As access to antiretroviral therapy (ART) improves, the population living with HIV increases as fewer people die from AIDS-related causes. In 2012, an estimated 35.3 million people were living with HIV – with 9.7 million people in low- and middle-income countries receiving ART. It has been estimated that during the

Figure 3. Impact of ART use on the estimated number of deaths due to HIV/AIDS (millions) that would otherwise have occurred in low- and middle-income countries, 1995–2012[1]

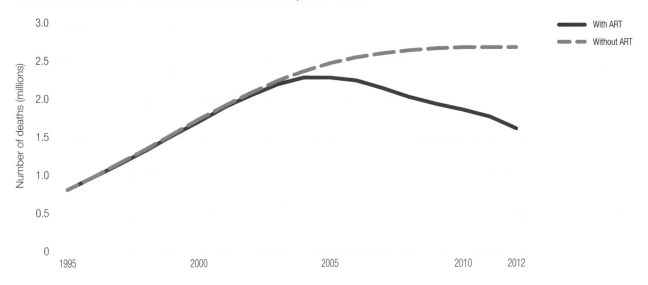

period 1995–2012, ART cumulatively averted 5.5 million deaths in such countries (**Fig. 3**). Globally, an estimated 1.6 million people died of HIV/AIDS in 2012; down from the peak of 2.3 million in 2005.

In 2012, an estimated 8.6 million people developed tuberculosis and 1.3 million died from the disease (including 320 000 deaths among HIV-positive people).[2] The rate of new tuberculosis cases worldwide has been falling for about a decade, thus achieving MDG target 6.C to reverse the spread of the disease by 2015. In addition, two WHO regions – the WHO Region of the Americas and the WHO Western Pacific Region – have also achieved related 2015 targets[3] to reduce tuberculosis incidence, prevalence and mortality rates (**Fig. 4**). Globally, the tuberculosis mortality rate has fallen by 45% since 1990 and the target of a

50% reduction by 2015 is within reach. Nevertheless, despite this decline in mortality rate, the number of tuberculosis deaths remains unacceptably high given that most are preventable.

Between 1995 and 2012, 56 million people were successfully treated for tuberculosis and 22 million lives were saved. However, multi-drug resistant tuberculosis (MDR-TB), which emerged primarily as a result of inadequate treatment, continues to pose problems. In 2012, an estimated 450 000 people worldwide developed MDR-TB, but only 94 000 were newly detected. Treatment options for MDR-TB are often limited and expensive, and recommended medicines are not always available or may cause numerous adverse side-effects.

Infection with HIV is the strongest risk factor for developing active tuberculosis disease. Many countries have made considerable progress in addressing the tuberculosis and HIV co-epidemic. However, less than half of notified tuberculosis patients had a documented HIV test result in 2012, with only 57% of those who tested positive being on ART or started on ART.

In 2012, almost half of the world's population – 3.4 billion people – was estimated to be at risk of malaria. Of these, 1.2 billion people were considered to be at high risk, with more than one case of malaria occur-

---

1. Global report: UNAIDS report on the global AIDS epidemic 2013. Geneva: Joint United Nations Programme on HIV/AIDS (UNAIDS); 2013.

2. **Table 2** in **Part III** presents data on mortality due to tuberculosis among HIV-negative people. Tuberculosis-related deaths among HIV-positive people are included in the mortality data for HIV/AIDS.

3. Stop TB Partnership targets linked to the MDG target 6.C of halting and beginning to reverse the incidence of major diseases such as tuberculosis by 2015, include reducing tuberculosis prevalence and deaths by 50% by 2015 compared with the 1990 baseline.

Figure 4. Reductions in tuberculosis incidence, prevalence and mortality, by WHO region, 1990–2012

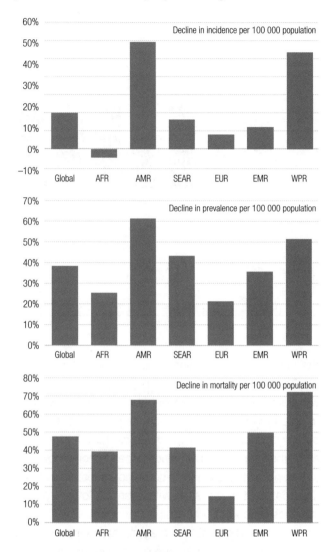

ring per 1000 population. The WHO African Region bears the highest burden of malaria, with 80% of the estimated 207 million cases and 90% of the estimated 627 000 malaria deaths worldwide occurring in this region in 2012. More than three quarters (77%) of all malaria deaths occur in children under 5 years of age (**Fig. 5**).

During the period 2000–2012, malaria incidence rates among populations at risk[1] are estimated to have fallen by 25% globally and by 31% in the WHO African Region. Over the same period, estimated malaria mortality rates[1] decreased by 42% globally, by 49% in the WHO African Region and by 48% in children under 5 years of age globally. An estimated 3.3 million lives were saved as a result of scaling-up malaria interventions during the same period. If the annual rate of decrease is maintained, malaria mortality rates are projected to decrease by 52% globally, and by 62% in the WHO African Region and by 60% in children under 5 years of age, by 2015. Of 103 countries that had ongoing malaria transmission in 2000, 62 have produced reliable trend data indicating that 59 are meeting the MDG target of reversing its incidence. In the other 41 countries – accounting for 80% of estimated cases of malaria – it is not possible to reliably assess national malaria trends using the data reported to WHO.

Neglected tropical diseases (NTDs)[2] are endemic in 149 countries, often cause multiple infections in a single individual, and can lead to severe pain, permanent disability and death. Many of these diseases can be prevented, eliminated or even eradicated with improved access to existing safe and cost-effective tools. The reported number of cases of human African trypanosomiasis dropped to less than 10 000 in 2009 – the lowest level in 50 years. In 2013, the number of cases of dracunculiasis worldwide

Figure 5. Estimated number of deaths due to malaria, 2012

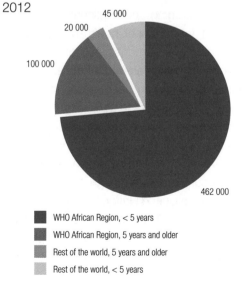

- WHO African Region, < 5 years
- WHO African Region, 5 years and older
- Rest of the world, 5 years and older
- Rest of the world, < 5 years

[1.] The percentage changes shown in this paragraph are based upon malaria incidence rates defined as cases per 1000 population at risk, and mortality rates as deaths per 100 000 population at risk. Elsewhere in this report, malaria incidence and mortality rates are calculated per 100 000 population.

[2.] The diseases concerned are: Buruli ulcer; Chagas disease; cysticercosis; dengue; dracunculiasis; echinococcosis; endemic treponematoses; foodborne trematode infections; human African trypanosomiasis; leishmaniasis; leprosy; lymphatic filariasis, onchocerciasis; rabies; schistosomiasis; soil-transmitted helminthiases; and trachoma.

fell below 150 for the first time. Leprosy has now been eliminated as a public health problem in 119 out of the 122 countries where it was previously endemic, and 728 million people worldwide were treated for at least one NTD through preventive chemotherapy in 2011. However, NTDs still affect more than one billion people worldwide, weaken impoverished populations, and frustrate the achievement of the health-related MDGs and other desirable global public health outcomes. In the case of dengue – the world's fastest growing viral infection – more than 2.5 billion people are estimated to be at risk.

The MDG target 7.C in relation to drinking-water, as measured by the proxy indicator of access to improved drinking-water sources, was met in 2010. Nevertheless, despite 2.3 billion people gaining access over the last 22 years as part of attaining the target, 748 million people remain un-served. This number increases to the order of billions if water quality and service sustainability are taken into account. Additionally, despite impressive progress, wide disparities exist between different regions, between urban and rural areas and between different socioeconomic groups – particularly between the rich and the poor. With regard to basic sanitation, more than 1949 million people have gained access to an improved sanitation facility since 1990. However, in 2012, 2523 million people (more than one third of the global population) still lacked such access. The current rate of progress is not sufficient to meet the sanitation target globally, which is projected to be missed by the order of 620 million people. The WHO Western Pacific Region is the only WHO region where access to basic sanitation has increased for more than one third of the population since 1990 (**Fig. 6**). In this region, the proportion of population using improved sanitation increased from 36% in 1990 to 70% in 2012 representing an increase of 34 percentage points.

Increasing access to affordable essential medicines[1] is vitally important in achieving the health-related MDGs. However, several factors undermine the availability of such medicines in a number of countries, including poor medicine supply and distribution systems, insufficient health facilities and staff, low investment in health and

---

[1.] Essential medicines are medicines that help meet the priority health-care needs of a population. They are selected with regard to disease prevalence, and evidence of their efficacy, safety and comparative cost–effectiveness.

Figure 6. Proportion of population with access to improved sanitation in 2012 and corresponding percentage change 1990–2012 – globally and by WHO region

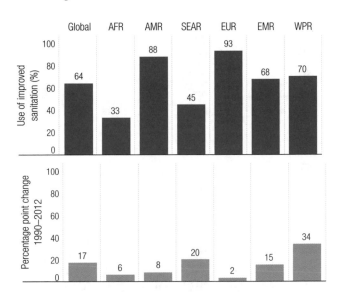

the high cost of medicines. Surveys undertaken from 2007 to 2012 indicated that selected generic medicines were only available in 56% of public outlets in low- and middle-income countries. Prices to patients of the lowest-priced generics in the private sector averaged five times the international reference prices, ranging upwards to around 14 times higher in some countries. As a result, the treatment of diseases with even the lowest-priced generics becomes impossible for many low-income households. The problem is aggravated when several household members become ill at the same time.

In conclusion, encouraging accomplishments across a broad range of international health-related goals and targets have clearly demonstrated that focused global actions can make a difference. At the same time, much remains to be done, and efforts continue to be needed to accelerate progress in achieving the MDGs and related objectives. Furthermore, efforts to improve health, and to achieve health equity, will continue well beyond 2015. This undertaking goes hand-in-hand with efforts to ensure universal health coverage – an aspiration backed by a United Nations General Assembly resolution adopted in December 2012 which urges governments to move towards providing all people with access to affordable good-quality health-care services.

Regional and country charts

Following the global and WHO regional summary shown in Figure 7, charts 1–13 provide country-by-country summaries of national trends in MDG indicators for which data are available.

Depending on the availability of data for each indicator, there are two types of chart:

Chart type I

For six indicators – under-five mortality rate; maternal mortality ratio; HIV prevalence; tuberculosis mortality rate; proportion of population without access to improved drinking-water sources; and proportion of population without access to improved sanitation – the charts show the average annual rate of decline (AARD) since 1990 up to the latest available year (or for the year range indicated), and the overall AARD required for the country to achieve the relevant MDG by 2015. The country figures show data for the latest available year.

Chart type II

For seven indicators – measles immunization coverage among 1-year-olds; births attended by skilled health personnel; antenatal care coverage; unmet need for family planning; antiretroviral therapy coverage among people eligible for treatment; children aged < 5 years sleeping under insecticide-treated nets; and children aged < 5 years with fever who received treatment with any antimalarial – the charts show only data for the latest available year, along with an indication of a WHO or partner agency target.

... indicates data not available or not applicable.

Further details can be found in the country tables shown in **Part III** as indicated below each chart.

Figure 7. Global and WHO regional progress towards the achievement of health-related MDGs

Key ■ On track ■ Insufficient progress

Target 1.C Halve, between 1990 and 2015, the proportion of people who suffer from hunger

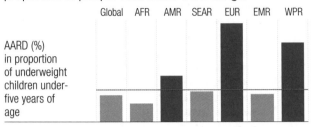

AARD (%) in proportion of underweight children under-five years of age

Target 4.A Reduce by two-thirds, between 1990 and 2015, the under-five mortality rate

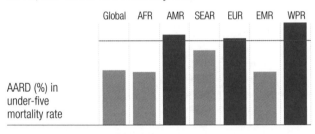

AARD (%) in under-five mortality rate

Target 5.A Reduce by three quarters, between 1990 and 2015, the maternal mortality ratio

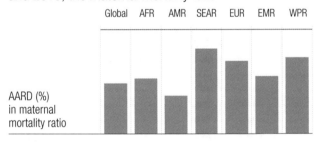

AARD (%) in maternal mortality ratio

Target 5.B Achieve, by 2015, universal access to reproductive health

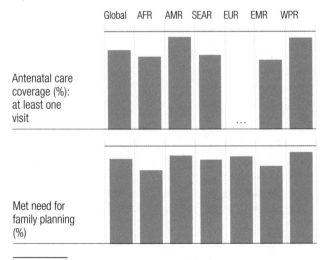

Antenatal care coverage (%): at least one visit

Met need for family planning (%)

Target 6.A Have halted by 2015 and begun to reverse the spread of HIV/AIDS

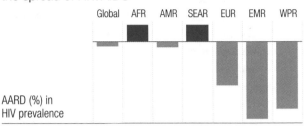

AARD (%) in HIV prevalence

Target 6.B Achieve, by 2010, universal access to treatment for HIV/AIDS for all those who need it

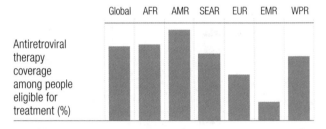

Antiretroviral therapy coverage among people eligible for treatment (%)

Target 6.C Have halted by 2015 and begun to reverse the incidence of malaria and other major diseases

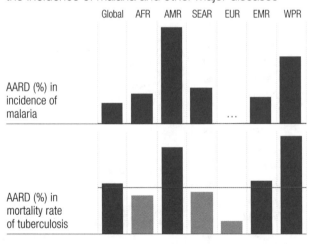

AARD (%) in incidence of malaria

AARD (%) in mortality rate of tuberculosis

Target 7.C Halve, by 2015, the proportion of people without sustainable access to safe drinking-water

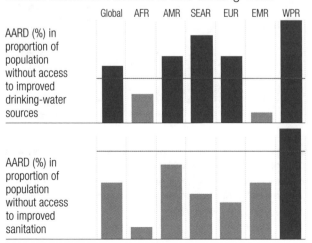

AARD (%) in proportion of population without access to improved drinking-water sources

AARD (%) in proportion of population without access to improved sanitation

Grey horizontal lines indicate either the MDG (where available) or relevant WHO or partner agency target. For more details, see the relevant country charts. For the AARD (%) in proportion of underweight children under 5 years of age (1990–2012) and the AARD (%) in the incidence of malaria (2000–2012), see **Part III: Table 5** and the *World Malaria Report 2013* respectively for more details.

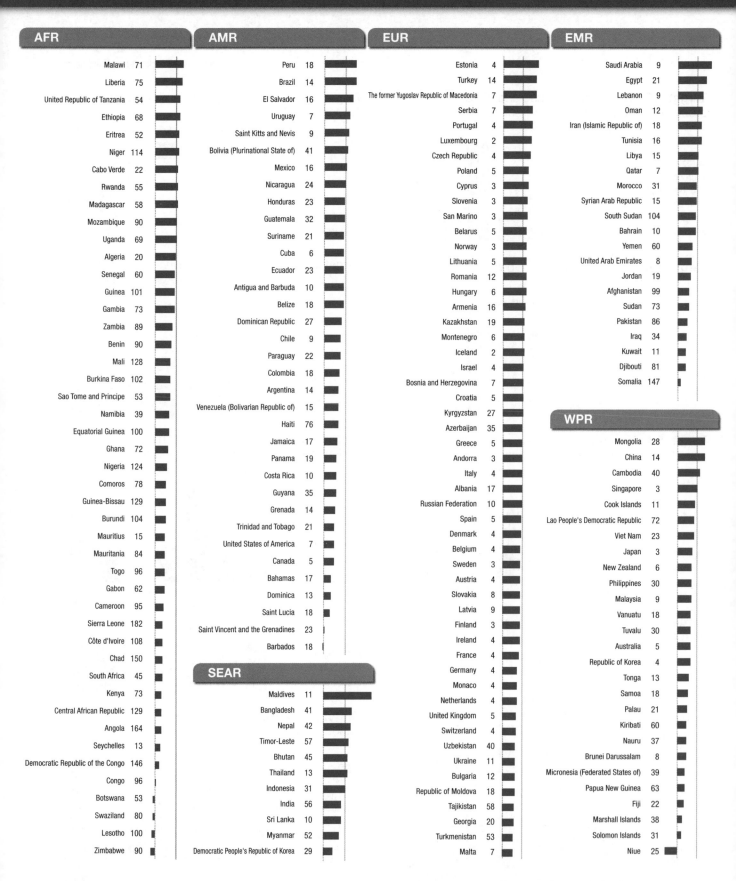

AFR

Malawi	71
Liberia	75
United Republic of Tanzania	54
Ethiopia	68
Eritrea	52
Niger	114
Cabo Verde	22
Rwanda	55
Madagascar	58
Mozambique	90
Uganda	69
Algeria	20
Senegal	60
Guinea	101
Gambia	73
Zambia	89
Benin	90
Mali	128
Burkina Faso	102
Sao Tome and Principe	53
Namibia	39
Equatorial Guinea	100
Ghana	72
Nigeria	124
Comoros	78
Guinea-Bissau	129
Burundi	104
Mauritius	15
Mauritania	84
Togo	96
Gabon	62
Cameroon	95
Sierra Leone	182
Côte d'Ivoire	108
Chad	150
South Africa	45
Kenya	73
Central African Republic	129
Angola	164
Seychelles	13
Democratic Republic of the Congo	146
Congo	96
Botswana	53
Swaziland	80
Lesotho	100
Zimbabwe	90

AMR

Peru	18
Brazil	14
El Salvador	16
Uruguay	7
Saint Kitts and Nevis	9
Bolivia (Plurinational State of)	41
Mexico	16
Nicaragua	24
Honduras	23
Guatemala	32
Suriname	21
Cuba	6
Ecuador	23
Antigua and Barbuda	10
Belize	18
Dominican Republic	27
Chile	9
Paraguay	22
Colombia	18
Argentina	14
Venezuela (Bolivarian Republic of)	15
Haiti	76
Jamaica	17
Panama	19
Costa Rica	10
Guyana	35
Grenada	14
Trinidad and Tobago	21
United States of America	7
Canada	5
Bahamas	17
Dominica	13
Saint Lucia	18
Saint Vincent and the Grenadines	23
Barbados	18

SEAR

Maldives	11
Bangladesh	41
Nepal	42
Timor-Leste	57
Bhutan	45
Thailand	13
Indonesia	31
India	56
Sri Lanka	10
Myanmar	52
Democratic People's Republic of Korea	29

EUR

Estonia	4
Turkey	14
The former Yugoslav Republic of Macedonia	7
Serbia	7
Portugal	4
Luxembourg	2
Czech Republic	4
Poland	5
Cyprus	3
Slovenia	3
San Marino	3
Belarus	5
Norway	3
Lithuania	5
Romania	12
Hungary	6
Armenia	16
Kazakhstan	19
Montenegro	6
Iceland	2
Israel	4
Bosnia and Herzegovina	7
Croatia	5
Kyrgyzstan	27
Azerbaijan	35
Greece	5
Andorra	3
Italy	4
Albania	17
Russian Federation	10
Spain	5
Denmark	4
Belgium	4
Sweden	3
Austria	4
Slovakia	8
Latvia	9
Finland	3
Ireland	4
France	4
Germany	4
Monaco	4
Netherlands	4
United Kingdom	5
Switzerland	4
Uzbekistan	40
Ukraine	11
Bulgaria	12
Republic of Moldova	18
Tajikistan	58
Georgia	20
Turkmenistan	53
Malta	7

EMR

Saudi Arabia	9
Egypt	21
Lebanon	9
Oman	12
Iran (Islamic Republic of)	18
Tunisia	16
Libya	15
Qatar	7
Morocco	31
Syrian Arab Republic	15
South Sudan	104
Bahrain	10
Yemen	60
United Arab Emirates	8
Jordan	19
Afghanistan	99
Sudan	73
Pakistan	86
Iraq	34
Kuwait	11
Djibouti	81
Somalia	147

WPR

Mongolia	28
China	14
Cambodia	40
Singapore	3
Cook Islands	11
Lao People's Democratic Republic	72
Viet Nam	23
Japan	3
New Zealand	6
Philippines	30
Malaysia	9
Vanuatu	18
Tuvalu	30
Australia	5
Republic of Korea	4
Tonga	13
Samoa	18
Palau	21
Kiribati	60
Nauru	37
Brunei Darussalam	8
Micronesia (Federated States of)	39
Papua New Guinea	63
Fiji	22
Marshall Islands	38
Solomon Islands	31
Niue	25

The under-five mortality rate is defined as the probability of dying by age 5 expressed as the total number of such deaths per 1000 live births. Within each WHO region countries are sorted in descending order based on the AARD in this rate.

In order to reach the MDG target of reducing by two thirds the under-five mortality rate between 1990 and 2015, an AARD of 4.3% is needed and this is denoted by the vertical line. The numerical values show the estimated under-five mortality rate in each country in 2012. For countries with low levels of under-five mortality, the target AARD may not be applicable.

Further details may be found in **Part III**: **Table 1**.

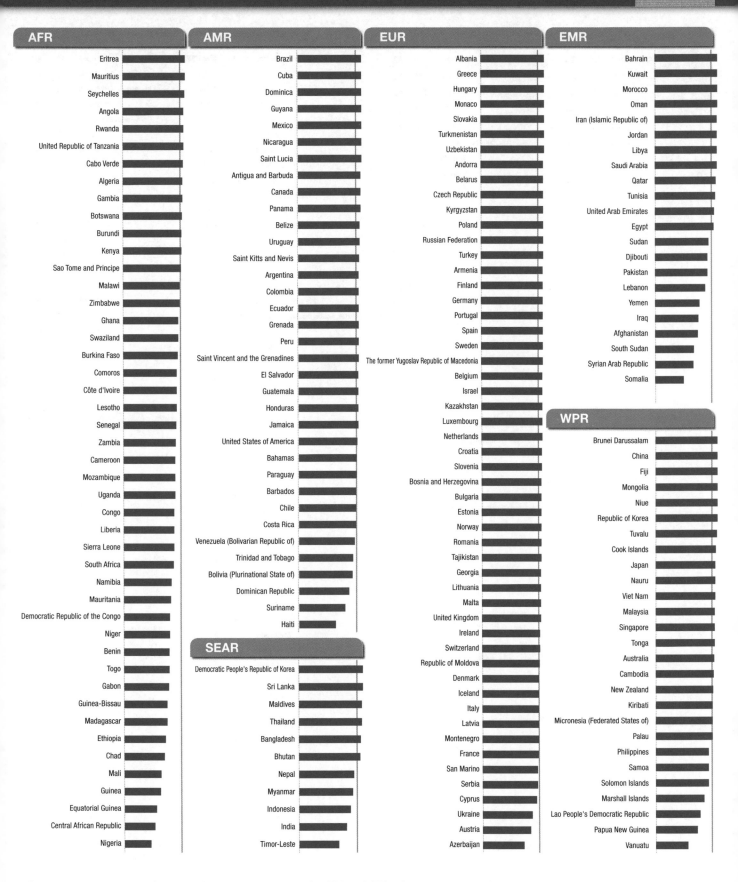

AFR

Eritrea
Mauritius
Seychelles
Angola
Rwanda
United Republic of Tanzania
Cabo Verde
Algeria
Gambia
Botswana
Burundi
Kenya
Sao Tome and Principe
Malawi
Zimbabwe
Ghana
Swaziland
Burkina Faso
Comoros
Côte d'Ivoire
Lesotho
Senegal
Zambia
Cameroon
Mozambique
Uganda
Congo
Liberia
Sierra Leone
South Africa
Namibia
Mauritania
Democratic Republic of the Congo
Niger
Benin
Togo
Gabon
Guinea-Bissau
Madagascar
Ethiopia
Chad
Mali
Guinea
Equatorial Guinea
Central African Republic
Nigeria

AMR

Brazil
Cuba
Dominica
Guyana
Mexico
Nicaragua
Saint Lucia
Antigua and Barbuda
Canada
Panama
Belize
Uruguay
Saint Kitts and Nevis
Argentina
Colombia
Ecuador
Grenada
Peru
Saint Vincent and the Grenadines
El Salvador
Guatemala
Honduras
Jamaica
United States of America
Bahamas
Paraguay
Barbados
Chile
Costa Rica
Venezuela (Bolivarian Republic of)
Trinidad and Tobago
Bolivia (Plurinational State of)
Dominican Republic
Suriname
Haiti

SEAR

Democratic People's Republic of Korea
Sri Lanka
Maldives
Thailand
Bangladesh
Bhutan
Nepal
Myanmar
Indonesia
India
Timor-Leste

EUR

Albania
Greece
Hungary
Monaco
Slovakia
Turkmenistan
Uzbekistan
Andorra
Belarus
Czech Republic
Kyrgyzstan
Poland
Russian Federation
Turkey
Armenia
Finland
Germany
Portugal
Spain
Sweden
The former Yugoslav Republic of Macedonia
Belgium
Israel
Kazakhstan
Luxembourg
Netherlands
Croatia
Slovenia
Bosnia and Herzegovina
Bulgaria
Estonia
Norway
Romania
Tajikistan
Georgia
Lithuania
Malta
United Kingdom
Ireland
Switzerland
Republic of Moldova
Denmark
Iceland
Italy
Latvia
Montenegro
France
San Marino
Serbia
Cyprus
Ukraine
Austria
Azerbaijan

EMR

Bahrain
Kuwait
Morocco
Oman
Iran (Islamic Republic of)
Jordan
Libya
Saudi Arabia
Qatar
Tunisia
United Arab Emirates
Egypt
Sudan
Djibouti
Pakistan
Lebanon
Yemen
Iraq
Afghanistan
South Sudan
Syrian Arab Republic
Somalia

WPR

Brunei Darussalam
China
Fiji
Mongolia
Niue
Republic of Korea
Tuvalu
Cook Islands
Japan
Nauru
Viet Nam
Malaysia
Singapore
Tonga
Australia
Cambodia
New Zealand
Kiribati
Micronesia (Federated States of)
Palau
Philippines
Samoa
Solomon Islands
Marshall Islands
Lao People's Democratic Republic
Papua New Guinea
Vanuatu

This chart shows the percentage of 1-year-olds fully immunized against measles. Within each WHO region countries are sorted by the 2012 level.

The vertical line denotes the target of 90% coverage by 2015 set at the 2010 World Health Assembly.

Further details may be found in **Part III: Table 4**.

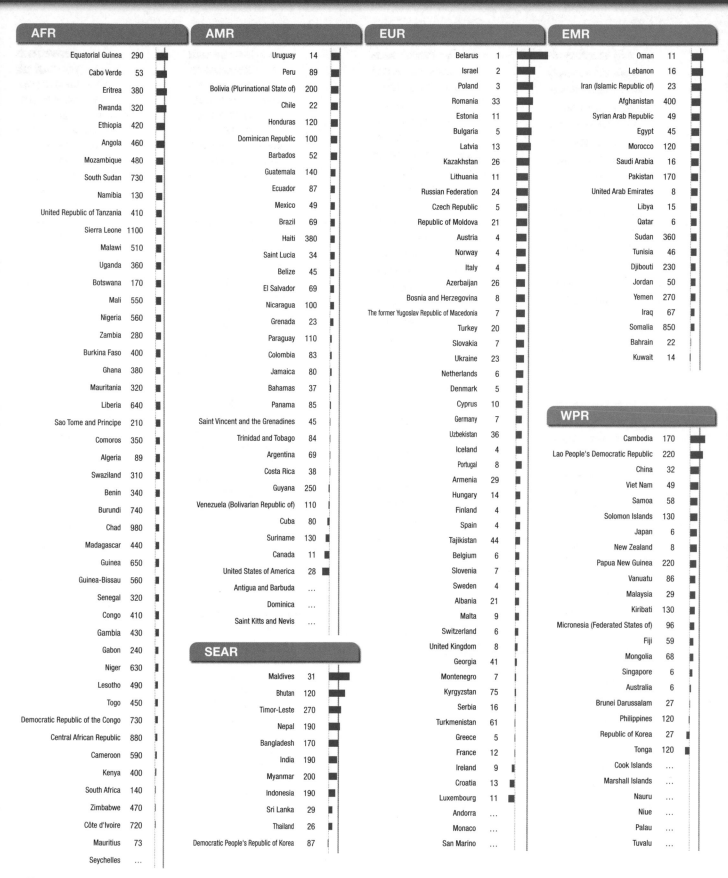

AFR

Country	Value
Equatorial Guinea	290
Cabo Verde	53
Eritrea	380
Rwanda	320
Ethiopia	420
Angola	460
Mozambique	480
South Sudan	730
Namibia	130
United Republic of Tanzania	410
Sierra Leone	1100
Malawi	510
Uganda	360
Botswana	170
Mali	550
Nigeria	560
Zambia	280
Burkina Faso	400
Ghana	380
Mauritania	320
Liberia	640
Sao Tome and Principe	210
Comoros	350
Algeria	89
Swaziland	310
Benin	340
Burundi	740
Chad	980
Madagascar	440
Guinea	650
Guinea-Bissau	560
Senegal	320
Congo	410
Gambia	430
Gabon	240
Niger	630
Lesotho	490
Togo	450
Democratic Republic of the Congo	730
Central African Republic	880
Cameroon	590
Kenya	400
South Africa	140
Zimbabwe	470
Côte d'Ivoire	720
Mauritius	73
Seychelles	…

AMR

Country	Value
Uruguay	14
Peru	89
Bolivia (Plurinational State of)	200
Chile	22
Honduras	120
Dominican Republic	100
Barbados	52
Guatemala	140
Ecuador	87
Mexico	49
Brazil	69
Haiti	380
Saint Lucia	34
Belize	45
El Salvador	69
Nicaragua	100
Grenada	23
Paraguay	110
Colombia	83
Jamaica	80
Bahamas	37
Panama	85
Saint Vincent and the Grenadines	45
Trinidad and Tobago	84
Argentina	69
Costa Rica	38
Guyana	250
Venezuela (Bolivarian Republic of)	110
Cuba	80
Suriname	130
Canada	11
United States of America	28
Antigua and Barbuda	…
Dominica	…
Saint Kitts and Nevis	…

SEAR

Country	Value
Maldives	31
Bhutan	120
Timor-Leste	270
Nepal	190
Bangladesh	170
India	190
Myanmar	200
Indonesia	190
Sri Lanka	29
Thailand	26
Democratic People's Republic of Korea	87

EUR

Country	Value
Belarus	1
Israel	2
Poland	3
Romania	33
Estonia	11
Bulgaria	5
Latvia	13
Kazakhstan	26
Lithuania	11
Russian Federation	24
Czech Republic	5
Republic of Moldova	21
Austria	4
Norway	4
Italy	4
Azerbaijan	26
Bosnia and Herzegovina	8
The former Yugoslav Republic of Macedonia	7
Turkey	20
Slovakia	7
Ukraine	23
Netherlands	6
Denmark	5
Cyprus	10
Germany	7
Uzbekistan	36
Iceland	4
Portugal	8
Armenia	29
Hungary	14
Finland	4
Spain	4
Tajikistan	44
Belgium	6
Slovenia	7
Sweden	4
Albania	21
Malta	9
Switzerland	6
United Kingdom	8
Georgia	41
Montenegro	7
Kyrgyzstan	75
Serbia	16
Turkmenistan	61
Greece	5
France	12
Ireland	9
Croatia	13
Luxembourg	11
Andorra	…
Monaco	…
San Marino	…

EMR

Country	Value
Oman	11
Lebanon	16
Iran (Islamic Republic of)	23
Afghanistan	400
Syrian Arab Republic	49
Egypt	45
Morocco	120
Saudi Arabia	16
Pakistan	170
United Arab Emirates	8
Libya	15
Qatar	6
Sudan	360
Tunisia	46
Djibouti	230
Jordan	50
Yemen	270
Iraq	67
Somalia	850
Bahrain	22
Kuwait	14

WPR

Country	Value
Cambodia	170
Lao People's Democratic Republic	220
China	32
Viet Nam	49
Samoa	58
Solomon Islands	130
Japan	6
New Zealand	8
Papua New Guinea	220
Vanuatu	86
Malaysia	29
Kiribati	130
Micronesia (Federated States of)	96
Fiji	59
Mongolia	68
Singapore	6
Australia	6
Brunei Darussalam	27
Philippines	120
Republic of Korea	27
Tonga	120
Cook Islands	…
Marshall Islands	…
Nauru	…
Niue	…
Palau	…
Tuvalu	…

The maternal mortality ratio is defined as the number of maternal deaths per 100 000 live births. Within each WHO region countries are sorted in descending order based on the AARD in this ratio. Unrounded values have been used to calculate the AARD.

In order to reach the MDG target of reducing the maternal mortality ratio by three quarters between 1990 and 2015, an AARD of 5.5% is needed and this is denoted by the vertical line. For countries with low levels of maternal mortality, the target AARD may not be applicable.

The numerical values show the estimated maternal mortality ratio for 2013. South Sudan was reassigned to the WHO African Region in May 2013 and is therefore listed accordingly in the above chart.

Further details may be found in **Part III: Table 2**.

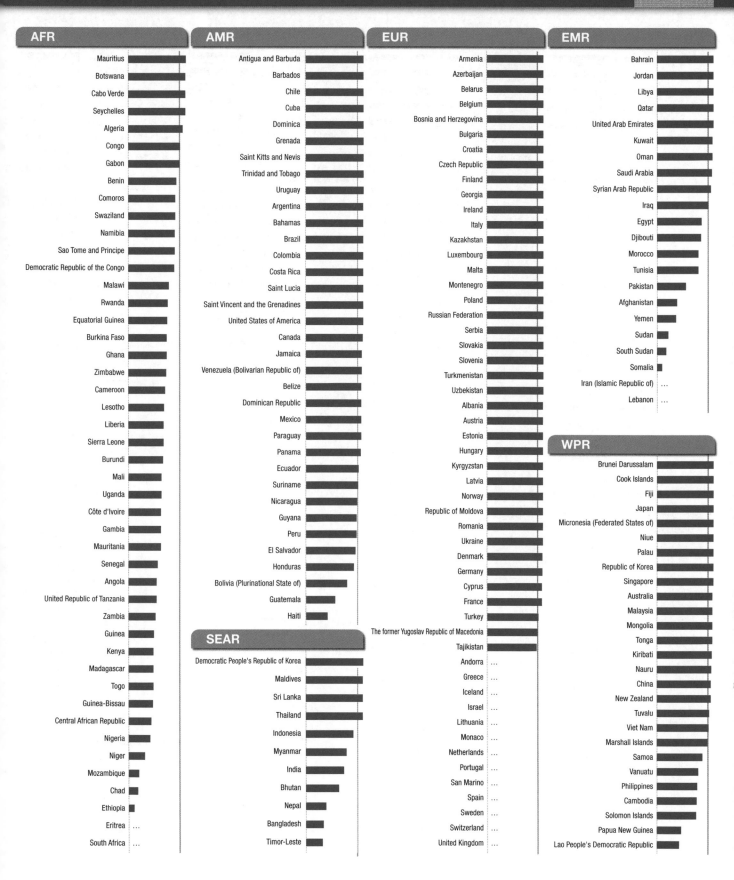

This chart shows the percentage of births attended by skilled health personnel. Within each WHO region countries are sorted by the latest available data since 2006.

The vertical line denotes the global target of 90% coverage by 2015 set by the International Conference on Population and Development (ICPD+5).

Further details may be found in **Part III Table 4**.

5 | Antenatal care coverage (%): at least one visit and at least four visits

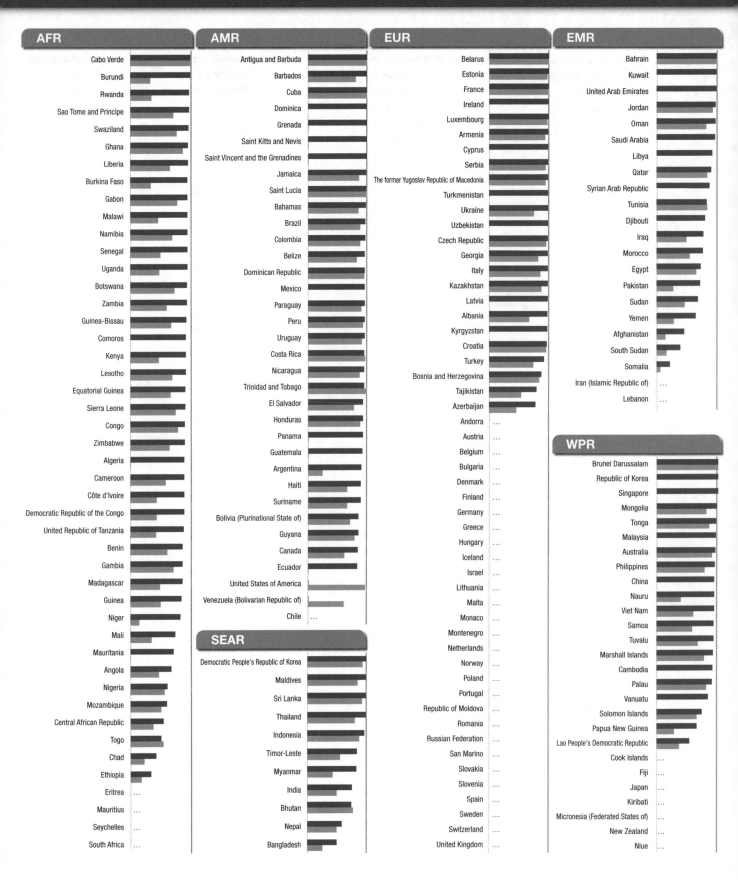

This chart shows the percentage of women who received antenatal care from skilled health personnel at least once and at least four times during pregnancy. Within each WHO region countries are sorted by the latest available data since 2006 for at least one visit.

■ At least one visit
■ At least four visits

The vertical line denotes the global target of 100% coverage by 2015 set by the International Conference on Population and Development (ICPD+5). South Sudan was reassigned to the WHO African Region in May 2013 and is therefore grouped accordingly in the above chart. Further details may be found in **Part III**: **Table 4**.

AFR

Guinea-Bissau	
Swaziland	
Zimbabwe	
Niger	
Madagascar	
Nigeria	
Namibia	
Rwanda	
Gambia	
Lesotho	
Cameroon	
Democratic Republic of the Congo	
Burkina Faso	
United Republic of Tanzania	
Ethiopia	
Kenya	
Malawi	
Benin	
Sierra Leone	
Zambia	
Chad	
Mali	
Senegal	
Burundi	
Uganda	
Ghana	
Liberia	
Togo	
Sao Tome and Principe	
Algeria	...
Angola	...
Botswana	...
Cabo Verde	...
Central African Republic	...
Comoros	...
Congo	...
Côte d'Ivoire	...
Equatorial Guinea	...
Eritrea	...
Gabon	...
Guinea	...
Mauritania	...
Mauritius	...
Mozambique	...
Seychelles	...
South Africa	...

AMR

Paraguay	
Brazil	
Peru	
Colombia	
United States of America	
Dominican Republic	
Nicaragua	
Mexico	
Belize	
Honduras	
Bolivia (Plurinational State of)	
Guyana	
Haiti	
Antigua and Barbuda	...
Argentina	...
Bahamas	...
Barbados	...
Canada	...
Chile	...
Costa Rica	...
Cuba	...
Dominica	...
Ecuador	...
El Salvador	...
Grenada	...
Guatemala	...
Jamaica	...
Panama	...
Saint Kitts and Nevis	...
Saint Lucia	...
Saint Vincent and the Grenadines	...
Suriname	...
Trinidad and Tobago	...
Uruguay	...
Venezuela (Bolivarian Republic of)	...

SEAR

Thailand	
Sri Lanka	
Indonesia	
Bhutan	
Bangladesh	
India	
Nepal	
Maldives	
Timor-Leste	
Democratic People's Republic of Korea	...
Myanmar	...

EUR

Cyprus	
Turkey	
Serbia	
Bosnia and Herzegovina	
Croatia	
Ukraine	
Georgia	
Kazakhstan	
Albania	
Armenia	
Azerbaijan	
Andorra	...
Austria	...
Belarus	...
Belgium	...
Bulgaria	...
Czech Republic	...
Denmark	...
Estonia	...
Finland	...
France	...
Germany	...
Greece	...
Hungary	...
Iceland	...
Ireland	...
Israel	...
Italy	...
Kyrgyzstan	...
Latvia	...
Lithuania	...
Luxembourg	...
Malta	...
Monaco	...
Montenegro	...
Netherlands	...
Norway	...
Poland	...
Portugal	...
Republic of Moldova	...
Romania	...
Russian Federation	...
San Marino	...
Slovakia	...
Slovenia	...
Spain	...
Sweden	...
Switzerland	...
Tajikistan	...
The former Yugoslav Republic of Macedonia	...
Turkmenistan	...
United Kingdom	...
Uzbekistan	...

EMR

Tunisia	
Iraq	
Egypt	
Morocco	
Jordan	
Pakistan	
Sudan	
Afghanistan	...
Bahrain	...
Djibouti	...
Iran (Islamic Republic of)	...
Kuwait	...
Lebanon	...
Libya	...
Oman	...
Qatar	...
Saudi Arabia	...
Somalia	...
South Sudan	...
Syrian Arab Republic	...
United Arab Emirates	...
Yemen	...

WPR

Viet Nam	
Marshall Islands	
Solomon Islands	
Cambodia	
Mongolia	
Philippines	
Nauru	
Tuvalu	
Papua New Guinea	
Kiribati	
Samoa	
Australia	...
Brunei Darussalam	...
China	...
Cook Islands	...
Fiji	...
Japan	...
Lao People's Democratic Republic	...
Malaysia	...
Micronesia (Federated States of)	...
New Zealand	...
Niue	...
Palau	...
Republic of Korea	...
Singapore	...
Tonga	...
Vanuatu	...

This chart shows the percentage of women who are fecund and sexually active but who want to stop or delay childbearing and are not using any method of contraception. Within each WHO region countries are sorted by the latest available data since 2006.

Achieving the MDG target of universal access to reproductive-health services by 2015 can be interpreted as 0% unmet need. The vertical line corresponds to 0% with the percentage of unmet need shown to the left of this line with a range of 50%.

Further details may be found in **Part III**: **Table 4**.

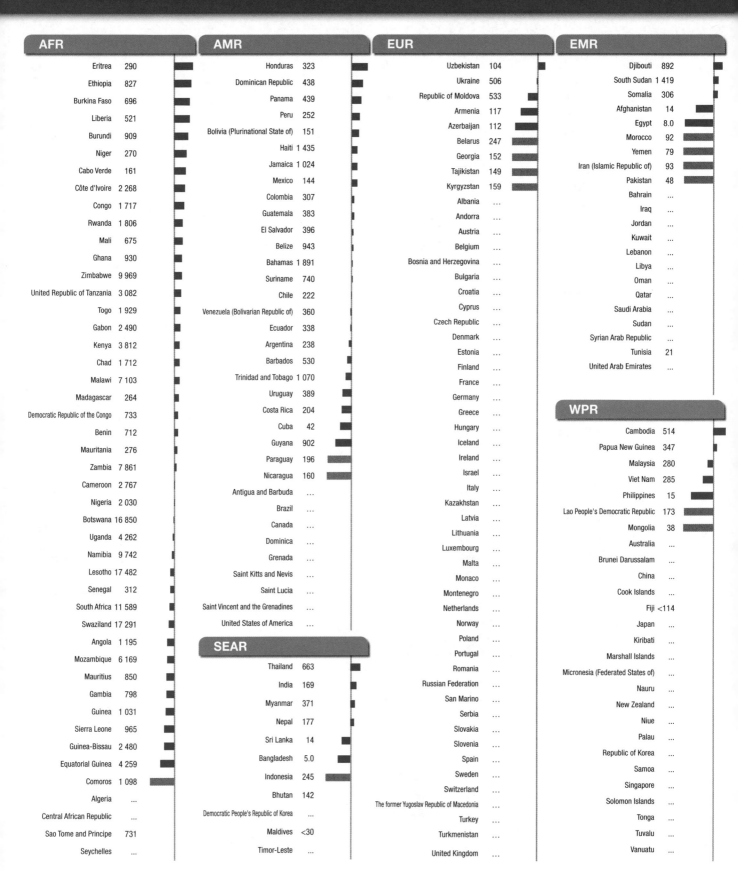

AFR			AMR			EUR			EMR		
Eritrea	290		Honduras	323		Uzbekistan	104		Djibouti	892	
Ethiopia	827		Dominican Republic	438		Ukraine	506		South Sudan	1 419	
Burkina Faso	696		Panama	439		Republic of Moldova	533		Somalia	306	
Liberia	521		Peru	252		Armenia	117		Afghanistan	14	
Burundi	909		Bolivia (Plurinational State of)	151		Azerbaijan	112		Egypt	8.0	
Niger	270		Haiti	1 435		Belarus	247		Morocco	92	
Cabo Verde	161		Jamaica	1 024		Georgia	152		Yemen	79	
Côte d'Ivoire	2 268		Mexico	144		Tajikistan	149		Iran (Islamic Republic of)	93	
Congo	1 717		Colombia	307		Kyrgyzstan	159		Pakistan	48	
Rwanda	1 806		Guatemala	383		Albania	...		Bahrain	...	
Mali	675		El Salvador	396		Andorra	...		Iraq	...	
Ghana	930		Belize	943		Austria	...		Jordan	...	
Zimbabwe	9 969		Bahamas	1 891		Belgium	...		Kuwait	...	
United Republic of Tanzania	3 082		Suriname	740		Bosnia and Herzegovina	...		Lebanon	...	
Togo	1 929		Chile	222		Bulgaria	...		Libya	...	
Gabon	2 490		Venezuela (Bolivarian Republic of)	360		Croatia	...		Oman	...	
Kenya	3 812		Ecuador	338		Cyprus	...		Qatar	...	
Chad	1 712		Argentina	238		Czech Republic	...		Saudi Arabia	...	
Malawi	7 103		Barbados	530		Denmark	...		Sudan	...	
Madagascar	264		Trinidad and Tobago	1 070		Estonia	...		Syrian Arab Republic	...	
Democratic Republic of the Congo	733		Uruguay	389		Finland	...		Tunisia	21	
Benin	712		Costa Rica	204		France	...		United Arab Emirates	...	
Mauritania	276		Cuba	42		Germany	...				
Zambia	7 861		Guyana	902		Greece	...				
Cameroon	2 767		Paraguay	196		Hungary	...		WPR		
Nigeria	2 030		Nicaragua	160		Iceland	...		Cambodia	514	
Botswana	16 850		Antigua and Barbuda	...		Ireland	...		Papua New Guinea	347	
Uganda	4 262		Brazil	...		Israel	...		Malaysia	280	
Namibia	9 742		Canada	...		Italy	...		Viet Nam	285	
Lesotho	17 482		Dominica	...		Kazakhstan	...		Philippines	15	
Senegal	312		Grenada	...		Latvia	...		Lao People's Democratic Republic	173	
South Africa	11 589		Saint Kitts and Nevis	...		Lithuania	...		Mongolia	38	
Swaziland	17 291		Saint Lucia	...		Luxembourg	...		Australia	...	
Angola	1 195		Saint Vincent and the Grenadines	...		Malta	...		Brunei Darussalam	...	
Mozambique	6 169		United States of America	...		Monaco	...		China	...	
Mauritius	850					Montenegro	...		Cook Islands	...	
Gambia	798		SEAR			Netherlands	...		Fiji	<114	
Guinea	1 031		Thailand	663		Norway	...		Japan	...	
Sierra Leone	965		India	169		Poland	...		Kiribati	...	
Guinea-Bissau	2 480		Myanmar	371		Portugal	...		Marshall Islands	...	
Equatorial Guinea	4 259		Nepal	177		Romania	...		Micronesia (Federated States of)	...	
Comoros	1 098		Sri Lanka	14		Russian Federation	...		Nauru	...	
Algeria	...		Bangladesh	5.0		San Marino	...		New Zealand	...	
Central African Republic	...		Indonesia	245		Serbia	...		Niue	...	
Sao Tome and Principe	731		Bhutan	142		Slovakia	...		Palau	...	
Seychelles	...		Democratic People's Republic of Korea	...		Slovenia	...		Republic of Korea	...	
			Maldives	<30		Spain	...		Samoa	...	
			Timor-Leste	...		Sweden	...		Singapore	...	
						Switzerland	...		Solomon Islands	...	
						The former Yugoslav Republic of Macedonia	...		Tonga	...	
						Turkey	...		Tuvalu	...	
						Turkmenistan	...		Vanuatu	...	
						United Kingdom	...				

This chart shows the AARD in the estimated prevalence of HIV infections per 100 000 population per year for the period 2001–2012. Within each WHO region countries are sorted in descending order based on the AARD in this rate.

The MDG target to halt by 2015 and begin to reverse the spread of HIV/AIDS can be interpreted as any AARD greater than 0%. The vertical line corresponds to an AARD of 0% with cut-off points of ±10% on either side. Grey bars indicate countries in which the AARD was less than -10%. The numerical values show estimated HIV prevalence per 100 000 population for 2012.

Further details may be found in **Part III**: **Table 2**.

WORLD HEALTH STATISTICS 2014

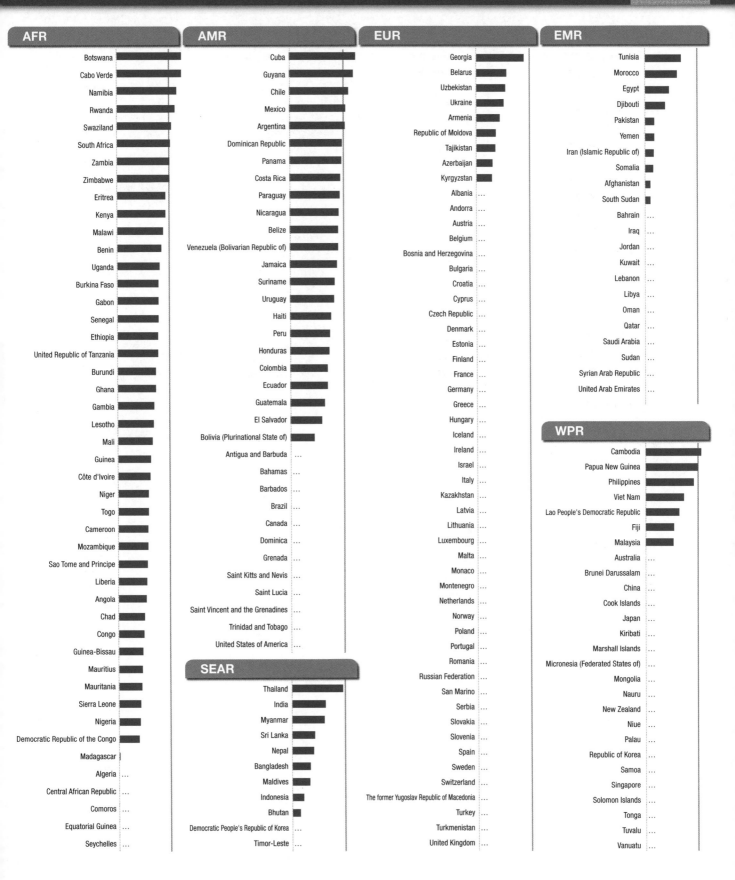

This chart shows estimated antiretroviral therapy coverage in 2012 based on the standards for treatment set out in the 2010 guidelines of the Joint United Nations Programme on HIV/AIDS. Within each WHO region countries are sorted in descending order by the level of coverage achieved.

The vertical line denotes the target of universal access to antiretroviral therapy, defined as providing antiretroviral therapy to at least 80% of patients in need.

Further details may be found in **Part III**: **Table 4**.

9 | Children aged < 5 years sleeping under insecticide-treated nets (%)

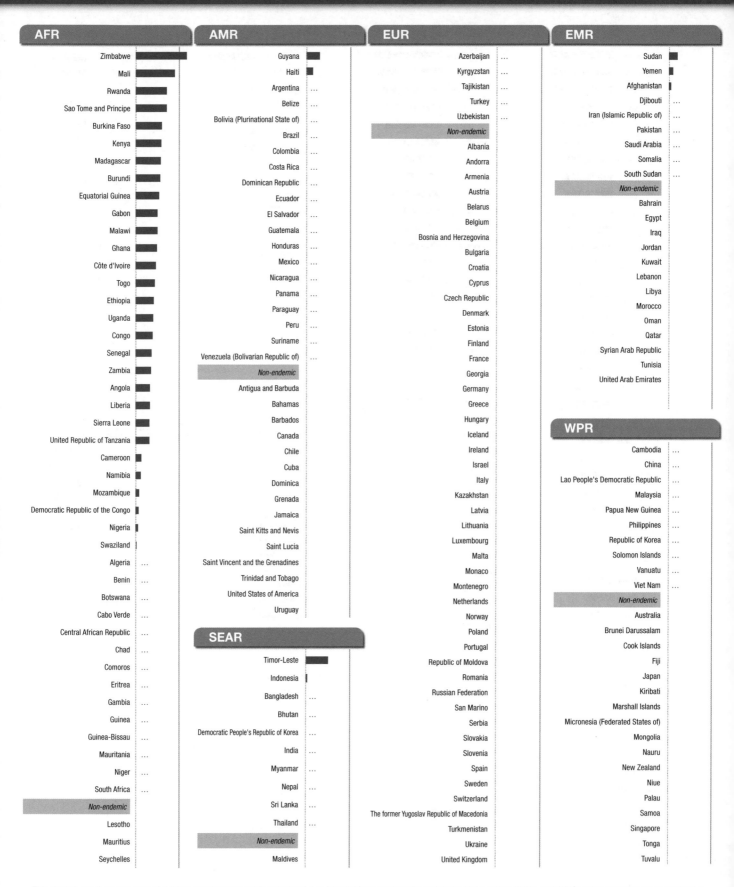

This chart shows the percentage of children under 5 years old that slept under an insecticide-treated net the night prior to the survey. Within each WHO region countries are sorted by the latest available data since 2006.

The vertical line denotes the target of 80% coverage set by WHO and the Roll Back Malaria Partnership.

Further details may be found in **Part III: Table 4**.

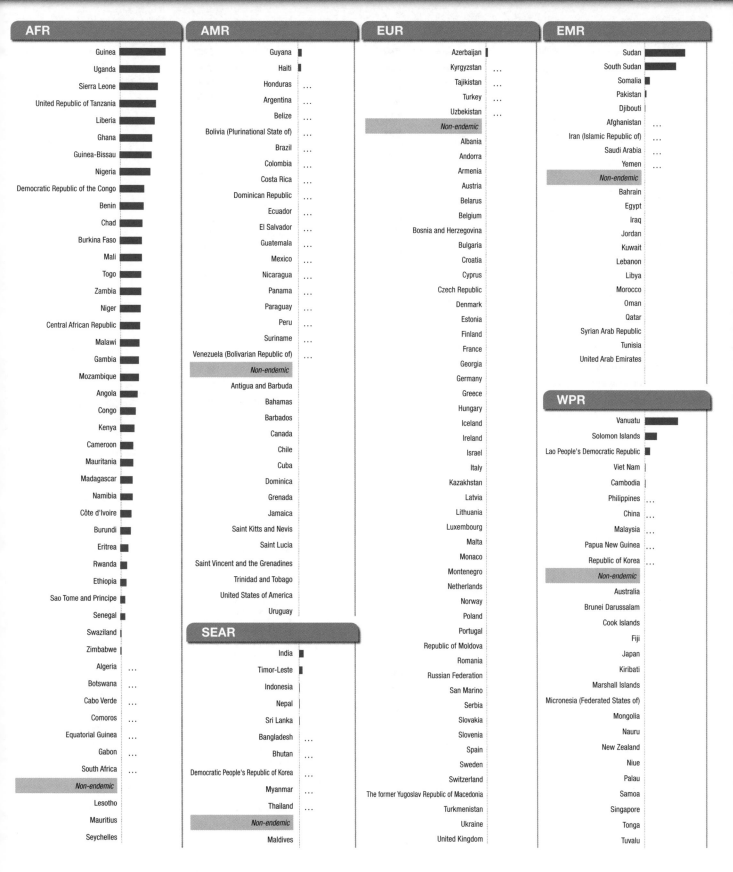

AFR
- Guinea
- Uganda
- Sierra Leone
- United Republic of Tanzania
- Liberia
- Ghana
- Guinea-Bissau
- Nigeria
- Democratic Republic of the Congo
- Benin
- Chad
- Burkina Faso
- Mali
- Togo
- Zambia
- Niger
- Central African Republic
- Malawi
- Gambia
- Mozambique
- Angola
- Congo
- Kenya
- Cameroon
- Mauritania
- Madagascar
- Namibia
- Côte d'Ivoire
- Burundi
- Eritrea
- Rwanda
- Ethiopia
- Sao Tome and Principe
- Senegal
- Swaziland
- Zimbabwe
- Algeria ...
- Botswana ...
- Cabo Verde ...
- Comoros ...
- Equatorial Guinea ...
- Gabon ...
- South Africa ...
- *Non-endemic*
- Lesotho
- Mauritius
- Seychelles

AMR
- Guyana
- Haiti
- Honduras ...
- Argentina ...
- Belize ...
- Bolivia (Plurinational State of) ...
- Brazil ...
- Colombia ...
- Costa Rica ...
- Dominican Republic ...
- Ecuador ...
- El Salvador ...
- Guatemala ...
- Mexico ...
- Nicaragua ...
- Panama ...
- Paraguay ...
- Peru ...
- Suriname ...
- Venezuela (Bolivarian Republic of) ...
- *Non-endemic*
- Antigua and Barbuda
- Bahamas
- Barbados
- Canada
- Chile
- Cuba
- Dominica
- Grenada
- Jamaica
- Saint Kitts and Nevis
- Saint Lucia
- Saint Vincent and the Grenadines
- Trinidad and Tobago
- United States of America
- Uruguay

SEAR
- India
- Timor-Leste
- Indonesia
- Nepal
- Sri Lanka
- Bangladesh ...
- Bhutan ...
- Democratic People's Republic of Korea ...
- Myanmar ...
- Thailand ...
- *Non-endemic*
- Maldives

EUR
- Azerbaijan
- Kyrgyzstan ...
- Tajikistan ...
- Turkey ...
- Uzbekistan ...
- *Non-endemic*
- Albania
- Andorra
- Armenia
- Austria
- Belarus
- Belgium
- Bosnia and Herzegovina
- Bulgaria
- Croatia
- Cyprus
- Czech Republic
- Denmark
- Estonia
- Finland
- France
- Georgia
- Germany
- Greece
- Hungary
- Iceland
- Ireland
- Israel
- Italy
- Kazakhstan
- Latvia
- Lithuania
- Luxembourg
- Malta
- Monaco
- Montenegro
- Netherlands
- Norway
- Poland
- Portugal
- Republic of Moldova
- Romania
- Russian Federation
- San Marino
- Serbia
- Slovakia
- Slovenia
- Spain
- Sweden
- Switzerland
- The former Yugoslav Republic of Macedonia
- Turkmenistan
- Ukraine
- United Kingdom

EMR
- Sudan
- South Sudan
- Somalia
- Pakistan
- Djibouti
- Afghanistan ...
- Iran (Islamic Republic of) ...
- Saudi Arabia ...
- Yemen ...
- *Non-endemic*
- Bahrain
- Egypt
- Iraq
- Jordan
- Kuwait
- Lebanon
- Libya
- Morocco
- Oman
- Qatar
- Syrian Arab Republic
- Tunisia
- United Arab Emirates

WPR
- Vanuatu
- Solomon Islands
- Lao People's Democratic Republic
- Viet Nam
- Cambodia
- Philippines ...
- China ...
- Malaysia ...
- Papua New Guinea
- Republic of Korea ...
- *Non-endemic*
- Australia
- Brunei Darussalam
- Cook Islands
- Fiji
- Japan
- Kiribati
- Marshall Islands
- Micronesia (Federated States of)
- Mongolia
- Nauru
- New Zealand
- Niue
- Palau
- Samoa
- Singapore
- Tonga
- Tuvalu

This chart shows the percentage of children under 5 years old with fever in the two weeks prior to the survey who received any antimalarial medicine. Within each WHO region countries are sorted by the latest available data since 2006.

The vertical line denotes the target of 100% coverage set by WHO and the Roll Back Malaria Partnership.

Further details may be found in **Part III**: **Table 4**.

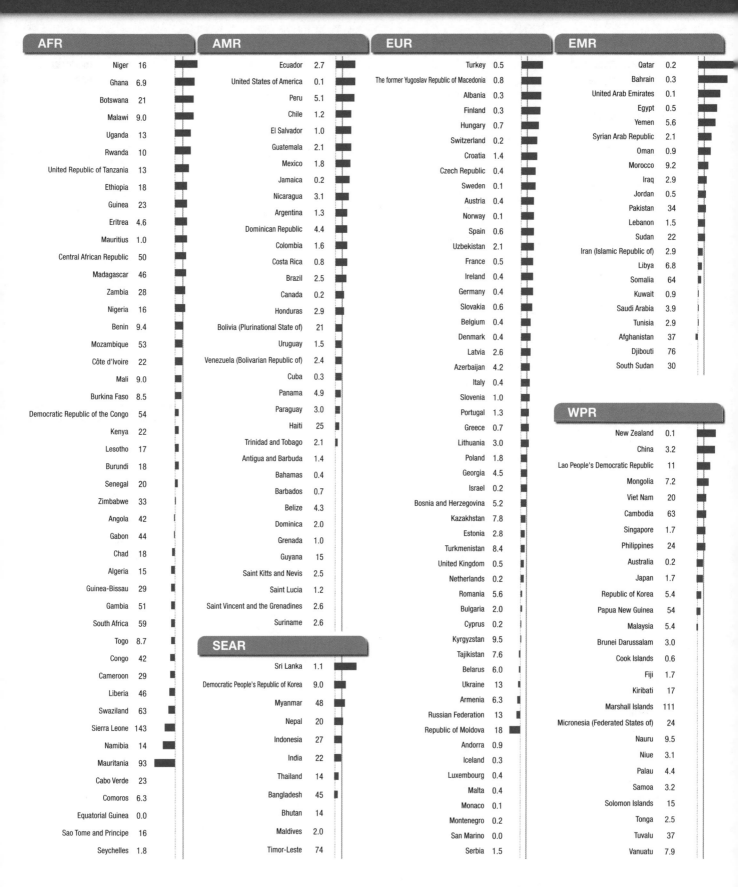

AFR

Country	Value
Niger	16
Ghana	6.9
Botswana	21
Malawi	9.0
Uganda	13
Rwanda	10
United Republic of Tanzania	13
Ethiopia	18
Guinea	23
Eritrea	4.6
Mauritius	1.0
Central African Republic	50
Madagascar	46
Zambia	28
Nigeria	16
Benin	9.4
Mozambique	53
Côte d'Ivoire	22
Mali	9.0
Burkina Faso	8.5
Democratic Republic of the Congo	54
Kenya	22
Lesotho	17
Burundi	18
Senegal	20
Zimbabwe	33
Angola	42
Gabon	44
Chad	18
Algeria	15
Guinea-Bissau	29
Gambia	51
South Africa	59
Togo	8.7
Congo	42
Cameroon	29
Liberia	46
Swaziland	63
Sierra Leone	143
Namibia	14
Mauritania	93
Cabo Verde	23
Comoros	6.3
Equatorial Guinea	0.0
Sao Tome and Principe	16
Seychelles	1.8

AMR

Country	Value
Ecuador	2.7
United States of America	0.1
Peru	5.1
Chile	1.2
El Salvador	1.0
Guatemala	2.1
Mexico	1.8
Jamaica	0.2
Nicaragua	3.1
Argentina	1.3
Dominican Republic	4.4
Colombia	1.6
Costa Rica	0.8
Brazil	2.5
Canada	0.2
Honduras	2.9
Bolivia (Plurinational State of)	21
Uruguay	1.5
Venezuela (Bolivarian Republic of)	2.4
Cuba	0.3
Panama	4.9
Paraguay	3.0
Haiti	25
Trinidad and Tobago	2.1
Antigua and Barbuda	1.4
Bahamas	0.4
Barbados	0.7
Belize	4.3
Dominica	2.0
Grenada	1.0
Guyana	15
Saint Kitts and Nevis	2.5
Saint Lucia	1.2
Saint Vincent and the Grenadines	2.6
Suriname	2.6

SEAR

Country	Value
Sri Lanka	1.1
Democratic People's Republic of Korea	9.0
Myanmar	48
Nepal	20
Indonesia	27
India	22
Thailand	14
Bangladesh	45
Bhutan	14
Maldives	2.0
Timor-Leste	74

EUR

Country	Value
Turkey	0.5
The former Yugoslav Republic of Macedonia	0.8
Albania	0.3
Finland	0.3
Hungary	0.7
Switzerland	0.2
Croatia	1.4
Czech Republic	0.4
Sweden	0.1
Austria	0.4
Norway	0.1
Spain	0.6
Uzbekistan	2.1
France	0.5
Ireland	0.4
Germany	0.4
Slovakia	0.6
Belgium	0.4
Denmark	0.4
Latvia	2.6
Azerbaijan	4.2
Italy	0.4
Slovenia	1.0
Portugal	1.3
Greece	0.7
Lithuania	3.0
Poland	1.8
Georgia	4.5
Israel	0.2
Bosnia and Herzegovina	5.2
Kazakhstan	7.8
Estonia	2.8
Turkmenistan	8.4
United Kingdom	0.5
Netherlands	0.2
Romania	5.6
Bulgaria	2.0
Cyprus	0.2
Kyrgyzstan	9.5
Tajikistan	7.6
Belarus	6.0
Ukraine	13
Armenia	6.3
Russian Federation	13
Republic of Moldova	18
Andorra	0.9
Iceland	0.3
Luxembourg	0.4
Malta	0.4
Monaco	0.1
Montenegro	0.2
San Marino	0.0
Serbia	1.5

EMR

Country	Value
Qatar	0.2
Bahrain	0.3
United Arab Emirates	0.1
Egypt	0.5
Yemen	5.6
Syrian Arab Republic	2.1
Oman	0.9
Morocco	9.2
Iraq	2.9
Jordan	0.5
Pakistan	34
Lebanon	1.5
Sudan	22
Iran (Islamic Republic of)	2.9
Libya	6.8
Somalia	64
Kuwait	0.9
Saudi Arabia	3.9
Tunisia	2.9
Afghanistan	37
Djibouti	76
South Sudan	30

WPR

Country	Value
New Zealand	0.1
China	3.2
Lao People's Democratic Republic	11
Mongolia	7.2
Viet Nam	20
Cambodia	63
Singapore	1.7
Philippines	24
Australia	0.2
Japan	1.7
Republic of Korea	5.4
Papua New Guinea	54
Malaysia	5.4
Brunei Darussalam	3.0
Cook Islands	0.6
Fiji	1.7
Kiribati	17
Marshall Islands	111
Micronesia (Federated States of)	24
Nauru	9.5
Niue	3.1
Palau	4.4
Samoa	3.2
Solomon Islands	15
Tonga	2.5
Tuvalu	37
Vanuatu	7.9

This chart shows the AARD in the estimated tuberculosis mortality rate per 100 000 population (excluding deaths among HIV-positive people) for the period 1990–2012. Within each WHO region countries are sorted in descending order based on the AARD in estimated tuberculosis mortality rates.

In order to reach the target of a 50% reduction between 1990 and 2015 set by the Stop TB Partnership, an AARD of 2.7% is needed and this is denoted by the vertical line. The numerical values shown are estimated tuberculosis mortality rates per 100 000 population in 2012. For countries with small populations, the AARD may not be applicable and only the 2012 estimated mortality rate is shown.

Further details may be found in **Part III: Table 2**.

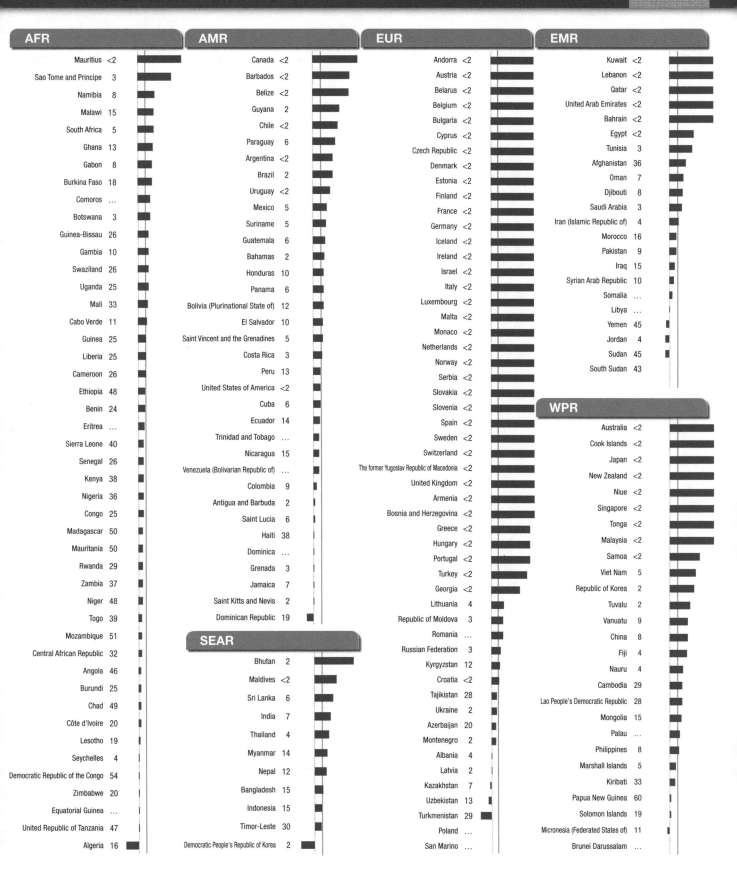

AFR

Mauritius	<2
Sao Tome and Principe	3
Namibia	8
Malawi	15
South Africa	5
Ghana	13
Gabon	8
Burkina Faso	18
Comoros	...
Botswana	3
Guinea-Bissau	26
Gambia	10
Swaziland	26
Uganda	25
Mali	33
Cabo Verde	11
Guinea	25
Liberia	25
Cameroon	26
Ethiopia	48
Benin	24
Eritrea	...
Sierra Leone	40
Senegal	26
Kenya	38
Nigeria	36
Congo	25
Madagascar	50
Mauritania	50
Rwanda	29
Zambia	37
Niger	48
Togo	39
Mozambique	51
Central African Republic	32
Angola	46
Burundi	25
Chad	49
Côte d'Ivoire	20
Lesotho	19
Seychelles	4
Democratic Republic of the Congo	54
Zimbabwe	20
Equatorial Guinea	...
United Republic of Tanzania	47
Algeria	16

AMR

Canada	<2
Barbados	<2
Belize	<2
Guyana	2
Chile	<2
Paraguay	6
Argentina	<2
Brazil	2
Uruguay	<2
Mexico	5
Suriname	5
Guatemala	6
Bahamas	2
Honduras	10
Panama	6
Bolivia (Plurinational State of)	12
El Salvador	10
Saint Vincent and the Grenadines	5
Costa Rica	3
Peru	13
United States of America	<2
Cuba	6
Ecuador	14
Trinidad and Tobago	...
Nicaragua	15
Venezuela (Bolivarian Republic of)	...
Colombia	9
Antigua and Barbuda	2
Saint Lucia	6
Haiti	38
Dominica	...
Grenada	3
Jamaica	7
Saint Kitts and Nevis	2
Dominican Republic	19

SEAR

Bhutan	2
Maldives	<2
Sri Lanka	6
India	7
Thailand	4
Myanmar	14
Nepal	12
Bangladesh	15
Indonesia	15
Timor-Leste	30
Democratic People's Republic of Korea	2

EUR

Andorra	<2
Austria	<2
Belarus	<2
Belgium	<2
Bulgaria	<2
Cyprus	<2
Czech Republic	<2
Denmark	<2
Estonia	<2
Finland	<2
France	<2
Germany	<2
Iceland	<2
Ireland	<2
Israel	<2
Italy	<2
Luxembourg	<2
Malta	<2
Monaco	<2
Netherlands	<2
Norway	<2
Serbia	<2
Slovakia	<2
Slovenia	<2
Spain	<2
Sweden	<2
Switzerland	<2
The former Yugoslav Republic of Macedonia	<2
United Kingdom	<2
Armenia	<2
Bosnia and Herzegovina	<2
Greece	<2
Hungary	<2
Portugal	<2
Turkey	<2
Georgia	<2
Lithuania	4
Republic of Moldova	3
Romania	...
Russian Federation	3
Kyrgyzstan	12
Croatia	<2
Tajikistan	28
Ukraine	2
Azerbaijan	20
Montenegro	2
Albania	4
Latvia	2
Kazakhstan	7
Uzbekistan	13
Turkmenistan	29
Poland	...
San Marino	...

EMR

Kuwait	<2
Lebanon	<2
Qatar	<2
United Arab Emirates	<2
Bahrain	<2
Egypt	<2
Tunisia	3
Afghanistan	36
Oman	7
Djibouti	8
Saudi Arabia	3
Iran (Islamic Republic of)	4
Morocco	16
Pakistan	9
Iraq	15
Syrian Arab Republic	10
Somalia	...
Libya	...
Yemen	45
Jordan	4
Sudan	45
South Sudan	43

WPR

Australia	<2
Cook Islands	<2
Japan	<2
New Zealand	<2
Niue	<2
Singapore	<2
Tonga	<2
Malaysia	<2
Samoa	<2
Viet Nam	5
Republic of Korea	2
Tuvalu	2
Vanuatu	9
China	8
Fiji	4
Nauru	4
Cambodia	29
Lao People's Democratic Republic	28
Mongolia	15
Palau	...
Philippines	8
Marshall Islands	5
Kiribati	33
Papua New Guinea	60
Solomon Islands	19
Micronesia (Federated States of)	11
Brunei Darussalam	...

The AARD in the proportion of the population without access to improved drinking-water sources was calculated using the complement of the estimated proportion using an improved drinking-water source, for the period 1990–2012 (or any minimum mperiod of five years since 1990). Within each WHO region countries are sorted in descending order based on this rate of decline.

In order to reach the MDG target of halving, by 2015, the proportion of people without sustainable access to safe drinking-water, an AARD of 2.7% will be required and is denoted by the vertical line. Countries with sustained low levels of proportion of population without access to improved drinking-water sources (< 2%) can be considered to have met the target and are shown with the maximum AARD at the beginning of their respective regional listing. The numerical values show the estimated percentage of the population not using improved drinking-water sources in 2012.

Further details may be found in **Part III: Table 5**.

13 | AARD (%) in proportion of population without access to improved sanitation

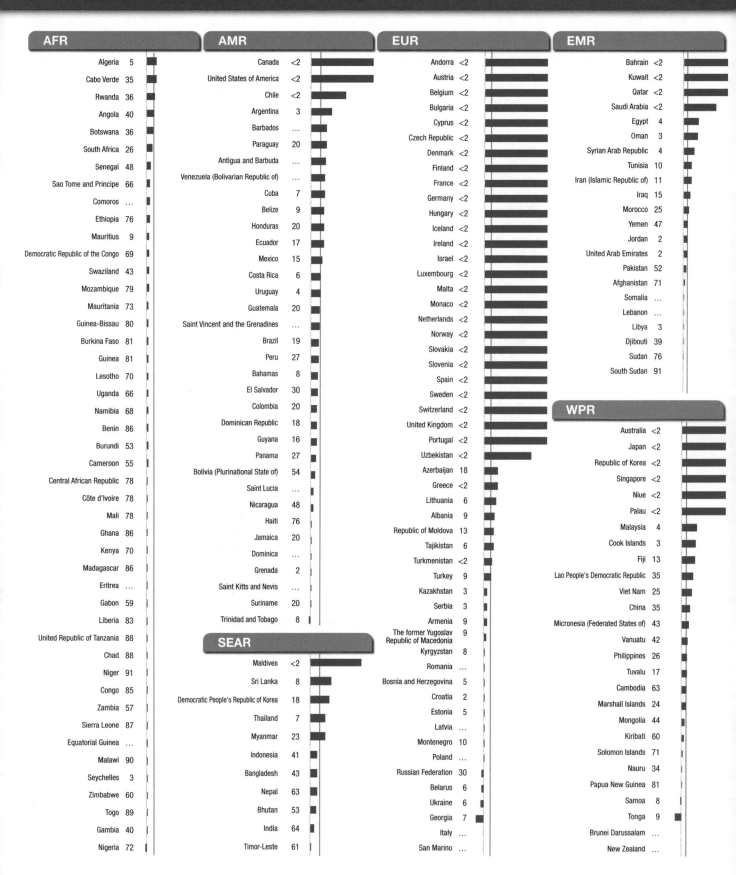

AFR

Country	Value
Algeria	5
Cabo Verde	35
Rwanda	36
Angola	40
Botswana	36
South Africa	26
Senegal	48
Sao Tome and Principe	66
Comoros	...
Ethiopia	76
Mauritius	9
Democratic Republic of the Congo	69
Swaziland	43
Mozambique	79
Mauritania	73
Guinea-Bissau	80
Burkina Faso	81
Guinea	81
Lesotho	70
Uganda	66
Namibia	68
Benin	86
Burundi	53
Cameroon	55
Central African Republic	78
Côte d'Ivoire	78
Mali	78
Ghana	86
Kenya	70
Madagascar	86
Eritrea	...
Gabon	59
Liberia	83
United Republic of Tanzania	88
Chad	88
Niger	91
Congo	85
Zambia	57
Sierra Leone	87
Equatorial Guinea	...
Malawi	90
Seychelles	3
Zimbabwe	60
Togo	89
Gambia	40
Nigeria	72

AMR

Country	Value
Canada	<2
United States of America	<2
Chile	<2
Argentina	3
Barbados	...
Paraguay	20
Antigua and Barbuda	...
Venezuela (Bolivarian Republic of)	...
Cuba	7
Belize	9
Honduras	20
Ecuador	17
Mexico	15
Costa Rica	6
Uruguay	4
Guatemala	20
Saint Vincent and the Grenadines	...
Brazil	19
Peru	27
Bahamas	8
El Salvador	30
Colombia	20
Dominican Republic	18
Guyana	16
Panama	27
Bolivia (Plurinational State of)	54
Saint Lucia	...
Nicaragua	48
Haiti	76
Jamaica	20
Dominica	...
Grenada	2
Saint Kitts and Nevis	...
Suriname	20
Trinidad and Tobago	8

SEAR

Country	Value
Maldives	<2
Sri Lanka	8
Democratic People's Republic of Korea	18
Thailand	7
Myanmar	23
Indonesia	41
Bangladesh	43
Nepal	63
Bhutan	53
India	64
Timor-Leste	61

EUR

Country	Value
Andorra	<2
Austria	<2
Belgium	<2
Bulgaria	<2
Cyprus	<2
Czech Republic	<2
Denmark	<2
Finland	<2
France	<2
Germany	<2
Hungary	<2
Iceland	<2
Ireland	<2
Israel	<2
Luxembourg	<2
Malta	<2
Monaco	<2
Netherlands	<2
Norway	<2
Slovakia	<2
Slovenia	<2
Spain	<2
Sweden	<2
Switzerland	<2
United Kingdom	<2
Portugal	<2
Uzbekistan	<2
Azerbaijan	18
Greece	<2
Lithuania	6
Albania	9
Republic of Moldova	13
Tajikistan	6
Turkmenistan	<2
Turkey	9
Kazakhstan	3
Serbia	3
Armenia	9
The former Yugoslav Republic of Macedonia	9
Kyrgyzstan	8
Romania	...
Bosnia and Herzegovina	5
Croatia	2
Estonia	5
Latvia	...
Montenegro	10
Poland	...
Russian Federation	30
Belarus	6
Ukraine	6
Georgia	7
Italy	...
San Marino	...

EMR

Country	Value
Bahrain	<2
Kuwait	<2
Qatar	<2
Saudi Arabia	<2
Egypt	4
Oman	3
Syrian Arab Republic	4
Tunisia	10
Iran (Islamic Republic of)	11
Iraq	15
Morocco	25
Yemen	47
Jordan	2
United Arab Emirates	2
Pakistan	52
Afghanistan	71
Somalia	...
Lebanon	...
Libya	3
Djibouti	39
Sudan	76
South Sudan	91

WPR

Country	Value
Australia	<2
Japan	<2
Republic of Korea	<2
Singapore	<2
Niue	<2
Palau	<2
Malaysia	4
Cook Islands	3
Fiji	13
Lao People's Democratic Republic	35
Viet Nam	25
China	35
Micronesia (Federated States of)	43
Vanuatu	42
Philippines	26
Tuvalu	17
Cambodia	63
Marshall Islands	24
Mongolia	44
Kiribati	60
Solomon Islands	71
Nauru	34
Papua New Guinea	81
Samoa	8
Tonga	9
Brunei Darussalam	...
New Zealand	...

The AARD in the proportion of the population without access to improved sanitation was calculated using the complement of the estimated proportion using improved sanitation, for the period 1990–2012 (or any minimum period of five years since 1990). Within each WHO region countries are sorted in descending order based on this rate of decline.

In order to reach the MDG target of halving, by 2015, the proportion of people without sustainable access to basic sanitation, an AARD of 2.7% will be required and is denoted by the vertical line. Countries with sustained low levels of proportion of population without access to improved sanitation (< 2%) can be considered to have met the target and are shown with the maximum AARD at the beginning of their respective regional listing. The numerical values show the estimated percentage of the population not using improved sanitation in 2012.

Further details may be found in **Part III**: **Table 5**.

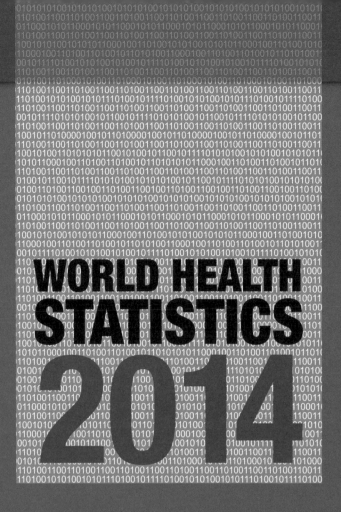

WORLD HEALTH STATISTICS 2014

Part II

Highlighted topics

Putting an ending to preventable maternal mortality – the next steps

A major catalyst in the progress made to date in reducing the number of maternal deaths has been the explicitly stated objective of MDG target 5.A to reduce the maternal mortality ratio by three quarters between 1990 and 2015. In addition, the setting of MDG target 5.B on achieving universal access to reproductive-health services has contributed to an accelerated rate of progress. Between the MDG baseline year of 1990 and 2000, the annual rate of decline in the global maternal mortality ratio was 1.4% – between 2000 and 2013 this figure increased to 3.5%. As a result, there were an estimated 289 000 maternal deaths globally in 2013, a decline of 45% from the level in 1990.[1]

[1.] WHO, UNICEF, UNFPA, United Nations Population Division and the World Bank. Trends in Maternal Mortality: 1990-2013. Geneva: World Health Organization; 2014. In preparation at the time of printing of this report.

Nevertheless, despite the stated aspiration to achieve MDG5 by 2015, it is clear that a number of countries will not reach this goal on time if their currently insufficient rate of progress – or lack of progress – continues (see **Part I: Chart 3**). Recent estimates of national maternal mortality ratios continue to highlight both ongoing global variations (**Fig. 8**) and stark regional inequalities in the lifetime risk of maternal death (**Table 2**).

As 2015 approaches, countries and the international maternal health community are reflecting on the progress made, while at the same time elaborating upon the new targets in the post-2015 landscape that would best encapsulate the ending of preventable maternal deaths. This ambitious but realistic vision to make further significant reductions in maternal mortality ratios is expected to be a key element of the discourse on global development goals beyond 2015. If successful, such a

Figure 8. Variations in national maternal mortality ratio (maternal deaths per 100 000 live births), 2013

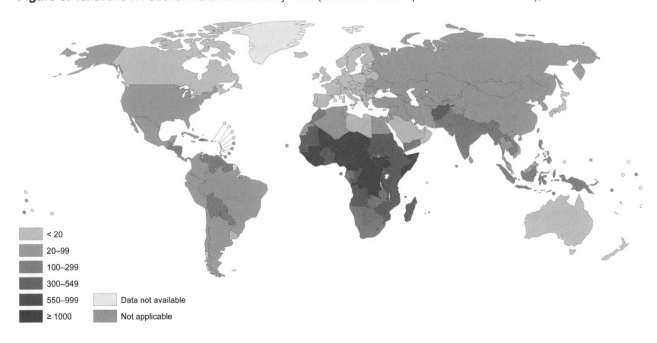

< 20	
20–99	
100–299	
300–549	
550–999	Data not available
≥ 1000	Not applicable

Table 2. Estimated maternal mortality ratio (maternal deaths per 100 000 live births), number of maternal deaths and lifetime risk, by WHO region, 2013[1]

| Region | Maternal mortality ratio (MMR) | Range of MMR uncertainty | | Number of maternal deaths | Lifetime risk of maternal deaths: 1 in |
		Lower estimate	Upper estimate		
AFR	500	370	720	171 000	40
AMR	68	52	92	11 000	680
SEAR	190	130	270	68 000	210
EUR	17	14	22	1 900	3300
EMR	170	120	260	26 000	180
WPR	45	32	66	12 000	1200
Global	210	160	290	289 000	190

vision would translate into a maternal mortality ratio of less than 90 per 100 000 live births by 2025, less than 70 by 2030 and less than 50 by 2035 (**Fig. 9**). With recent demonstrable reductions having being achieved in maternal mortality even in challenging settings, such a target is attainable worldwide.

Strategies for achieving and sustaining further reductions in maternal mortality are now needed. Vital to the development of these strategies will be the improved measurement of maternal mortality – documenting not only how many maternal deaths occur but also data on the causes and circumstances leading to each of these deaths. Such information, obtained for example through confidential enquiries or maternal death surveillance and response activities, will enable the coherent development of strategies to respond to needs, target monitoring efforts and ensure collective accountability

and action. Too often, the data that are being collected are of poor quality, bringing only limited returns on the resources used while severely constraining the informed development of programmes and policies. Efforts to understand the causes of maternal death have also been hampered by inconsistency in death attribution, reporting and resultant coding; even within high-quality data sources such as vital registration systems. In 1990, a "checkbox" was added to International Classification of Diseases (ICD) death certificates to indicate whether or not a woman was pregnant, or had recently delivered or terminated a pregnancy. And yet the ongoing misclassification and underreporting of deaths continues to introduce bias into activities aimed at understanding the magnitude and causes of maternal deaths.

In 2010, the Secretary-General of the United Nations launched the Global Strategy for Women's and Children's Health to mobilize the commitment of governments, civil society organizations and development partners to accelerate progress towards achieving MDGs 4 and 5. Subsequently, the Commission on Information and Accountability for Women's and Children's Health was established to:

---

[1] WHO, UNICEF, UNFPA, United Nations Population Division and The World Bank. Trends in Maternal Mortality: 1990–2013. Geneva: World Health Organization; 2014. In preparation at the time of printing of this report. See report for regional groupings used.

Figure 9. Estimated and target reductions in global maternal mortality ratio, 1990–2035[1]

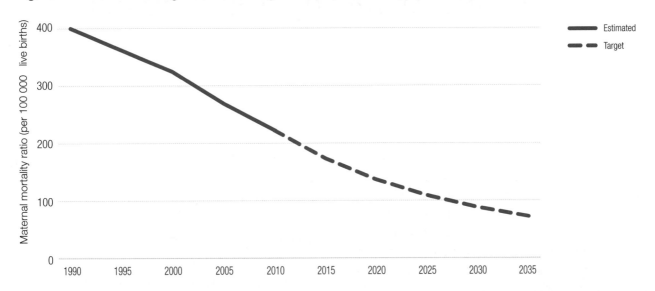

... determine the most effective international institutional arrangements for global reporting, oversight and accountability on women's and children's health.[2]

One of the 10 recommendations of the Commission specifically focused on improving the measurement of maternal (and child) deaths. This recommendation requires that:

... by 2015, all countries have taken significant steps to establish a system for registration of births, deaths and causes of death, and have well-functioning health information systems that combine data from facilities, administrative sources and surveys.[2]

The increased use of innovative approaches such as mobile Health (mHealth) technologies to strengthen the capture, analysis and application of data will be a vital element in meeting this goal. Improvements in the measurement of maternal deaths must then be used to complement strategies for implementing targeted interventions to reduce maternal mortality.

As part of further reducing the levels of maternal mortality, efforts to ensure equity and maintain a human-rights-based approach will be vital. At the same time, there will be a need to respond to changing demographics, meet the specific needs of women in respect of their reproductive health and strengthen health-care systems. Universal access to high-quality health services, including family planning and information and services for reproductive health (especially for vulnerable and at-risk populations), should be placed at the centre of efforts to achieve the vision of ending preventable maternal deaths.

1. Bustreo F, Say L, Koblinsky M, Pullum TW, Temmerman M, Pablos-Mendez A. Ending preventable maternal deaths: the time is now. Lancet, Global Health. October 2013;1(4):e176–7. doi:10.1016/S2214-109X(13)70059-7 (http://www.thelancet.com/journals/langlo/article/PIIS2214-109X%2813%2970059-7/fulltext, accessed 12 March 2014).

2. Commission on Information and Accountability for Women's and Children's Health. Keeping promises, measuring results. Geneva: World Health Organization; 2011 (http://www.everywomaneverychild.org/images/content/files/accountability_commission/final_report/Final_EN_Web.pdf, accessed 9 March 2014).

Rising childhood obesity – time to act

Historically, a heavy child was regarded as a healthy child and there was widespread acceptance of the concept of "bigger is better". Today, such perceptions are changing in the face of evidence that obesity in childhood is associated with a wide range of serious health complications and an increased risk of premature illness. Beyond the increased risk of becoming an overweight adult, overweight children are often diagnosed with at least one additional risk factor for cardiovascular disease, such as elevated blood pressure or raised blood cholesterol. In addition, Type 2 diabetes is increasingly prevalent in young children, with lack of physical exercise and unhealthy diet among the typical risk factors. Further health complications can arise, including joint problems and breathing difficulties. In addition to these physical problems a number of potential psychological health issues are also associated with overweight and obese children. Such children often suffer from poor self-image, low self-confidence and even depression – all of which are health problems that can track into adolescence and adult life.

Since its inception in 1986, the WHO Global Database on Child Growth and Malnutrition[1] has been monitoring patterns and trends in overweight and obese children. One of the objectives of this database is to compile, standardize and disseminate the results of nutritional surveys conducted worldwide. For the last several years a UNICEF, WHO and World Bank initiative has been using the data obtained to derive joint global and regional prevalence and number estimates of child stunting, underweight, wasting and overweight. Resulting from the harmonization of survey data and statistical methods, prevalence estimates are derived based on the WHO Child Growth Standards[2] median for:

- stunting – proportion of children with height-for-age below –2 standard deviations (SD);
- underweight – proportion of children with weight-for-age below –2 SD;
- wasting – proportion of children with weight-for-height below –2 SD;
- overweight – proportion of children with weight-for-height above +2 SD and including obesity which is defined as above +3 SD.

In 2012, an estimated 44 million (6.7%) of children under 5 years of age were overweight or obese worldwide (**Fig. 10**). Based on this latest figure, the global prevalence of overweight and obese children has grown from around 5% in 1990 to 7% in 2012. In the WHO African Region alone the number of overweight children increased from 4 to 10 million over the same period.

Although such overall estimates give an indication of general direction, overweight trends can vary at country level. As long as the majority of national trends remain moderate and the prevalences of overweight children relatively low (**Fig. 11**) there will be a window of opportunity for preventing further increases. For that reason WHO has proposed to its Member States that efforts now be undertaken to halt any further increase in the prevalence of overweight children globally. This objective was one of the six global nutrition targets for 2025 endorsed by the World Health Assembly in 2012.

[1] WHO Global Database on Child Growth and Malnutrition [online database]. Geneva: World Health Organization; 2012 (http://www.who.int/nutgrowthdb, accessed 15 January 2014).

[2] WHO Multicentre Growth Reference Study Group. WHO Child Growth Standards: Length/height-for-age, weight-for-age, weight-for-length, weight-for-height and body mass index-for-age: Methods and development. Geneva: World Health Organization; 2006 (http://www.who.int/childgrowth/standards/technical_report/en/, accessed 10 March 2014).

Figure 10. Number and prevalence of overweight or obese children – globally, 1990–2012[1]

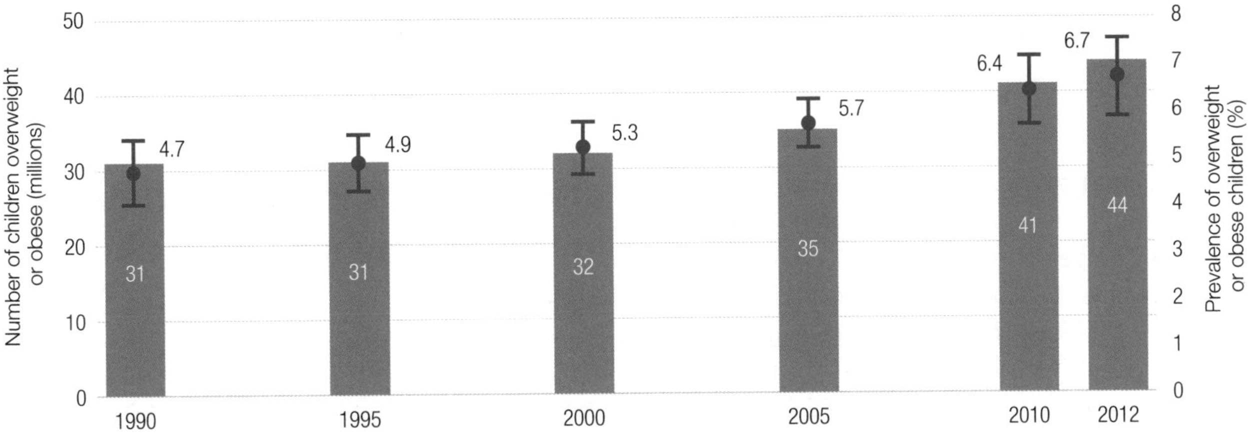

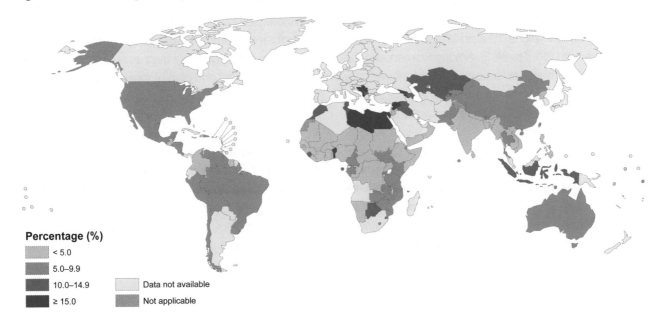

Figure 11. Children aged < 5 years overweight (%), latest available year, 2006–2012

Percentage (%)
- < 5.0
- 5.0–9.9
- 10.0–14.9
- ≥ 15.0
- Data not available
- Not applicable

Countries shown without available data may have survey estimates prior to 2006 or use national reference data instead of WHO standards.

Exclusive breastfeeding from birth to 6 months of age is one way to help prevent early child overweight. The WHO Child Growth Standards were based on exclusively breastfed infants to develop a comparison group that reflected good practices. The children included in this cohort were found to be leaner compared with the former international reference used until then. The application of these new standards will thus play an important role in efforts to prevent increases in the levels of overweight and obese children. Furthermore the application of the WHO standards and associated tools will allow for a comprehensive assessment of child growth to be made. This is important as the use of single indicators alone carries the risk of only partially reflecting the true picture of child nutritional status. Challenges to be tackled include ensuring the availability of adequate equipment and skills for accurately measuring length and height, as this is the key to a comprehensive assessment of childhood undernutrition, overnutrition and stunting.

[1] 2012 Joint child malnutrition estimates – Levels and trends [online database]. New York: UNICEF, Geneva: WHO and Washington, DC: The World Bank (http://www.who.int/nutgrowthdb/estimates2012).

Life expectancy in the world in 2012

In 2012, global life expectancy at birth was 68.1 years for men and 72.7 years for women. Among men, life expectancy ranged from a high of 75.8 years in high-income countries to a low of 60.2 years in low-income countries – a difference of 15.6 years (**Fig. 12**). For women, a gap of 18.9 years separates the life expectancy figures in high-income countries (82.0 years) and low-income countries (63.1 years).

As shown in **Table 3**, life expectancy among men is 80 years or higher in nine countries with populations over 250 000, with the highest found in Australia, Iceland and Switzerland (80.5 to 81.2). Among women, the top 10 countries all have life expectancies of 84 years or longer. Women in Japan have the highest life expectancy in the world at 87.0 years, followed by Spain, Switzerland and Singapore.

At the lower end, there are nine countries where both male and female life expectancies are still estimated to be below 55 years. All of these countries are located in sub-Saharan Africa. It should also be noted that estimates of life expectancies in the poorest countries are associated with much greater uncertainty levels due to a lack of reliable data, especially on levels of adult mortality.

Life expectancy at birth has increased by six years since 1990

At the global level both male and female life expectancies have increased by six years since 1990, with gains recorded across all country-income groups (**Fig. 13**). Recent increases have been largest in low-income countries, where both male and female life expectancies increased by around nine years – from 51.2 to 60.2 years for men and from 54.0 to 63.1 years for women. This is more than twice as high as recent gains in high-income countries, and also higher than the gains made in both upper- and lower-middle-income countries.

In low-income countries such gains in life expectancy are equivalent to an average increase of 3 days per week – or 10 hours every day. This has been achieved despite the ongoing HIV/AIDS pandemic affecting many low-income countries in sub-Saharan Africa during this same period. The main driver of this improvement in life expectancy at birth has been the rapid decrease in child mortality seen in many countries over the last decade.

Figure 12. Life expectancy at birth for men and women in 2012, by country income group

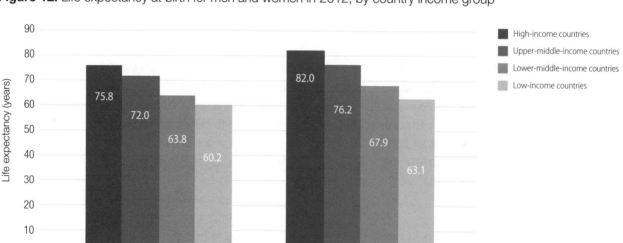

Table 3. Life expectancy at birth among men and women in 2012 in the 10 top-ranked countries

	Men				Women	
Rank	Country	Life expectancy		Rank	Country	Life expectancy
1	Iceland	81.2		1	Japan	87.0
2	Switzerland	80.7		2	Spain	85.1
3	Australia	80.5		3	Switzerland	85.1
4	Israel	80.2		4	Singapore	85.1
5	Singapore	80.2		5	Italy	85.0
6	New Zealand	80.2		6	France	84.9
7	Italy	80.2		7	Australia	84.6
8	Japan	80.0		8	Republic of Korea	84.6
9	Sweden	80.0		9	Luxembourg	84.1
10	Luxembourg	79.7		10	Portugal	84.0

Countries with a population below 250 000 are omitted due to uncertainty in life-expectancy estimates.

Figure 13. Years gained in life expectancy 1990–2012, by sex and country income group

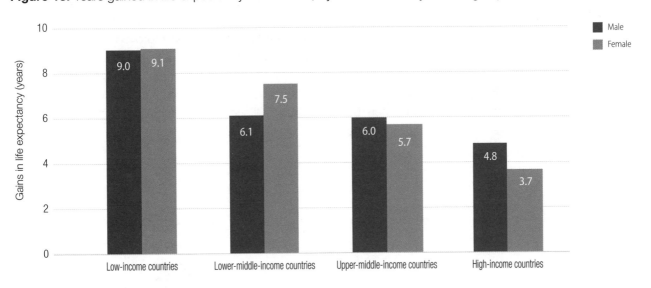

At the national level, 24 countries gained more than 10 years in life expectancy (both sexes combined) between 1990 and 2012. Of these countries, 12 were in the WHO African Region and five in the WHO South-East Asia Region, along with Afghanistan, Cambodia, the Islamic Republic of Iran, the Lao People's Democratic Republic, Lebanon, South Sudan and Turkey.

The top six individual gains recorded were in Liberia (19.7 years) followed by Ethiopia, Maldives, Cambodia, Timor-Leste and Rwanda. Among high-income countries, the average gain was 5.1 years, ranging from 0.2 years in the Russian Federation to 9.2 years in the Republic of Korea.

Women continue to live longer than men

Women live longer than men all around the world. The gap in life expectancy between the sexes was 4.6 years in 1990 and had remained the same by 2012. As shown in **Fig. 14**, this gap is much larger in high-income countries (more than six years) than in low-income countries (around three years). There are also differences in trends across different country income groups. Among high-income countries, the gap narrowed by one year; mainly due to larger reductions in recent decades in male smoking rates than in female smoking rates. The experience in low- and middle-income countries has been mixed. Among lower-middle-income countries the gap is widening. However, due to lower-quality data, the reasons for this change are unclear. Potential contributing factors include historical increases in tobacco smoking rates among men but not women, and recent decreases in the maternal mortality ratio.

Older adults are also living longer

Globally, between 1990 and 2012, life expectancy at age 60 increased from 16.6 years to 18.5 years for men and from 19.7 years to 21.5 years for women. Life expectancies at age 60 were longer and the increases larger in high-income countries. In such countries, life expectancy at age 60 had increased by almost as much as life expectancy at birth – around three years for both men and women. By 2012, a 60-year–old Japanese woman could expect to live another 29.1 years, which is a 4.4 year increase on what her prospects would have been in 1990. Much of the impressive gain seen in male life expectancy at birth in Australia stems from reductions in older-age mortality levels. Australian male life expectancy at age 60 increased from 19.0 years in 1990 to 23.8 years in 2012.

Almost all high-income countries collect data on causes of death. These data indicate that falls in mortality from cardiovascular diseases are the main driver of rising life expectancy at age 60 for both men and women. For women, this reduction can probably be attributed in approximately equal measure to improved prevention and management of the metabolic risk factors for cardiovascular disease, such as hypertension, and to improved treatment of cardiovascular conditions. Men have also benefited from declining rates of tobacco use. In low- and middle-income countries, life expectancy at age 60 has improved, but not as quickly as in high-income countries. These increases ranged from one to two years since 1990. Nevertheless, the experience of high-income countries demonstrates that substantial scope exists for improving life expectancy at age 60 in these countries.

Figure 14. Gap in life expectancy between women and men, by country income group, 1990–2012

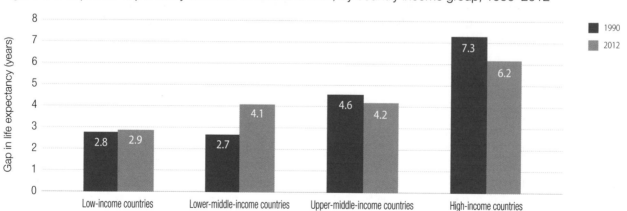

Years of life lost due to premature mortality – trends and causes

The total number of deaths from specific causes does not provide a good metric for informing public health priorities. Such a measure, for example, assigns the same weight to a death at age 80 as it does at age 30 or even at 1 year of age. The preponderance of noncommunicable diseases (NCDs) such as ischaemic heart disease and cerebrovascular disease in cause-of-death rankings is therefore potentially misleading and may not appropriately reflect the impact of premature mortality.

In **Part III: Table 2**, estimates are presented of the years of life lost (YLL) in 2012 in three broad disease categories. YLL is a measure of premature mortality that takes into account both the frequency of deaths and the age at which it occurs. YLL are calculated from the number of deaths at each age multiplied by

a global standard life expectancy for the age at which death occurs (**Box 1**). The overall patterns of premature mortality at global and regional levels are summarized below in terms of YLL.

What were the leading causes of YLL in 2012?

The top three causes of YLL in 2012 were ischaemic heart disease, lower respiratory infections (such as pneumonia) and stroke. **Fig. 15** summarizes the 20 leading causes of YLL in that year for both sexes combined. Half of the top-20 causes comprise infectious diseases, and maternal, neonatal and nutritional causes (referred to as "MDG conditions") while the other half consist of NCDs or injuries.

Box 1: YLL due to premature mortality

YLL due to premature mortality are calculated from the number of deaths at each age multiplied by a global standard life expectancy of the age at which death occurs. For the YLL reported in *World Health Statistics 2014*, the standard life table is based on the projected frontier life expectancy for 2050, with a life expectancy at birth of 92 years.[1] The standard reference life table is intended to represent the potential maximum life expectancy of an individual at a given age, and is used for both males and females. A death at birth will thus result in 92.0 YLL, a death

at age 30 in 62.1 YLL and a death at age 70 in 23.2 YLL.

This standard differs from the previous WHO standard which was based on separate life tables for males and females, with life expectancy at birth of 82.5 and 80.0 years respectively. The age weighting and time discounting previously applied in the calculation of YLL are also no longer done. Detailed estimates of YLL for 2000 and 2012 are available by country, region, age, sex and cause of death in the Global Health Observatory.[2]

[1] WHO methods and data sources for global burden of disease estimates 2000–2011. Global Health Estimates Technical Paper WHO/HIS/HSI/GHE/2013.4. Geneva: World Health Organization; 2013 (http://www.who.int/healthinfo/statistics/GlobalDALYmethods.pdf?ua=1, accessed 11 March 2014).

[2] Global Health Observatory [online database]. Geneva: World Health Organization (http://apps.who.int/gho/data/node.main.686?lang=en, accessed 6 March 2014).

Figure 15. The 20 leading causes of YLL – globally, 2012

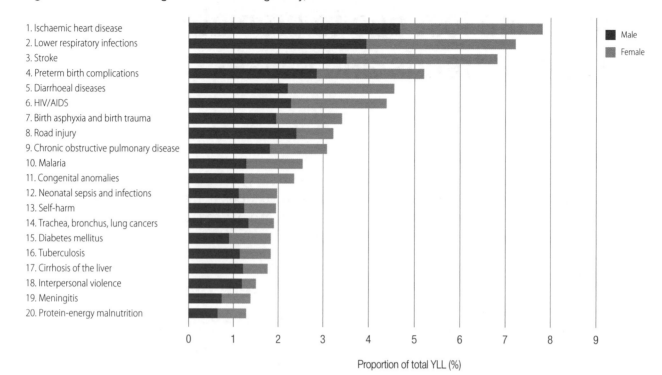

Proportion of total YLL (%)

What causes changed most between 2000 and 2012?

During the period 2000–2012, a major shift occurred in the main causes of YLL, away from MDG conditions and towards NCDs and injuries, with the proportion of YLL due to MDG conditions declining in almost every country in the world. Countries in which MDG conditions were responsible for the most YLL in 2000 are generally those in which the greatest reductions have taken place, including many African countries. Countries are, however, in very different stages of this epidemiological transition (**Fig. 16**). For example, there are 22 African countries in which MDG conditions are still responsible for more than 70% of all YLL. At the other end of this epidemiological shift, there are 47 countries in which MDG conditions cause less than 10% of all YLL.

What are the main contributors to change?

As outlined in the previous highlight section, the world has witnessed major gains in life expectancy in recent decades. This has resulted from a substantial decline in YLL for almost all of the leading causes for the year

2000 (**Fig. 17**). The biggest declines have been observed for measles (79% lower in 2012 than in 2000) followed by diarrhoeal diseases (40% lower), malaria (32% lower) and tuberculosis (32% lower).

Globally, the proportion of YLL resulting from NCDs has increased from 38% in 2000 to 47% in 2012. This reflects the successes achieved in reducing mortality from a number of leading communicable diseases. Combined with reduced levels of neonatal, infant, child and maternal mortality, and the resulting substantial increases in life expectancy now seen in many developing countries, people are increasingly surviving to ages at which NCDs are the primary causes of death. Of the leading 15 causes of YLL shown in **Fig. 17**, ischaemic heart disease and stroke were two of the three causes for which YLL increased between 2000 and 2012. Such changes also have implications for overall rankings as ischaemic heart disease overtook lower respiratory infections as the leading cause of YLL in the world. The 14% increase in YLL due to road injury deaths reflects increasing levels of motorization in developing countries which more than outweighs reductions in YLL caused by road injuries in developed countries. In contrast, global YLL decreased for several other important causes of injury, for example suicide (–12%) and drowning (–23%).

Figure 16. Countries are at different stages of the epidemiological transition away from MDG conditions as the main causes of YLL

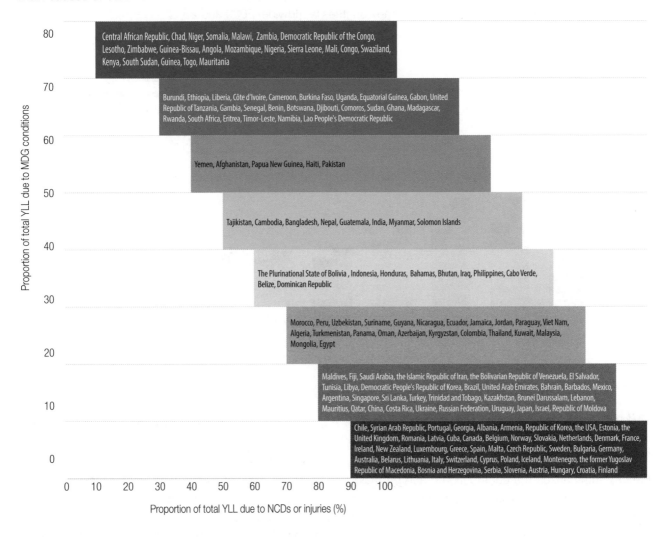

Figure 17. Changes in YLL due to leading causes – globally, 2000–2012

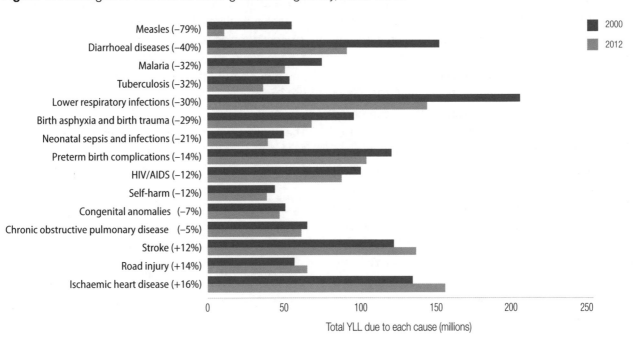

Figure 18. Contribution of major causes of death to YLL per 100 000 population in low- and middle-income countries in each WHO region and in high-income countries worldwide, 2000 and 2012

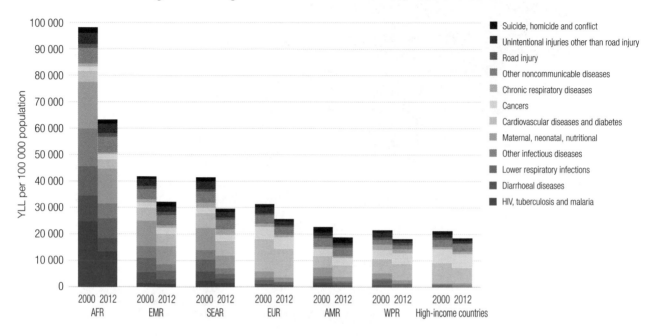

What are the patterns of YLL in different WHO regions?

Fig. 18 summarizes the contribution made by major causes of death to premature mortality rates (measured in terms of YLL per 100 000 population) in low- and middle-income countries in each of the six WHO regions, as well as in high-income countries worldwide. In the WHO African Region, the level of YLL due to communicable diseases alone exceeds the level due to all causes combined in each of the other regions. When maternal, neonatal and nutritional conditions are added, these causes account for around 70% of all YLL in the WHO African Region in 2012, compared with less than 50% in the WHO South-East Asia Region and WHO Eastern Mediterranean Region. In even greater contrast, such causes account for only 8% of YLL in high-income countries. Also clearly shown in Fig. 18 is the continuing impact of HIV, tuberculosis and malaria on YLL in the WHO African Region, despite recent substantial reductions in these and other MDG conditions. Despite a 36% fall in the overall YLL rate for the WHO African Region following such reductions the level of YLL in this region remains twice that of the next-highest region.

The impact of cardiovascular diseases as a cause of premature mortality in eastern Europe is apparent in **Fig. 18**, especially compared with high-income countries. Recent research has highlighted the role of alcohol and alcohol-drinking patterns in contributing to this very high level of premature mortality,[1] which results in male YLL rates for this region being 40% higher than those for males in high-income countries. in 2012. The impact of high levels of cardiovascular diseases and injuries in males results in a male–female YLL ratio of 1.54 in eastern Europe – higher than that observed in any other part of the world except Latin America and the Caribbean.

The contribution made by injuries to YLL rates ranges from a high of 21% of YLLs in 2012 in Latin America and the Caribbean to a low of 10% in the WHO African

---

1. Zaridze D, Lewington S, Boroda A, Scélo G, Karpov R, Lazarev A et al. Alcohol and mortality in Russia: prospective observational study of 151 000 adults. *Lancet*, Early Online Publication. 31 January 2014. doi:10.1016/S0140-6736(13)62247-3 (http://www.thelancet.com/journals/lancet/article/PIIS0140-6736%2813%2962247-3/abstract, accessed 12 March 2014).

Region. This two-fold variation across regions conceals much higher variations for some of the specific causes of injuries. For example, there is a 17-fold variation in interpersonal violence (highest in Latin America and the Caribbean; lowest in eastern Europe) and a 29-fold variation in burns (highest in the WHO African Region; lowest in Latin America and the Caribbean).

The YLL metric clearly highlights that, despite the considerable gains made, the global aspiration to substantially reduce mortality from MDG conditions has not yet been achieved in parts of the world – particularly in Africa, the Middle East and South Asia. This same metric provides compelling evidence of the need to now accelerate efforts to address the substantial and growing burden of premature mortality caused by NCDs as the world moves towards the post-2015 global health agenda.

Civil registration and vital statistics – the key to national and global advancement

Complete information from a civil registration and vital statistics (CRVS) system – that is, the registering of all births and all deaths and the recording of causes of death – represents one of the most valuable assets a country can have. Not only does the registration of births, deaths and other vital events provide individuals with critical documentation that enables them to realize a range of economic and social rights, the production of reliable information on fertility, mortality and causes of death in a population is central to governance, and to health, economic and social policy-making. Cause-specific mortality statistics by age, sex and geographical location derived from civil registration systems are instrumental in guiding national, regional and global health priorities.

Reporting cause-of-death statistics

Although reliable cause-of-death reporting is crucially important in health policy development and planning, cause-of-death reporting remains one of the most challenging aspects of CRVS. Overall, only around one third of all deaths worldwide are recorded in civil registries along with cause-of-death information.[1]

In order to produce globally comparable cause-of-death statistics, countries should use the International Classification of Diseases (ICD) as the standard for classifying causation. The ICD is updated and revised to reflect the latest knowledge available on the etiology of major diseases and health conditions. **Fig. 19** shows the number of reporting countries over time along with an indication of which revision of the ICD

was used. One striking feature has been the variable time lag between the introduction of a new revision of the ICD and its roll-out in countries. From ICD-7 to ICD-8 and from ICD-8 to ICD-9 the adoption of each new revision happened relatively quickly. However, the corresponding rate of change from ICD-9 to ICD-10[2] was slower, and it took until 2005 (around a decade) to achieve a level of 90% of countries using ICD-10. Some countries – including Denmark, Switzerland and Turkey – never adopted ICD-9, moving instead directly from ICD-8 to ICD-10. WHO is currently developing the 11th revision of the ICD. From a statistical perspective, ICD revision presents a number of challenges due to breaks in the statistical series. Although WHO recommends that countries maintain dual systems for a period of transfer from one revision to the next, this represents a considerable burden for coders and is not always done. Moreover, interim updates of the ICD between major revisions also occur, making the tasks of coders even more complex.

As is also shown in **Fig. 19**, only around 32 countries regularly reported cause-of-death information in the mid-1950s. This number increased to 66 countries in the mid-1970s and to 90 countries in the mid-1990s. Since then, however, the average number of countries annually reporting cause-of-death information in line with the ICD has virtually stagnated at 97 out of a total of 194 countries.

There is also a huge disparity among countries in the production of cause-of-death statistics. Whilst high-income countries have been generating such information on a routine basis for many years, the majority of low- and middle-income countries continue to struggle

[1] World Health Statistics 2012. Geneva: World Health Organization; 2012 (http://apps.who.int/iris/bitstream/10665/44844/1/9789241564441_eng.pdf?ua=1&ua=1, accessed 12 March 2014).

[2] International Statistical Classification of Diseases and Health Related Problems, Tenth Revision, 2010 Edition. Geneva: World Health Organization; 2012 (http://apps.who.int/classifications/icd10/browse/2010/en, accessed 31 March 2014.)

Figure 19. Trends in cause-of-death data reporting, by country income group and by ICD revision

By income group
Number of countries

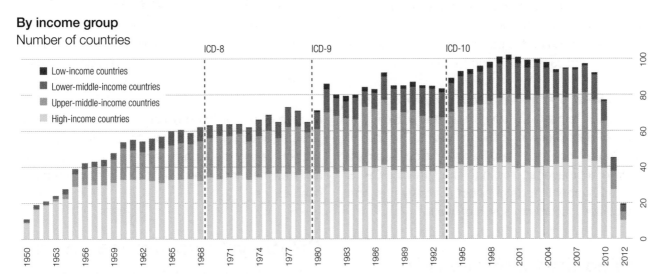

By ICD
Number of countries

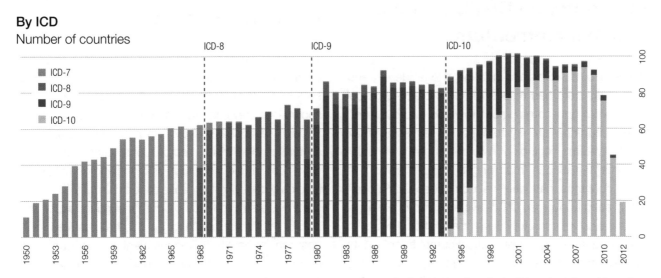

Because of the typically observed lag of 18–24 months before countries report finalized latest data, it should not be inferred from these charts that reporting for the most recent years has decreased.

The implementation year of the ICD revisions are indicated by the dashed lines.

to produce cause-of-death statistics due to dysfunctional CRVS systems, outdated legal frameworks, lack of awareness and capacities for accurate cause-of-death certification on the part of physicians, and lack of training and capacities among statistical coders.

Nevertheless, over the last decade several countries have made remarkable progress in the collection of cause-of-death data, including the Islamic Republic of Iran, South Africa and, lately, Turkey. This development is part of a broader approach to strengthening CRVS systems in order to register all births and deaths, and to accurately record all causes of death.

Laying the foundations for strengthened CRVS systems – a global momentum

Demand for CRVS as a foundation of legal identity and vital policy data has resulted in an increased global momentum and commitment towards improvement. Many countries are systematically assessing their CRVS systems, including in terms of the role health systems can play in improving them (see below). In some countries, national-level committees have been established to oversee CRVS systems improvement in accordance with carefully developed national plans. In many countries high-level political commitment exists for the strengthening of CRVS systems, and for the reporting of progress through regional structures. For example:

- In Africa, ministers with responsibility for civil registration have endorsed CRVS systems strengthening as a priority, and will meet with ministers of health at the end of 2014 to consider the best way forward.

- In Asia-Pacific, senior officials have endorsed a regional approach to CRVS, and ministers for civil registration, health and statistics will meet in late 2014 to endorse a regional plan. In addition, Pacific health ministers have twice endorsed the importance of CRVS systems strengthening as a priority activity.

- In the WHO Eastern Mediterranean Region, health ministers have endorsed a plan for country-level improvement of CRVS systems, with most countries

in the region having now completed comprehensive national CRVS systems assessments.

- In Latin America, significant work has been undertaken to strengthen both civil registration and vital statistics, with progress reported annually to health ministers on a regional committee.

It is clear that global political commitment to CRVS systems strengthening is growing, and that countries are now taking the further steps necessary to assess and plan the improvements that continue to be urgently needed.

CRVS systems strengthening – creating strong foundations for a global resource

The health sector is not only a beneficiary of CRVS information – it is also a strong contributor to the CRVS system. Several countries, including Mozambique, have shown that they can make progress in improving CRVS through their health sector. In many well-functioning systems, the health sector contributes information which confirms events such as births and deaths, while medically certifying the cause of death. In less-functional systems, a strong focus on demonstrating results and accountability for health outcomes has resulted in an upsurge in health-sector interventions to track vital events – notably births, deaths and causes of death – in order to better understand the scale of the challenges in areas such as maternal and under-five mortality, and to develop and monitor interventions for addressing them.[1]

Some countries report partial cause-of-death information using interim approaches such as Sample Registration with Verbal Autopsy (SAVVY), mortality surveillance in selected sites, or through hospital-reporting systems – as occurs, for example in the Lao People's Democratic Republic. Trials of new technologies, such as maternal and child health tracking systems and mobile phone notifications of births and deaths, are being

---

[1] World Health Statistics 2012. Geneva: World Health Organization; 2012 (http://apps.who.int/iris/bitstream/10665/44844/1/9789241564441_eng.pdf?ua=1&ua=1, accessed 12 March 2014).

tested using community health structures. These and other approaches and developments will be crucially important in the provision of future support for CRVS system improvements in countries.

In December 2013, a joint technical meeting was organized by WHO and partner agencies on strengthening CRVS systems through innovative approaches in the health sector. The outcome report of this meeting[1] highlighted the role of the health sector in this endeavour, and identified a range of principles and good practices by which it could best contribute to broader CRVS system strengthening. Meeting participants also acknowledged the growing global momentum towards improving CRVS systems and highlighted the means by which the health sector could play its full part in this effort.

CRVS systems and the data and information they generate are increasingly being acknowledged as invaluable assets in driving forward national and global advancement. In the past three years, greater global awareness and national political commitment has been achieved in this area than has ever been the case previously. Recently, a United Nations Economic and Social Commission for Asia and the Pacific (UNESCAP) regional steering group declared a "CRVS decade" with the explicit target of achieving universal civil registration and generating high-quality vital statistics.[2]

It is clear that without well-functioning CRVS systems that capture all births, all deaths and all causes of death there will be no "data revolution" to drive the

health aspirations of the post-MDG agenda.[3] With an ever-increasing focus now being placed on sustainable results, the role of the health sector in strengthening CRVS systems will only become more prominent, and will involve the harnessing of technological and other innovations as key enablers of progress. Building on current commitments and on the progress already made, the systematic strengthening of CRVS systems must become a crucial focus of action for 2015 and beyond.

1. Using innovative approaches in the health sector to strengthen and modernize civil and vital statistics (CRVS) systems: guiding principles and good practices. Report of a technical meeting sponsored by WHO in collaboration with Canada, UNICEF, USAID and the World Bank, 17–18 December 2013, Geneva (http://www.who.int/healthinfo/civil_registration/crvs_meeting_dec2013_report.pdf?ua=1, accessed 13 March 2014).

2. UNESCAP Regional Steering Group for CRVS 2014 [Communiqué]. First Meeting of the Regional Steering Group for Civil Registration and Vital Statistics (CRVS) in Asia and the Pacific. 11 December 2013, Bangkok (http://www.unescap.org/sites/default/files/RSG%20CRVS%20Communique.pdf, accessed 13 March 2014).

3. A New Global Partnership: Eradicate Poverty and Transform Economies through Sustainable Development. The Report of the High-Level Panel of Eminent Persons on the Post-2015 Development Agenda, 2013 (http://www.post2015hlp.org/wp-content/uploads/2013/05/UN-Report.pdf, accessed 13 March 2014).

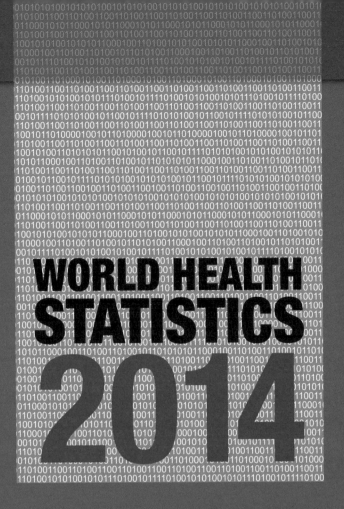

WORLD HEALTH STATISTICS 2014

Part III

Global health indicators

General notes

The following summary tables represent the best estimates of WHO for a broad range of key public health indicators – based on evidence available in 2013. These best estimates have wherever possible been computed by WHO using standardized categories and methods in order to enhance cross-national comparability. This approach may result in some cases in differences between the estimates presented here and the official national statistics prepared and endorsed by individual Member States.

It is also important to stress that these estimates are subject to considerable uncertainty, especially for countries with weak statistical and health information systems where the quality of underlying empirical data is limited.

For indicators with a reference period expressed as a range in Tables 4, 5, 6 and 9, figures refer to the latest available year in the range unless otherwise noted. For survey data, the year of the report is used to determine the latest available year to be consistent across indicators. For more information on specific years, indicator definitions and metadata, please refer to: http://www.who.int/gho.

The WHO regional, income-group and global aggregates for rates and ratios are weighted averages when relevant, while for absolute numbers they are the sums. Aggregates are calculated only if data are available for at least 50% of the population within an indicated group. For indicators with a reference period expressed as a range, aggregates are for the reference period shown in the heading unless otherwise noted. Unless otherwise noted, income-group aggregates are calculated using the World Bank analytical income classification of economies for fiscal year 2014, which is based on the 2012 Atlas gross national income per capita estimates.[1]

... indicates data not available or not applicable.

---

[1] See Annex 1 below.

1. Life expectancy and mortality

The indicators of life expectancy and mortality presented in Table 1 are: life expectancy at birth; life expectancy at age 60; healthy life expectancy (HALE) at birth; neonatal mortality rate (the probability of death occurring during the first 28 days of life); infant and under-five mortality rates (the probability of dying between birth and 1 year of age, and before 5 years of age, respectively); and adult mortality rate (the probability of dying between 15 and 60 years of age).

The estimates of mortality presented here have been derived wherever possible from death-registration data reported annually to WHO. For countries where such data are not available or are of poor quality, household surveys and censuses are used to prepare estimates of mortality rates and life expectancy. Life expectancy is derived from life tables and is based on sex- and age-specific death rates. Life expectancy at birth reflects the overall mortality level of a population and summarizes the mortality pattern that prevails across all age groups – children and adolescents, adults and the elderly. HALE represents the average number of years that a person in a population can expect to live "in full health" by taking into account years lived in less than full health due to disease and/or injury.

In recent years, WHO has liaised more closely with the United Nations Population Division in producing life tables for countries in order to maximize the consistency of United Nations and WHO life tables, and to minimize differences in the use and interpretation of available data on mortality levels.

In the case of child mortality, WHO is part of the Inter-agency Group for Child Mortality Estimation (IGME) which carries out annual updates of estimates for infant and child mortality for UNICEF, WHO and other international agencies. As well as harmonizing the child mortality estimates used by its members, the IGME monitors progress towards the achievement of the relevant MDG target.[1] Child mortality rates measure child survival, and reflect the social, economic and environmental conditions in which children (and others in society) live, including their health care.

---

[1] MDG 4; Target 4.A: Reduce by two thirds, between 1990 and 2015, the under-five mortality rate.

1. Life expectancy and mortality

| Member State | Life expectancy at birth[a] (years) | | | | | | Life expectancy at age 60[a] (years) | | | | | |
| | Both sexes | | Male | | Female | | Both sexes | | Male | | Female | |
	1990	2012	1990	2012	1990	2012	1990	2012	1990	2012	1990	2012
Afghanistan	49	60	49	58	50	61	14	16	13	15	15	17
Albania	69	74	67	73	71	75	16	19	15	18	18	20
Algeria	68	72	66	70	69	73	17	18	16	17	18	19
Andorra	77	83	74	79	81	86	22	25	19	23	24	28
Angola	43	51	41	50	45	52	14	16	13	15	14	16
Antigua and Barbuda	71	75	70	73	72	77	17	22	17	21	18	23
Argentina	73	76	69	73	76	79	20	21	17	19	22	24
Armenia	67	71	63	67	71	75	16	17	14	15	18	19
Australia	77	83	74	81	80	85	21	25	19	24	23	27
Austria	76	81	72	78	79	83	21	24	18	22	22	25
Azerbaijan	63	72	60	69	66	75	16	19	15	17	17	20
Bahamas	72	75	69	72	74	78	19	21	17	19	20	23
Bahrain	73	77	72	76	74	78	18	20	17	19	19	21
Bangladesh	60	70	60	69	59	71	17	18	17	18	17	19
Barbados	74	78	71	75	77	81	20	23	18	21	22	25
Belarus	71	72	66	67	76	78	19	19	16	15	21	21
Belgium	76	80	73	78	79	83	21	23	18	21	23	25
Belize	71	75	69	72	74	78	19	21	18	19	20	23
Benin	53	59	51	57	56	60	15	16	14	15	16	16
Bhutan	53	68	53	68	53	69	16	19	16	19	16	19
Bolivia (Plurinational State of)	58	68	56	65	60	70	17	19	16	18	18	20
Bosnia and Herzegovina	73	77	70	75	75	80	18	21	16	19	19	22
Botswana	65	62	65	61	66	63	17	18	18	18	17	18
Brazil	66	74	63	70	70	77	18	21	16	19	19	22
Brunei Darussalam	73	77	71	76	75	78	18	21	17	20	20	21
Bulgaria	71	74	68	71	75	78	18	19	16	17	19	21
Burkina Faso	50	58	48	57	51	59	15	15	14	15	15	15
Burundi	49	56	48	54	51	57	15	16	14	15	16	17
Cabo Verde	66	74	63	71	68	78	17	20	16	17	18	22
Cambodia	54	72	51	70	57	75	17	24	16	22	18	25
Cameroon	54	56	53	55	56	57	16	16	15	16	16	17
Canada	77	82	74	80	81	84	22	25	19	23	24	26
Central African Republic	48	51	46	50	50	52	15	16	14	15	15	16
Chad	45	51	43	50	47	52	14	15	13	14	15	15
Chile	73	80	69	77	76	83	19	24	17	22	21	26
China	69	75	67	74	71	77	18	19	16	18	19	21
Colombia	71	79	67	76	75	83	21	25	19	23	22	27
Comoros	56	62	54	60	58	63	15	16	14	15	16	17
Congo	56	59	55	57	58	60	16	17	16	17	17	18
Cook Islands	69	76	67	73	72	78	17	21	17	20	18	22
Costa Rica	77	79	75	77	78	81	22	23	21	22	22	25
Côte d'Ivoire	51	53	50	52	54	54	16	16	15	15	17	16
Croatia	73	78	69	74	76	81	18	21	16	19	20	23
Cuba	74	79	73	76	76	81	20	22	19	21	21	24
Cyprus	76	82	74	80	79	84	20	24	19	23	22	26
Czech Republic	71	78	68	75	75	81	17	21	15	19	19	23
Democratic People's Republic of Korea	70	70	66	66	73	73	17	17	14	14	20	19
Democratic Republic of the Congo	49	52	48	50	51	53	15	15	14	15	16	16
Denmark	75	80	72	78	78	82	20	23	18	21	22	24

Healthy life expectancy at birth[a] (years)	Neonatal mortality rate[b] (per 1000 live births) Both sexes		Infant mortality rate[b] (probability of dying by age 1 per 1000 live births) Both sexes			Under-five mortality rate[b] (probability of dying by age 5 per 1000 live births) Both sexes			Adult mortality rate[a] (probability of dying between 15 and 60 years of age per 1000 population) Male		Female		Member State
2012	1990	2012	1990	2000	2012	1990	2000	2012	1990	2012	1990	2012	
49	50	36	120	94	71	176	134	99	412	294	368	242	Afghanistan
65	17	8	37	25	15	43	29	17	158	121	104	87	Albania
62	23	12	42	30	17	50	35	20	199	165	152	122	Algeria
72	2	1	7	4	3	8	5	3	144	92	60	43	Andorra
44	52	45	126	121	100	213	203	164	505	376	409	336	Angola
64	12	6	20	14	9	24	16	10	205	203	143	147	Antigua and Barbuda
67	16	8	24	18	13	28	20	14	198	152	103	84	Argentina
62	24	10	42	27	15	49	30	16	280	228	135	96	Armenia
73	5	3	8	5	4	9	6	5	124	75	66	44	Australia
71	5	2	8	5	3	10	6	4	154	91	74	47	Austria
63	29	15	74	59	31	93	72	35	289	169	162	82	Azerbaijan
64	10	8	20	14	14	23	17	17	193	153	120	100	Bahamas
66	8	4	20	11	8	23	13	10	117	70	103	55	Bahrain
60	54	24	100	64	33	144	88	41	195	159	212	129	Bangladesh
66	9	10	16	16	17	18	18	18	188	118	109	66	Barbados
64	7	3	14	11	4	17	14	5	283	287	107	98	Belarus
71	5	2	8	5	3	10	6	4	139	99	75	57	Belgium
63	17	9	35	21	16	43	25	18	162	160	104	86	Belize
50	41	28	109	91	59	181	147	90	318	284	246	240	Benin
59	42	21	92	59	36	131	80	45	381	221	403	217	Bhutan
59	38	19	85	58	33	123	78	41	299	238	245	175	Bolivia (Plurinational State of)
68	11	4	16	9	6	18	10	7	181	140	86	65	Bosnia and Herzegovina
53	25	29	38	55	41	48	85	53	243	370	242	327	Botswana
64	28	9	52	29	13	62	33	14	272	210	150	107	Brazil
68	7	4	9	8	7	12	10	8	151	104	112	71	Brunei Darussalam
66	12	7	18	18	11	22	21	12	217	188	97	83	Bulgaria
50	40	28	102	96	66	202	186	102	371	301	313	259	Burkina Faso
48	46	36	100	92	67	164	150	104	417	370	356	313	Burundi
64	21	10	47	31	19	62	38	22	240	149	167	70	Cabo Verde
61	37	18	85	82	34	116	111	40	400	212	317	161	Cambodia
48	35	28	84	92	61	135	150	95	340	371	287	349	Cameroon
72	4	4	7	5	5	8	6	5	132	83	71	52	Canada
43	47	41	113	109	91	171	164	129	447	445	376	430	Central African Republic
44	47	40	114	105	89	209	189	150	501	413	401	385	Chad
70	8	5	16	9	8	19	11	9	196	110	98	56	Chile
68	25	9	42	30	12	54	37	14	173	106	127	79	China
68	20	11	29	21	15	35	25	18	230	147	115	74	Colombia
53	41	31	87	71	58	124	99	78	347	283	283	236	Comoros
50	33	32	65	75	62	100	118	96	379	325	325	284	Congo
64	12	6	21	15	9	25	17	11	253	166	155	74	Cook Islands
69	9	7	14	11	9	17	13	10	129	113	86	65	Costa Rica
46	48	40	104	99	76	152	145	108	412	409	351	396	Côte d'Ivoire
68	8	3	11	7	4	13	8	5	224	143	89	60	Croatia
67	7	3	11	7	4	13	8	6	155	124	111	74	Cuba
74	5	2	10	6	3	11	7	3	110	77	61	36	Cyprus
69	9	2	13	6	3	15	7	4	230	126	95	58	Czech Republic
62	21	16	33	45	23	44	60	29	168	188	105	115	Democratic People's Republic of Korea
44	47	44	112	112	100	171	171	146	401	382	345	323	Democratic Republic of the Congo
70	5	3	7	5	3	9	6	4	152	102	99	61	Denmark

Member State	Life expectancy at birth[a] (years)						Life expectancy at age 60[a] (years)					
	Both sexes		Male		Female		Both sexes		Male		Female	
	1990	2012	1990	2012	1990	2012	1990	2012	1990	2012	1990	2012
Djibouti	57	61	55	60	59	63	15	16	15	15	16	17
Dominica	74	75	72	72	76	77	20	21	19	21	21	22
Dominican Republic	69	77	68	76	70	78	19	23	19	23	20	23
Ecuador	69	75	67	73	72	78	20	22	19	21	21	23
Egypt	65	71	63	69	67	74	17	17	16	16	18	19
El Salvador	65	72	61	68	70	77	19	22	18	20	20	23
Equatorial Guinea	48	55	46	54	49	57	15	16	14	16	15	17
Eritrea	48	63	46	61	50	66	12	15	11	13	13	17
Estonia	70	77	64	71	75	81	18	21	15	18	20	24
Ethiopia	45	64	42	62	48	65	15	18	14	17	15	19
Fiji	66	69	64	67	68	73	15	17	14	15	16	19
Finland	75	81	71	78	79	84	20	24	17	22	22	26
France	78	82	73	79	82	85	22	25	20	23	25	27
Gabon	61	63	60	62	63	64	17	18	17	18	18	19
Gambia	52	61	50	59	53	63	16	17	15	16	16	17
Georgia	71	74	67	70	75	78	19	20	17	17	20	22
Germany	76	81	72	78	79	83	20	24	18	22	22	25
Ghana	57	62	55	61	58	64	16	17	16	17	17	18
Greece	77	81	75	78	80	83	21	24	20	22	23	26
Grenada	70	73	67	69	74	77	18	19	15	16	20	23
Guatemala	62	72	60	68	65	75	18	21	17	20	19	23
Guinea	47	58	46	57	48	59	15	16	15	16	16	17
Guinea-Bissau	49	54	47	53	52	56	14	15	14	14	15	15
Guyana	63	63	59	60	67	67	16	15	14	13	18	17
Haiti	54	62	52	61	56	64	15	17	15	16	16	18
Honduras	67	74	65	72	69	77	19	22	18	21	20	23
Hungary	69	75	65	71	74	79	17	20	15	17	19	22
Iceland	78	82	75	81	81	84	22	25	20	24	24	25
India	58	66	57	64	58	68	15	17	14	16	16	18
Indonesia	62	71	60	69	64	73	16	18	15	17	17	19
Iran (Islamic Republic of)	64	74	63	72	64	76	16	20	16	19	16	20
Iraq	69	70	67	66	71	74	18	18	17	16	19	20
Ireland	75	81	72	79	78	83	19	24	17	22	21	25
Israel	77	82	75	80	79	84	21	24	20	23	22	26
Italy	77	83	74	80	80	85	21	25	19	23	23	27
Jamaica	71	74	69	72	74	77	20	21	19	20	21	23
Japan	79	84	76	80	82	87	23	26	20	23	25	29
Jordan	70	74	68	72	71	75	17	19	17	18	18	20
Kazakhstan	66	68	61	63	70	72	17	16	15	13	19	18
Kenya	60	61	58	59	62	62	17	18	16	17	18	18
Kiribati	60	66	57	64	62	69	16	17	15	16	17	18
Kuwait	73	78	73	78	74	79	18	21	19	21	18	21
Kyrgyzstan	66	69	62	66	69	73	18	17	16	15	19	19
Lao People's Democratic Republic	53	66	51	64	54	67	15	17	14	16	16	18
Latvia	69	74	64	69	74	79	18	20	15	16	20	22
Lebanon	67	80	64	78	71	82	17	22	16	21	18	25
Lesotho	61	50	59	49	62	52	17	16	16	15	17	17
Liberia	42	62	39	60	46	63	14	16	13	15	15	17
Libya	68	75	67	73	70	77	17	20	16	18	18	21

Healthy life expectancy at birth[a] (years)	Neonatal mortality rate[b] (per 1000 live births) Both sexes		Infant mortality rate[b] (probability of dying by age 1 per 1000 live births) Both sexes			Under-five mortality rate[b] (probability of dying by age 5 per 1000 live births) Both sexes			Adult mortality rate[a] (probability of dying between 15 and 60 years of age per 1000 population) Male		Female		Member State
2012	1990	2012	1990	2000	2012	1990	2000	2012	1990	2012	1990	2012	
52	40	31	93	85	66	119	108	81	324	293	269	250	Djibouti
63	12	9	14	14	12	17	16	13	194	225	145	118	Dominica
66	27	15	46	32	23	60	40	27	183	137	156	93	Dominican Republic
66	20	10	44	28	20	56	34	23	219	159	141	87	Ecuador
61	33	12	63	36	18	86	45	21	232	196	145	120	Egypt
63	17	6	46	26	14	59	32	16	330	294	162	138	El Salvador
47	47	34	123	99	72	182	143	100	411	379	353	336	Equatorial Guinea
54	35	18	92	58	37	150	89	52	534	313	447	245	Eritrea
67	11	2	17	9	3	20	11	4	301	199	107	68	Estonia
55	54	29	121	90	47	204	146	68	478	250	366	212	Ethiopia
60	13	10	26	21	19	31	24	22	266	242	194	146	Fiji
71	4	2	6	4	2	7	4	3	183	108	70	51	Finland
72	4	2	7	4	3	9	5	4	162	109	67	52	France
54	33	25	60	56	42	92	86	62	267	285	221	273	Gabon
53	46	28	80	63	49	170	116	73	348	296	300	244	Gambia
65	23	15	30	30	18	35	34	20	217	176	86	66	Georgia
71	4	2	7	4	3	9	5	4	157	94	77	50	Germany
54	40	28	80	66	49	128	103	72	299	263	260	227	Ghana
71	9	3	11	7	4	13	8	5	117	105	56	46	Greece
63	10	7	18	13	11	22	16	14	215	195	150	121	Grenada
62	29	15	60	40	27	80	51	32	320	240	205	129	Guatemala
49	54	34	142	104	65	241	171	101	355	306	307	277	Guinea
47	58	46	122	105	81	206	174	129	365	354	286	307	Guinea-Bissau
55	28	19	46	37	29	60	46	35	372	379	231	259	Guyana
52	37	25	100	75	57	144	105	76	352	268	299	227	Haiti
64	23	12	46	31	19	59	38	23	239	176	179	122	Honduras
66	13	4	17	10	5	19	11	6	305	203	133	92	Hungary
72	3	1	5	3	2	6	4	2	112	67	69	34	Iceland
57	51	31	88	67	44	126	92	56	288	242	242	160	India
62	30	15	62	41	26	84	52	31	266	178	204	124	Indonesia
64	26	11	44	28	15	56	35	18	239	156	217	84	Iran (Islamic Republic of)
61	26	19	42	36	28	53	45	34	170	223	117	107	Iraq
71	5	2	8	6	3	9	7	4	134	83	81	50	Ireland
72	6	2	10	6	3	12	7	4	107	72	71	39	Israel
73	6	2	8	5	3	10	6	4	129	70	60	39	Italy
64	17	11	25	20	14	30	23	17	191	177	122	107	Jamaica
75	3	1	5	3	2	6	5	3	109	82	53	43	Japan
64	19	12	30	23	16	37	28	19	175	132	135	97	Jordan
60	23	10	46	38	17	54	44	19	318	324	150	147	Kazakhstan
53	33	27	64	68	49	98	110	73	287	307	228	261	Kenya
58	29	22	68	54	46	94	71	60	299	210	222	138	Kiribati
68	9	6	14	11	10	16	13	11	128	59	81	43	Kuwait
61	29	14	58	42	24	71	50	27	291	275	156	131	Kyrgyzstan
57	44	27	112	85	54	163	120	72	358	202	309	163	Lao People's Democratic Republic
65	13	5	17	14	8	20	17	9	311	226	118	86	Latvia
69	16	5	27	17	8	33	20	9	280	72	150	47	Lebanon
43	45	45	68	80	74	85	114	100	297	560	247	503	Lesotho
52	51	27	165	120	56	248	176	75	544	282	376	246	Liberia
64	21	9	37	24	13	43	28	15	194	119	142	81	Libya

1. Life expectancy and mortality

Member State	Life expectancy at birth[a] (years)						Life expectancy at age 60[a] (years)					
	Both sexes		Male		Female		Both sexes		Male		Female	
	1990	2012	1990	2012	1990	2012	1990	2012	1990	2012	1990	2012
Lithuania	71	74	66	68	76	80	19	21	16	17	21	23
Luxembourg	76	82	72	80	79	84	20	25	18	23	22	26
Madagascar	51	64	50	62	53	65	15	17	15	16	16	17
Malawi	45	59	43	58	46	60	15	16	14	16	15	17
Malaysia	71	74	68	72	73	76	17	19	16	18	18	20
Maldives	58	77	60	76	57	78	13	20	14	20	12	21
Mali	46	57	46	57	46	57	14	15	14	15	14	16
Malta	76	81	74	79	78	83	19	24	18	22	21	25
Marshall Islands	63	70	61	68	65	72	16	18	15	17	17	20
Mauritania	58	63	57	61	60	65	16	16	15	16	16	17
Mauritius	70	74	66	70	74	78	17	20	15	18	19	22
Mexico	71	76	68	73	75	79	21	22	20	21	22	23
Micronesia (Federated States of)	66	69	65	68	67	70	17	17	16	16	17	18
Monaco	78	82	74	79	81	86	22	25	20	23	25	27
Mongolia	61	67	58	64	64	72	15	16	14	14	16	18
Montenegro	76	76	73	73	79	78	22	20	19	18	23	21
Morocco	64	71	63	69	66	73	17	18	16	17	18	19
Mozambique	43	53	41	52	45	54	14	16	14	16	15	17
Myanmar	59	66	57	64	61	68	16	17	15	16	16	17
Namibia	63	67	62	64	64	69	16	18	16	18	16	19
Nauru	73	79	69	75	77	83	20	23	17	20	23	27
Nepal	54	68	54	67	55	69	15	17	14	16	16	18
Netherlands	77	81	74	79	80	83	21	24	18	22	23	25
New Zealand	76	82	73	80	78	84	20	25	18	24	22	26
Nicaragua	71	73	68	70	74	76	22	21	20	20	24	22
Niger	43	59	43	59	43	59	15	15	14	15	15	16
Nigeria	46	54	45	53	47	55	15	16	14	15	15	16
Niue	71	74	69	72	75	78	17	19	16	17	19	21
Norway	77	82	74	80	80	84	21	24	18	22	23	25
Oman	68	76	66	74	70	78	17	20	16	19	18	22
Pakistan	60	65	59	64	61	66	17	17	17	17	18	18
Palau	66	73	65	71	68	75	16	18	15	17	17	19
Panama	74	77	72	74	76	80	21	23	20	22	22	25
Papua New Guinea	56	62	53	60	59	65	13	15	12	13	15	16
Paraguay	73	75	71	72	76	78	21	21	19	20	22	23
Peru	70	77	68	75	72	79	21	23	20	21	22	24
Philippines	66	69	63	65	70	72	18	17	17	15	19	19
Poland	71	77	67	73	76	81	18	21	15	19	20	24
Portugal	74	81	71	77	78	84	20	24	18	22	22	26
Qatar	75	79	74	79	76	80	19	22	19	22	20	22
Republic of Korea	72	81	68	78	76	85	18	24	15	21	20	27
Republic of Moldova	68	71	65	66	72	75	17	17	15	15	19	19
Romania	70	74	66	71	73	78	18	20	17	17	19	22
Russian Federation	69	69	63	63	74	75	18	17	15	14	20	20
Rwanda	48	65	46	63	50	66	15	18	14	17	15	19
Saint Kitts and Nevis	68	74	65	71	71	78	17	19	16	17	19	21
Saint Lucia	72	75	70	71	74	79	20	21	19	19	21	23
Saint Vincent and the Grenadines	72	74	69	72	75	76	19	21	18	20	21	22
Samoa	66	73	63	70	69	77	15	19	14	16	18	21

Healthy life expectancy at birth[a] (years)	Neonatal mortality rate[b] (per 1000 live births)		Infant mortality rate[b] (probability of dying by age 1 per 1000 live births)			Under-five mortality rate[b] (probability of dying by age 5 per 1000 live births)			Adult mortality rate[a] (probability of dying between 15 and 60 years of age per 1000 population)				Member State
	Both sexes		Both sexes			Both sexes			Male		Female		
2012	1990	2012	1990	2000	2012	1990	2000	2012	1990	2012	1990	2012	
65	9	2	14	10	4	17	12	5	288	266	107	93	Lithuania
72	4	1	7	4	2	9	5	2	160	81	79	51	Luxembourg
55	40	22	97	69	41	159	109	58	370	263	320	213	Madagascar
50	50	24	143	103	46	244	174	71	467	376	407	330	Malawi
64	8	5	14	9	7	17	10	9	209	172	129	89	Malaysia
67	34	6	68	36	9	94	45	11	259	91	327	59	Maldives
48	59	42	130	116	80	253	220	128	348	282	340	277	Mali
71	7	5	10	7	6	11	8	7	108	77	62	45	Malta
59	19	16	39	33	31	49	41	38	268	155	217	106	Marshall Islands
53	43	34	82	75	65	128	111	84	270	235	223	188	Mauritania
65	16	9	20	16	13	23	19	15	264	204	121	96	Mauritius
67	16	7	37	22	14	46	25	16	215	177	120	90	Mexico
60	21	16	43	42	31	55	54	39	210	182	187	155	Micronesia (Federated States of)
72	4	2	6	4	3	8	5	4	155	107	67	49	Monaco
60	25	10	76	48	23	107	63	28	269	314	183	150	Mongolia
66	11	4	15	13	6	17	14	6	165	152	73	80	Montenegro
61	35	18	63	42	27	80	50	31	224	172	172	124	Morocco
45	54	30	155	112	63	233	166	90	459	466	384	453	Mozambique
57	41	26	76	59	41	106	79	52	316	242	248	184	Myanmar
57	29	18	49	48	28	73	73	39	268	293	230	204	Namibia
66	28	21	45	34	30	58	42	37	154	90	78	45	Nauru
59	53	24	99	61	34	142	82	42	340	197	308	164	Nepal
71	5	3	7	5	3	8	6	4	116	72	67	54	Netherlands
72	4	3	9	6	5	11	7	6	143	81	93	53	New Zealand
64	25	12	50	33	21	66	40	24	171	204	122	118	Nicaragua
50	48	28	137	101	63	326	227	114	317	257	295	246	Niger
46	52	39	126	112	78	213	188	124	408	371	364	346	Nigeria
64	7	12	12	20	21	14	23	25	222	166	124	85	Niue
71	4	2	7	4	2	9	5	3	128	73	65	44	Norway
66	18	7	32	15	10	39	17	12	215	119	151	74	Oman
56	56	42	106	88	69	138	112	86	220	190	197	157	Pakistan
62	15	10	30	22	15	34	28	21	268	159	217	109	Palau
67	13	9	26	22	16	32	26	19	146	152	101	83	Panama
53	30	24	65	58	48	89	79	63	437	321	333	245	Papua New Guinea
65	22	12	36	27	19	46	33	22	138	178	99	97	Paraguay
67	28	9	56	30	14	79	40	18	163	118	123	91	Peru
60	23	14	41	30	24	59	40	30	272	258	154	138	Philippines
67	11	3	15	8	4	17	9	5	263	180	102	69	Poland
71	7	2	12	6	3	15	7	4	176	114	80	49	Portugal
68	10	4	18	11	6	21	12	7	94	73	82	51	Qatar
73	3	2	6	5	3	7	6	4	237	98	102	40	Republic of Korea
63	14	9	27	25	15	32	30	18	285	269	155	110	Republic of Moldova
66	18	8	31	23	11	38	27	12	239	207	114	82	Romania
61	14	6	22	20	9	26	23	10	318	339	117	127	Russian Federation
55	38	21	92	108	39	151	182	55	487	253	406	212	Rwanda
63	18	7	23	14	7	29	18	9	272	166	193	80	Saint Kitts and Nevis
63	13	10	18	15	15	22	18	18	204	178	147	85	Saint Lucia
63	15	15	21	19	21	25	22	23	217	169	140	111	Saint Vincent and the Grenadines
64	11	7	25	18	15	30	22	18	300	170	194	100	Samoa

Member State	Life expectancy at birth[a] (years)						Life expectancy at age 60[a] (years)					
	Both sexes		Male		Female		Both sexes		Male		Female	
	1990	2012	1990	2012	1990	2012	1990	2012	1990	2012	1990	2012
San Marino	79	83	76	82	83	84	23	25	20	24	25	25
Sao Tome and Principe	61	67	59	65	63	69	17	18	17	17	18	19
Saudi Arabia	69	76	67	74	71	78	17	19	16	18	18	21
Senegal	57	64	56	63	59	66	16	16	15	15	16	17
Serbia	72	75	69	72	75	77	19	19	17	17	20	20
Seychelles	69	74	64	69	75	78	17	20	14	17	21	23
Sierra Leone	38	46	38	45	38	46	11	13	11	12	11	13
Singapore	75	83	73	80	78	85	20	25	18	23	21	27
Slovakia	71	76	66	72	75	80	18	21	15	18	20	23
Slovenia	74	80	70	77	78	83	19	23	17	21	21	25
Solomon Islands	62	69	61	67	63	70	15	17	15	16	16	18
Somalia	47	53	45	51	50	55	15	16	14	15	15	17
South Africa	62	59	59	56	66	62	15	16	13	14	17	18
South Sudan	42	55	41	54	44	56	14	16	13	16	14	17
Spain	77	82	73	79	81	85	22	25	19	22	24	27
Sri Lanka	69	75	65	71	75	78	19	20	18	18	21	22
Sudan	55	63	54	61	57	65	16	17	16	17	17	18
Suriname	73	77	71	75	76	80	21	23	19	22	22	25
Swaziland	61	54	62	52	61	55	16	17	16	17	15	17
Sweden	78	82	75	80	81	84	21	24	19	23	23	25
Switzerland	78	83	74	81	81	85	22	25	19	24	24	27
Syrian Arab Republic	70	68	69	62	71	76	18	19	17	18	18	22
Tajikistan	64	68	62	67	65	69	18	17	17	17	18	17
Thailand	69	75	66	71	72	79	18	21	16	19	19	23
The former Yugoslav Republic of Macedonia	72	76	70	73	75	78	19	19	18	18	20	20
Timor-Leste	50	66	48	65	51	68	14	17	13	16	15	18
Togo	55	58	54	57	57	59	16	17	16	16	17	17
Tonga	68	71	64	74	74	69	17	18	14	18	19	18
Trinidad and Tobago	68	70	65	67	71	74	17	18	15	16	18	20
Tunisia	70	76	69	74	72	78	19	21	18	19	19	22
Turkey	65	75	62	72	68	78	18	21	16	18	20	23
Turkmenistan	62	63	59	60	65	67	16	16	14	15	17	17
Tuvalu	62	68	59	66	64	70	14	16	13	15	16	18
Uganda	47	57	44	56	49	58	15	16	14	16	16	17
Ukraine	70	71	65	66	75	76	18	18	15	15	20	20
United Arab Emirates	72	76	71	76	73	78	17	20	17	19	18	20
United Kingdom	76	81	73	79	79	83	20	24	18	22	22	25
United Republic of Tanzania	51	61	49	59	52	63	16	18	15	17	16	18
United States of America	75	79	72	76	79	81	21	23	19	21	23	24
Uruguay	73	77	69	73	76	81	19	22	17	19	21	24
Uzbekistan	67	69	63	67	70	72	18	17	16	16	20	18
Vanuatu	66	72	64	70	67	74	16	18	15	17	17	19
Venezuela (Bolivarian Republic of)	72	76	70	72	74	80	19	23	18	21	20	24
Viet Nam	70	76	66	71	75	80	20	22	18	19	23	25
Yemen	58	64	56	62	59	65	16	16	15	15	16	17
Zambia	43	57	40	55	47	58	15	17	14	16	16	18
Zimbabwe	62	58	60	56	64	60	18	18	17	17	18	19

Healthy life expectancy at birth[a] (years)	Neonatal mortality rate[b] (per 1000 live births) Both sexes		Infant mortality rate[b] (probability of dying by age 1 per 1000 live births) Both sexes			Under-five mortality rate[b] (probability of dying by age 5 per 1000 live births) Both sexes			Adult mortality rate[a] (probability of dying between 15 and 60 years of age per 1000 population) Male		Female		Member State
2012	1990	2012	1990	2000	2012	1990	2000	2012	1990	2012	1990	2012	
73	5	1	10	5	3	11	6	3	80	55	40	47	San Marino
57	31	20	67	57	38	104	87	53	264	222	210	169	Sao Tome and Principe
65	21	5	37	19	7	47	22	9	178	90	131	68	Saudi Arabia
55	41	24	71	70	45	142	139	60	282	246	220	194	Senegal
65	17	4	24	11	6	28	13	7	184	173	94	85	Serbia
67	10	8	14	12	11	17	14	13	318	217	127	101	Seychelles
39	59	50	153	143	117	257	234	182	525	444	512	426	Sierra Leone
76	4	1	6	3	2	8	4	3	152	68	93	42	Singapore
67	12	4	16	10	6	18	12	8	269	170	104	67	Slovakia
70	6	2	9	5	3	10	6	3	207	114	82	50	Slovenia
59	16	14	31	29	26	39	35	31	318	205	290	165	Solomon Islands
45	50	46	107	103	91	177	171	147	473	382	364	299	Somalia
51	21	15	47	51	33	61	74	45	344	463	219	350	South Africa
48	57	36	149	109	67	251	181	104	448	373	391	349	South Sudan
73	7	3	9	5	4	11	7	5	146	86	60	40	Spain
65	13	6	18	15	8	21	17	10	294	186	125	75	Sri Lanka
53	40	29	80	68	49	128	106	73	342	276	276	214	Sudan
66	23	12	43	29	19	51	33	21	188	160	123	94	Suriname
46	29	30	54	80	56	71	121	80	253	494	288	411	Swaziland
72	4	2	6	3	2	7	4	3	114	68	66	44	Sweden
73	4	3	7	5	4	8	6	4	126	67	62	40	Switzerland
59	18	9	31	20	12	38	24	15	158	332	140	109	Syrian Arab Republic
60	33	23	82	73	49	105	91	58	217	178	180	154	Tajikistan
66	19	8	31	19	11	38	23	13	233	182	132	90	Thailand
66	17	6	33	14	7	37	16	7	153	135	87	73	The former Yugoslav Republic of Macedonia
57	47	24	129	83	48	171	106	57	424	214	361	170	Timor-Leste
50	41	33	89	77	62	143	122	96	304	318	259	293	Togo
62	11	7	20	16	11	23	18	13	314	117	128	248	Tonga
61	22	15	29	25	18	33	28	21	248	229	166	130	Trinidad and Tobago
66	24	10	40	25	14	51	30	16	146	133	102	71	Tunisia
65	30	9	55	31	12	74	37	14	232	150	133	75	Turkey
56	31	22	72	64	45	90	79	53	301	378	193	201	Turkmenistan
58	22	13	45	34	25	58	42	30	348	240	259	185	Tuvalu
49	39	23	107	89	45	178	147	69	503	389	418	360	Uganda
63	9	5	17	16	9	20	19	11	287	297	112	116	Ukraine
67	10	5	14	10	7	17	11	8	150	85	121	60	United Arab Emirates
71	5	3	8	6	4	9	7	5	129	90	78	56	United Kingdom
52	43	21	101	81	38	166	132	54	388	342	328	277	United Republic of Tanzania
70	6	4	9	7	6	11	8	7	173	130	91	77	United States of America
68	11	4	20	14	6	23	16	7	196	149	98	79	Uruguay
61	21	14	61	51	34	74	61	40	251	211	144	131	Uzbekistan
62	15	9	29	21	15	35	24	18	256	164	210	116	Vanuatu
66	15	9	25	18	13	30	21	15	178	200	117	89	Venezuela (Bolivarian Republic of)
66	22	12	36	25	18	51	32	23	212	191	95	69	Viet Nam
54	42	27	88	70	46	125	97	60	301	264	247	214	Yemen
49	44	29	114	99	56	192	169	89	634	398	452	353	Zambia
49	31	39	50	61	56	74	102	90	308	390	255	313	Zimbabwe

1. Life expectancy and mortality

	Life expectancy at birth[a] (years)						Life expectancy at age 60[a] (years)					
	Both sexes		Male		Female		Both sexes		Male		Female	
	1990	2012	1990	2012	1990	2012	1990	2012	1990	2012	1990	2012
Ranges of country values												
Minimum	38	46	38	45	38	46	11	13	11	12	11	13
Median	68	74	65	70	71	76	17	19	16	18	19	21
Maximum	79	84	76	82	83	87	23	26	21	24	25	29
WHO region												
African Region	50	58	48	56	52	59	15	17	14	16	16	17
Region of the Americas	71	76	68	74	75	79	20	22	18	21	22	24
South-East Asia Region	59	67	58	66	60	69	16	17	15	16	16	18
European Region	72	76	68	72	75	80	19	22	17	19	21	23
Eastern Mediterranean Region	62	68	61	66	63	70	17	18	16	17	18	19
Western Pacific Region	69	76	67	74	72	78	18	21	17	19	20	22
Income group												
Low income	53	62	51	60	54	63	16	17	15	16	16	18
Lower middle income	59	66	58	64	60	68	16	17	15	16	17	19
Upper middle income	68	74	66	72	71	76	18	20	17	18	19	21
High income	75	79	71	76	78	82	20	23	18	21	22	25
Global	64	70	62	68	67	73	18	20	17	18	20	21

a. Mortality Data [online database]. Geneva: World Health Organization; 2014 (http://www.who.int/gho/mortality_burden_disease/life_tables/en/index.html).

b. Levels & Trends in Child Mortality. Report 2013. Estimates Developed by the UN Inter-agency Group for Child Mortality Estimation. New York: UNICEF; 2013 (http://www.childinfo.org/files/Child_Mortality_Report_2013.pdf, accessed 14 March 2014).

Table 1

Healthy life expectancy at birth[a] (years)	Neonatal mortality rate[b] (per 1000 live births)		Infant mortality rate[b] (probability of dying by age 1 per 1000 live births)			Under-five mortality rate[b] (probability of dying by age 5 per 1000 live births)			Adult mortality rate[a] (probability of dying between 15 and 60 years of age per 1000 population)				
	Both sexes		Both sexes			Both sexes			Male		Female		
2012	1990	2012	1990	2000	2012	1990	2000	2012	1990	2012	1990	2012	
39	2	1	5	3	2	6	4	2	80	55	40	34	Minimum
63	21	10	37	26	16	46	32	19	246	187	145	107	Median
76	59	50	165	143	117	326	234	182	634	560	512	503	Maximum
50	44	32	105	94	63	173	154	95	395	343	326	298	African Region
67	18	8	34	22	13	42	26	15	205	161	115	89	Region of the Americas
59	47	27	83	61	39	118	84	50	276	222	226	149	South-East Asia Region
67	14	6	26	18	10	32	22	12	216	179	96	80	European Region
58	40	26	76	61	44	103	82	57	239	194	196	139	Eastern Mediterranean Region
68	23	9	40	28	14	52	35	16	174	116	119	78	Western Pacific Region
53	47	30	104	85	56	166	134	82	343	272	294	230	Low income
57	44	28	82	66	46	118	93	61	286	241	222	164	Lower middle income
66	24	10	42	30	16	54	38	20	199	143	133	92	Upper middle income
70	7	4	12	8	5	15	10	6	182	137	83	67	High income
62	33	21	63	53	35	90	75	48	233	187	161	124	Global

2. Cause-specific mortality and morbidity

Table 2 brings together indicators on the levels and distribution of the broad categories and more-specific causes of deaths. The three broad categories shown are communicable[1] and non-communicable conditions, and deaths caused by injury. The years of life lost (YLL) is a measure of premature mortality that takes into account the frequency of premature death and the ages at which deaths occur. Estimates are also provided of the number of deaths among children under 5 years old, and the percentage distributions of the major causes of such deaths. These causes include: HIV/AIDS; diarrhoea; other major communicable diseases such as measles, malaria and pneumonia; conditions arising in the perinatal period such as prematurity, birth asphyxia, neonatal sepsis and congenital anomalies; and deaths caused by other diseases and by injury. Table 2 also includes point estimates for key MDG-related indicators, including maternal mortality, and mortality and morbidity caused by HIV/AIDS, malaria and tuberculosis.

The cause-specific indicators presented in Table 2 have been derived from a range of sources of mortality, incidence and prevalence data. These include death-registration records, health-facility reports, household surveys, censuses, and special studies on deaths due to HIV and to conflict. Estimating cause-specific mortality is particularly difficult in developing countries where systems for counting deaths and accurately recording their causes are weak or non-existent. Due to resulting limitations in data availability, quality and timeliness, many of the indicators shown are associated with significant uncertainty, the margins of which are available on the Global Health Observatory website (http://www.who.int/gho).

[1.] Columns labelled "Communicable" show estimates pertaining to a group of conditions that includes communicable (infectious or contagious) diseases, maternal causes, conditions arising during the neonatal period and nutritional deficiencies. While the latter three conditions are not communicable, the term is used for practical purpose to refer to the entire group of conditions encompassing the primary mortality risks for countries still undergoing epidemiological transition.

Member State	Age-standardized mortality rates by cause[a] (per 100 000 population) 2012			Years of life lost[a] (per 100 000 population) 2012				MDG 4 Number of deaths among children aged <5 years[a] (000s)		Mortality Distribution of causes of death among children aged <5 years[a,b] (%)							
	Communicable	Non-communicable	Injuries	All causes	Communicable	Non-communicable	Injuries	2000	2012	HIV 2000	HIV 2012	Diarrhoea 2000	Diarrhoea 2012	Measles 2000	Measles 2012	Malaria 2000	Malaria 201
Afghanistan	363	846	169	53 252	31 128	12 324	9 801	135	103	0	0	18	14	8	3	0	0
Albania	46	672	48	21 581	1 927	17 284	2 370	2	1	0	0	2	1	0	0	0	0
Algeria	98	710	54	19 635	4 810	12 406	2 418	20	20	0	1	7	4	6	1	0	0
Andorra	…	…	…	…	…	…	…	0	0	…	…	…	…	…	…	…	…
Angola	873	768	138	102 199	75 280	17 031	9 887	133	149	1	1	19	15	1	1	15	13
Antigua and Barbuda	…	…	…	…	…	…	…	0	0	…	…	…	…	…	…	…	…
Argentina	69	467	51	18 693	2 917	13 363	2 413	14	10	0	0	2	1	0	0	0	0
Armenia	45	848	49	28 511	2 368	23 695	2 447	1	1	0	0	3	1	0	0	0	0
Australia	14	303	28	11 934	591	10 017	1 326	2	2	0	0	0	0	0	0	0	0
Austria	13	360	31	16 311	531	14 341	1 439	0	0	0	0	0	0	0	0	0	0
Azerbaijan	71	664	34	20 621	4 926	13 802	1 893	9	6	0	0	15	8	0	0	0	0
Bahamas	122	465	46	17 998	6 301	9 780	1 917	0	0	1	0	1	0	0	0	0	0
Bahrain	48	506	34	7 589	1 236	5 024	1 329	0	0	0	0	1	0	0	0	0	0
Bangladesh	235	549	64	22 389	10 015	9 632	2 742	312	127	0	0	13	6	4	2	0	0
Barbados	61	404	28	16 633	2 659	12 630	1 345	0	0	5	0	0	0	0	0	0	0
Belarus	28	683	91	31 213	1 543	24 934	4 737	1	1	0	0	2	1	0	0	0	0
Belgium	28	357	39	17 423	1 165	14 445	1 814	1	1	0	0	1	0	0	0	0	0
Belize	108	472	77	14 837	4 594	7 186	3 056	0	0	2	0	5	3	0	0	0	0
Benin	577	761	98	53 328	35 559	12 712	5 057	43	31	1	1	12	10	7	1	26	21
Bhutan	187	573	142	28 592	9 826	11 790	6 977	1	1	0	0	14	8	2	0	0	0
Bolivia (Plurinational State of)	226	635	100	30 515	11 727	13 300	5 488	20	11	1	0	16	8	0	0	0	0
Bosnia and Herzegovina	20	513	42	20 122	777	17 315	2 030	1	0	0	0	1	0	1	0	0	0
Botswana	555	612	88	39 743	26 187	9 111	4 444	4	3	46	5	5	7	8	1	1	0
Brazil	93	514	80	20 190	3 345	12 542	4 303	125	42	0	0	7	2	0	0	0	0
Brunei Darussalam	56	475	45	10 800	1 273	7 905	1 622	0	0	0	0	1	1	0	0	0	0
Bulgaria	33	638	36	30 280	1 553	26 901	1 826	1	1	0	0	2	1	0	0	0	0
Burkina Faso	648	784	119	62 658	42 924	13 422	6 312	96	66	2	1	13	11	5	1	29	23
Burundi	705	729	147	74 914	51 897	14 209	8 809	42	43	4	1	16	13	5	0	8	5
Cabo Verde	142	482	54	15 736	5 127	8 695	1 914	0	0	6	4	11	5	2	0	0	0
Cambodia	227	394	62	26 837	12 889	10 043	3 906	32	14	1	0	17	8	2	0	2	0
Cameroon	769	675	106	66 447	45 696	14 488	6 263	97	74	4	3	14	12	5	1	19	12
Canada	23	318	31	13 838	935	11 421	1 482	2	2	0	0	0	0	0	0	0	0
Central African Republic	1 212	551	108	86 460	69 308	10 575	6 577	24	19	6	3	10	9	10	1	23	25
Chad	1 071	713	114	94 968	75 598	12 700	6 670	73	82	3	2	14	13	5	0	24	19
Chile	36	367	41	13 209	1 317	9 887	2 006	3	2	0	0	1	0	0	0	0	0
China	41	576	50	17 541	1 858	13 475	2 208	629	258	0	0	7	4	1	0	0	0
Colombia	58	335	69	14 780	3 308	7 622	3 851	23	16	0	0	5	2	0	0	0	0
Comoros	495	695	132	47 196	29 959	11 603	5 634	2	2	0	1	12	9	0	0	15	15
Congo	667	632	89	62 710	45 395	11 739	5 576	14	15	6	3	10	8	5	0	22	25
Cook Islands	…	…	…	…	…	…	…	0	0	…	…	…	…	…	…	…	…
Costa Rica	31	392	46	12 179	1 274	8 695	2 211	1	1	0	0	3	1	0	0	0	0
Côte d'Ivoire	861	794	124	78 319	54 054	16 884	7 382	87	75	6	2	10	10	4	0	22	16
Croatia	12	496	40	22 859	575	20 431	1 853	0	0	0	0	0	0	0	0	0	0
Cuba	33	422	45	17 235	1 182	14 141	1 911	1	1	0	0	2	1	0	0	0	0
Cyprus	16	333	27	10 965	489	9 158	1 318	0	0	0	0	0	0	0	0	0	0
Czech Republic	27	461	39	20 032	1 068	17 096	1 868	0	0	0	0	0	1	0	0	0	0
Democratic People's Republic of Korea	117	751	92	27 438	4 657	18 529	4 252	24	10	0	0	13	6	0	0	0	0
Democratic Republic of the Congo	921	724	137	94 624	70 873	14 227	9 524	352	391	1	1	12	12	11	4	19	16
Denmark	29	406	23	17 859	1 114	15 722	1 023	0	0	0	0	1	1	0	0	0	0

Mortality

Distribution of causes of death among children aged <5 years[a,b] (%)

Acute respiratory infections		Prematurity		Intrapartum-related complications		Neonatal sepsis		Congenital anomalies		Other diseases		Injuries		Member State
2000	2012	2000	2012	2000	2012	2000	2012	2000	2012	2000	2012	2000	2012	
20	20	11	13	8	11	3	7	2	3	24	22	6	7	Afghanistan
17	11	20	19	6	7	3	4	20	27	20	21	11	10	Albania
15	12	23	20	11	13	6	8	11	20	15	14	6	8	Algeria
...	...	...	...	...	...	...	...	...	...	...	...	...	...	Andorra
18	17	9	11	7	9	3	5	2	5	21	19	4	5	Angola
...	...	...	...	...	...	...	...	...	...	...	...	...	...	Antigua and Barbuda
7	9	27	26	6	5	6	6	24	28	19	18	9	6	Argentina
19	9	23	25	7	8	4	5	18	26	18	18	9	8	Armenia
3	3	17	21	10	11	2	1	28	28	29	29	11	7	Australia
2	2	21	21	6	10	1	2	38	38	20	23	10	3	Austria
21	17	17	20	9	11	4	5	6	11	21	20	7	9	Azerbaijan
24	32	17	13	10	7	5	6	18	12	12	24	12	7	Bahamas
2	4	17	16	6	18	1	4	37	30	20	23	16	6	Bahrain
18	13	13	20	13	14	11	11	4	9	18	18	5	7	Bangladesh
0	10	36	14	18	14	1	2	8	26	26	33	5	2	Barbados
13	6	19	21	6	7	3	3	29	37	18	18	9	8	Belarus
2	2	18	21	8	9	2	3	29	28	30	28	9	9	Belgium
14	5	24	14	9	10	3	6	16	12	13	42	14	8	Belize
13	15	9	12	7	10	5	6	2	4	13	15	3	5	Benin
21	17	10	18	13	12	9	8	5	9	19	18	7	9	Bhutan
18	17	12	16	13	15	6	7	7	11	19	18	7	8	Bolivia (Plurinational State of)
8	6	29	30	9	9	4	4	27	29	16	16	5	4	Bosnia and Herzegovina
7	13	10	24	7	14	4	8	3	9	6	14	2	5	Botswana
11	7	24	23	9	11	8	9	14	21	21	22	4	5	Brazil
5	4	24	25	8	8	1	2	30	28	21	23	10	10	Brunei Darussalam
21	16	14	25	9	11	4	2	28	28	18	13	5	4	Bulgaria
14	15	8	11	6	9	3	5	2	4	15	16	3	5	Burkina Faso
19	19	10	12	8	11	4	7	2	4	19	20	5	7	Burundi
19	14	17	19	9	8	4	5	12	19	16	23	4	3	Cabo Verde
22	17	10	16	10	13	5	8	3	10	22	18	6	8	Cambodia
15	17	10	11	7	11	3	6	3	5	16	18	4	6	Cameroon
2	2	26	30	8	10	3	3	30	27	22	22	8	5	Canada
12	14	10	12	8	10	3	5	2	3	13	14	3	4	Central African Republic
14	17	8	11	7	8	2	3	2	3	18	19	3	5	Chad
10	6	24	27	5	4	3	3	34	37	14	15	10	8	Chile
28	14	14	16	18	15	3	2	6	13	10	23	12	13	China
12	9	27	24	10	9	6	8	15	23	19	20	6	6	Colombia
16	15	16	15	10	13	6	8	3	5	16	15	4	5	Comoros
12	12	13	14	10	10	4	6	3	5	12	12	3	4	Congo
...	...	...	...	...	...	...	...	...	...	...	...	...	...	Cook Islands
7	2	24	27	7	9	4	2	32	42	17	14	4	3	Costa Rica
12	15	12	13	10	12	6	8	3	5	12	15	3	5	Côte d'Ivoire
6	2	30	17	7	7	5	4	30	27	13	40	9	2	Croatia
6	11	16	15	11	11	7	6	27	21	22	28	8	8	Cuba
6	3	21	22	9	8	3	3	30	37	23	21	8	6	Cyprus
4	5	21	24	12	11	3	7	20	25	28	20	11	7	Czech Republic
20	16	20	22	10	11	5	6	6	12	20	19	7	8	Democratic People's Republic of Korea
14	16	11	12	8	9	3	5	2	3	16	17	3	5	Democratic Republic of the Congo
3	1	27	44	9	6	1	1	32	19	22	25	6	3	Denmark

73

Member State	Mortality							
	MDG 5 Maternal mortality ratio[c] (per 100 000 live births)			MDG 6 Cause-specific mortality rate (per 100 000 population)				
				HIV/AIDS[d]		Malaria[e]	Tuberculosis among HIV-negative people[f]	
	1990	2000	2013	2001	2012	2012	2000	2012
Afghanistan	1 200	1 100	400	<1	<2	0.1	53	37
Albania	31	28	21	...	...	...	0.8	0.3
Algeria	160	120	89	...	...	0.0	14	15
Andorra	...	...	...	...	...	...	1.3	0.9
Angola	1 400	1 100	460	59	60	99	42	42
Antigua and Barbuda	...	...	...	...	...	...	1.8	1.4
Argentina	71	63	69	7.7	8.9	0.0	2.3	1.3
Armenia	47	43	29	<3	<17	...	6.3	6.3
Australia	7	9	6	0.3[a]	0.2[a]	...	0.2	0.2
Austria	10	5	4	0.6[a]	0.5[a]	...	0.9	0.4
Azerbaijan	60	57	26	<2	<11	0.0	22	4.2
Bahamas	43	44	37	<165	<134	...	2.2	0.4
Bahrain	21	27	22	...	...	...	2.5	0.3
Bangladesh	550	340	170	<1	<1	0.9	58	45
Barbados	120	42	52	<37	<35	...	0.7	0.7
Belarus	37	32	1	0.7[a]	11[a]	...	8.1	6.0
Belgium	10	9	6	...	...	...	0.8	0.4
Belize	75	110	45	<82	<62	0.0	3.3	4.3
Benin	600	490	340	57	31	79	14	9.4
Bhutan	900	390	120	<17	<13	0.0	73	14
Bolivia (Plurinational State of)	510	330	200	<12	13	0.0	28	21
Bosnia and Herzegovina	19	11	8	...	...	...	5.9	5.2
Botswana	360	390	170	1 171	282	0.1	50	21
Brazil	120	85	69	8.4[a]	7.8[a]	0.1	4.4	2.5
Brunei Darussalam	26	24	27	...	...	...	4.3	3.0
Bulgaria	24	29	5	...	...	...	7.3	2.0
Burkina Faso	770	580	400	163	33	101	13	8.5
Burundi	1 300	1 000	740	191	48	33	40	18
Cabo Verde	230	84	53	<44	<20	...	34	23
Cambodia	1 200	540	170	48	18	1.8	128	63
Cameroon	720	740	590	176	159	56	51	29
Canada	6	7	11	1.5[a]	1.1[a]	...	0.3	0.2
Central African Republic	1 200	1 200	880	...	...	116	143	50
Chad	1 700	1 500	980	160	116	136	24	18
Chile	55	29	22	3.7[a]	2.4[a]	...	1.9	1.2
China	97	63	32	...	...	0.0	8.7	3.2
Colombia	100	130	83	21	14	0.2	3.2	1.6
Comoros	630	480	350	0.0	6.7	68	6.9	6.3
Congo	670	610	410	280	119	104	36	42
Cook Islands	...	...	...	...	...	...	0.5	0.6
Costa Rica	38	44	38	3.5[a]	2.9[a]	0.0	1.8	0.8
Côte d'Ivoire	740	670	720	283	157	71	56	22
Croatia	8	11	13	...	...	...	4.2	1.4
Cuba	63	63	80	1.1[a]	2.6[a]	...	0.4	0.3
Cyprus	18	16	10	0.2[a]	0.2[a]	...	0.0	0.2
Czech Republic	15	7	5	...	...	...	1.2	0.4
Democratic People's Republic of Korea	85	120	87	...	...	0.0	17	9.0
Democratic Republic of the Congo	1 000	1 100	730	65	48	105	61	54
Denmark	9	9	5	0.7[a]	0.5[a]	...	0.4	0.4

Morbidity — Member State

Incidence rate (per 100 000 population)					Prevalence (per 100 000 population)				Member State
HIV/AIDS[d]		Malaria[e]	Tuberculosis[g]		HIV/AIDS[d]		Tuberculosis[g]		
2001	2012	2012	2000	2012	2001	2012	2000	2012	
...	...	1 263	189	189	7.6	14	449	358	Afghanistan
...	...	...	23	16	...	...	30	22	Albania
...	...	0.2	87	89	...	...	148	152	Algeria
...	...	...	21	13	...	...	31	21	Andorra
133	134	18 241	250	316	894	1 195	421	474	Angola
...	...	...	5.9	3.9	...	...	9.3	4.8	Antigua and Barbuda
...	...	0.0	40	25	209	238	59	36	Argentina
<16	<17	...	61	52	56	117	93	79	Armenia
...	...	...	6.2	6.5	...	...	8.7	8.8	Australia
...	...	...	17	7.9	...	...	25	11	Austria
...	...	0.0	682	95	44	112	1 693	124	Azerbaijan
<330	<134	...	32	9.9	1 963	1 891	34	11	Bahamas
...	...	...	36	20	...	...	56	29	Bahrain
<1	<1	395	225	225	2.9	5.2	507	434	Bangladesh
<75	<35	...	1.3	1.6	428	530	2.1	1.8	Barbados
20	17	...	84	70	73	247	130	108	Belarus
...	...	...	14	9.7	...	...	20	13	Belgium
<204	<62	13	40	40	1 011	943	52	51	Belize
104	41	29 282	86	70	866	712	134	110	Benin
...	...	20	402	180	<86	142	754	225	Bhutan
27	10	101	184	127	209	151	299	215	Bolivia (Plurinational State of)
...	...	...	63	49	...	...	73	73	Bosnia and Herzegovina
1 518	616	30	918	408	16 694	16 850	720	343	Botswana
...	...	158	60	46	...	...	84	59	Brazil
...	...	...	106	68	...	...	165	90	Brunei Darussalam
...	...	...	58	32	...	...	88	43	Bulgaria
70	35	33 759	71	54	1 502	696	108	82	Burkina Faso
82	46	8 492	288	130	1 842	909	408	199	Burundi
...	...	22	160	144	285	161	311	237	Cabo Verde
48	9.2	1 070	577	411	848	514	1 619	764	Cambodia
381	206	16 877	310	238	2 955	2 767	504	319	Cameroon
...	...	...	6.5	4.6	...	...	8.5	6.1	Canada
...	...	34 675	1 071	367	...	...	1 495	520	Central African Republic
266	125	26 152	151	151	2 213	1 712	252	221	Chad
...	...	...	22	16	212	222	30	21	Chile
...	...	0.5	109	73	...	...	170	99	China
26	19	204	43	33	346	307	68	48	Colombia
...	...	22 419	39	34	0.1	1 098	64	62	Comoros
277	108	33 824	353	381	2 856	1 717	455	530	Congo
...	...	6.5	5.6	...	...	7.6	7.2	Cook Islands
...	...	0.2	35	11	129	204	63	12	Costa Rica
356	149	20 730	369	172	3 845	2 268	513	228	Côte d'Ivoire
...	...	...	42	14	...	...	57	20	Croatia
...	...	...	13	9.3	25	42	19	14	Cuba
...	...	...	4.0	5.4	...	...	4.8	6.1	Cyprus
...	...	...	16	5.3	...	...	21	7.2	Czech Republic
...	...	104	383	409	...	...	479	511	Democratic People's Republic of Korea
107	52	25 999	327	327	909	733	611	576	Democratic Republic of the Congo
...	...	...	13	7.4	...	...	19	10	Denmark

	Age-standardized mortality rates by cause[a] (per 100 000 population)			Years of life lost[a] (per 100 000 population)				MDG 4 Number of deaths among children aged <5 years[a] (000s)		Mortality Distribution of causes of death among children aged < years[a,b] (%)							
										HIV		Diarrhoea		Measles		Malaria	
Member State	Communicable	Non-communicable	Injuries	All causes	Communicable	Non-communicable	Injuries	2000	2012	2000	2012	2000	2012	2000	2012	2000	201
	2012			2012													
Djibouti	626	631	106	49 454	32 528	12 131	4 795	2	2	2	2	15	9	8	16	1	1
Dominica	…	…	…	…	…	…	…	0	0	…	…	…	…	…	…	…	…
Dominican Republic	77	396	66	16 888	5 127	8 525	3 236	8	6	4	1	8	5	0	0	0	0
Ecuador	97	410	84	17 885	4 586	9 122	4 176	11	8	1	0	9	4	0	0	0	0
Egypt	74	782	33	20 949	4 268	15 168	1 513	77	40	0	0	9	5	3	0	0	0
El Salvador	96	475	158	22 986	4 079	10 914	7 994	5	2	2	2	9	5	0	0	0	0
Equatorial Guinea	757	729	134	71 724	48 783	15 054	7 887	3	3	3	7	11	8	5	4	24	15
Eritrea	506	672	119	36 628	22 640	9 469	4 519	15	12	2	1	12	10	24	6	0	0
Estonia	36	496	44	24 216	1 810	20 218	2 189	0	0	0	0	2	1	0	0	0	0
Ethiopia	559	476	94	42 966	29 697	8 571	4 697	412	205	4	2	16	10	5	2	5	3
Fiji	105	804	64	24 231	4 602	16 839	2 791	0	0	0	0	6	4	2	0	0	0
Finland	9	367	39	17 271	413	15 028	1 830	0	0	0	0	1	0	0	0	0	0
France	21	313	35	15 435	936	12 899	1 600	4	3	0	0	2	1	0	0	0	0
Gabon	589	505	77	44 352	30 028	10 127	4 197	3	3	7	2	8	7	3	1	19	19
Gambia	590	630	96	53 070	35 805	11 970	5 295	6	5	1	1	11	7	4	0	23	20
Georgia	39	615	32	25 556	2 419	21 490	1 647	2	1	0	0	3	1	0	0	0	0
Germany	22	365	23	18 285	926	16 246	1 113	4	3	0	0	0	0	0	0	0	0
Ghana	476	670	76	45 576	28 629	12 863	4 084	65	56	3	1	8	7	10	1	21	19
Greece	24	365	27	17 792	1 027	15 467	1 298	1	1	0	0	0	0	0	0	0	0
Grenada	…	…	…	…	…	…	…	0	0	0	0	4	0	0	0	0	0
Guatemala	213	409	111	24 271	10 458	7 885	5 929	20	15	2	1	12	8	0	0	0	0
Guinea	680	681	96	64 439	45 952	12 912	5 574	68	42	1	2	11	8	15	2	24	27
Guinea-Bissau	870	765	112	75 954	56 025	13 835	6 094	9	8	2	3	11	10	8	1	23	18
Guyana	177	1 024	150	32 349	8 533	17 196	6 621	1	1	3	1	14	5	0	0	4	9
Haiti	405	725	89	43 976	25 017	13 728	5 232	28	20	4	1	17	11	0	0	1	1
Honduras	118	441	81	18 716	6 564	8 031	4 121	7	5	4	1	9	6	0	0	0	0
Hungary	18	602	44	27 112	795	24 235	2 081	1	1	0	0	0	0	0	0	0	0
Iceland	14	312	29	10 958	462	9 207	1 289	0	0	0	0	0	0	0	0	0	0
India	253	682	116	32 584	13 613	14 186	4 785	2 417	1 407	0	0	15	11	3	2	0	0
Indonesia	162	680	49	22 051	7 905	12 030	2 116	228	151	0	1	10	6	9	4	0	2
Iran (Islamic Republic of)	56	569	75	17 220	3 118	10 302	3 799	44	26	0	0	8	4	0	0	0	0
Iraq	87	715	128	23 080	7 823	9 610	5 647	38	35	0	0	9	6	1	0	0	0
Ireland	22	344	32	12 068	728	9 828	1 512	0	0	0	0	0	0	1	0	0	0
Israel	31	311	21	10 156	1 024	8 286	846	1	1	0	0	1	0	0	0	0	0
Italy	15	304	20	15 248	712	13 583	953	3	2	0	0	0	0	0	0	0	0
Jamaica	97	519	51	20 191	5 142	12 320	2 729	1	1	9	1	3	2	0	0	0	0
Japan	34	244	40	15 821	1 604	12 212	2 005	5	3	0	0	1	2	0	0	0	0
Jordan	53	640	53	14 574	3 691	8 584	2 299	4	4	0	0	7	4	0	0	0	0
Kazakhstan	59	947	101	30 421	3 834	21 333	5 254	9	6	0	0	10	5	0	0	0	0
Kenya	657	515	101	51 435	37 031	9 133	5 271	128	108	13	4	13	10	1	0	5	4
Kiribati	…	…	…	…	…	…	…	0	0	0	0	15	11	0	0	0	0
Kuwait	82	406	25	7 067	1 468	4 400	1 199	1	1	0	0	0	0	0	0	0	0
Kyrgyzstan	70	832	64	24 489	5 767	15 300	3 421	6	4	0	0	10	6	0	0	0	0
Lao People's Democratic Republic	329	680	75	35 081	21 052	10 183	3 846	20	14	0	0	17	12	6	0	2	1
Latvia	40	613	51	30 076	2 076	25 436	2 564	0	0	0	0	0	0	0	0	0	0
Lebanon	30	385	41	10 507	1 196	7 934	1 377	1	1	0	1	4	2	0	0	0	0
Lesotho	1 110	672	142	76 738	57 102	11 697	7 939	7	6	34	19	8	7	1	1	0	0
Liberia	609	657	83	47 041	32 485	10 525	4 030	23	11	1	1	11	8	17	1	23	21
Libya	53	550	63	13 193	2 305	8 377	2 511	3	2	0	0	4	2	0	0	0	0

Mortality

Distribution of causes of death among children aged <5 years[a,b] (%)

Member State

Acute respiratory infections		Prematurity		Intrapartum-related complications		Neonatal sepsis		Congenital anomalies		Other diseases		Injuries		Member State
2000	2012	2000	2012	2000	2012	2000	2012	2000	2012	2000	2012	2000	2012	
18	14	13	14	11	10	4	5	4	7	18	15	5	5	Djibouti
...	...	...	...	...	...	...	...	...	...	...	...	...	...	Dominica
15	13	25	23	11	12	6	7	12	17	13	13	6	9	Dominican Republic
16	12	19	19	7	7	3	4	15	21	19	22	10	10	Ecuador
15	10	28	29	13	13	2	2	12	21	16	15	3	4	Egypt
19	13	15	17	7	7	4	3	16	22	20	22	8	8	El Salvador
13	15	12	13	9	11	4	6	2	4	14	14	3	4	Equatorial Guinea
17	19	8	9	9	12	5	7	3	8	15	19	5	8	Eritrea
7	7	16	7	4	9	10	10	28	25	10	21	23	20	Estonia
19	18	10	13	10	15	4	8	2	5	21	18	5	6	Ethiopia
14	13	18	19	8	7	5	5	18	20	19	20	10	12	Fiji
2	5	21	19	8	6	2	3	40	30	19	30	7	6	Finland
2	2	17	16	12	12	3	3	28	26	28	33	9	6	France
12	12	18	17	9	12	5	7	5	8	11	12	3	5	Gabon
12	13	11	13	11	13	6	8	4	7	13	13	4	5	Gambia
15	8	28	30	8	9	6	7	15	22	18	17	7	6	Georgia
2	2	29	30	5	7	2	2	33	32	22	22	7	6	Germany
11	13	11	14	11	13	6	8	4	7	11	13	3	5	Ghana
3	2	38	32	6	6	2	0	36	45	9	11	6	4	Greece
9	1	25	15	23	15	13	7	2	17	16	42	8	3	Grenada
21	17	13	13	13	14	8	9	7	12	18	17	7	9	Guatemala
12	13	8	11	8	12	4	6	2	3	13	13	3	4	Guinea
13	14	11	11	8	12	4	7	3	4	15	15	3	4	Guinea-Bissau
10	5	21	19	13	12	6	6	10	9	15	28	5	6	Guyana
21	22	12	14	10	11	4	6	4	6	21	21	6	7	Haiti
15	13	21	23	9	9	5	6	12	17	23	21	3	3	Honduras
7	5	43	37	5	6	0	3	23	30	14	16	7	4	Hungary
0	0	30	36	10	0	0	0	19	12	32	49	8	3	Iceland
18	14	17	27	13	11	8	8	5	6	16	16	4	4	India
17	17	16	20	12	11	6	6	6	10	18	17	6	7	Indonesia
15	13	22	23	12	11	7	7	13	19	16	15	7	7	Iran (Islamic Republic of)
16	16	18	20	15	15	9	9	10	13	14	14	6	7	Iraq
3	2	25	23	3	7	0	1	45	42	20	20	3	5	Ireland
2	1	29	26	4	4	3	2	26	35	30	25	7	6	Israel
2	1	32	28	9	9	2	4	34	24	17	31	4	4	Italy
9	8	26	25	10	9	7	7	17	23	14	17	6	7	Jamaica
7	6	10	9	5	5	2	2	40	39	23	23	13	14	Japan
14	10	27	28	10	10	4	6	17	23	12	12	9	8	Jordan
17	13	22	19	10	13	4	6	11	20	18	16	8	8	Kazakhstan
17	18	10	13	10	14	5	7	3	6	16	18	5	7	Kenya
21	19	12	14	13	12	5	6	7	9	20	21	7	8	Kiribati
6	8	22	32	5	3	2	1	44	39	13	11	7	6	Kuwait
18	14	19	18	12	14	6	7	10	17	17	14	8	9	Kyrgyzstan
21	20	9	12	11	13	5	7	3	5	21	21	6	8	Lao People's Democratic Republic
5	2	18	10	16	32	2	7	34	30	15	14	11	5	Latvia
12	7	24	30	8	11	5	4	21	23	16	16	9	6	Lebanon
11	12	12	16	11	14	6	8	3	4	11	13	3	4	Lesotho
12	14	9	11	7	13	3	7	2	5	13	14	3	5	Liberia
12	8	22	23	11	9	4	5	20	27	18	18	9	8	Libya

Member State	Maternal mortality ratio[c] (per 100 000 live births)			Cause-specific mortality rate (per 100 000 population)				
	MDG 5			MDG 6				
				HIV/AIDS[d]		Malaria[e]	Tuberculosis among HIV-negative people[f]	
	1990	2000	2013	2001	2012	2012	2000	2012
Djibouti	400	360	230	<136	<116	7.3	57	76
Dominica	…	…	…	…	…	…	3.4	2.0
Dominican Republic	240	120	100	52	19	0.0	8.7	4.4
Ecuador	160	120	87	22	17	0.0	14	2.7
Egypt	120	75	45	<1	<1	…	1.7	0.5
El Salvador	110	80	69	27	<16	0.0	2.8	1.0
Equatorial Guinea	1 600	790	290	<187	194	69	0.0	0.0
Eritrea	1 700	670	380	66	19	3.2	7.7	4.6
Estonia	48	26	11	…	…	…	8.0	2.8
Ethiopia	1 400	990	420	148	51	17	41	18
Fiji	89	72	59	<12	<11	…	3.7	1.7
Finland	6	7	4	…	…	…	1.6	0.3
France	12	10	12	2.0[a]	0.7[a]	…	1.1	0.5
Gabon	380	330	240	187	143	67	81	44
Gambia	710	580	430	<39	<56	82	36	51
Georgia	50	60	41	<2	<5	0.0	7.7	4.5
Germany	13	7	7	…	…	…	0.6	0.4
Ghana	760	570	380	100	46	69	27	6.9
Greece	6	5	5	…	…	…	0.8	0.7
Grenada	34	29	23	…	…	…	0.0	1.0
Guatemala	270	160	140	17	23	0.0	5.1	2.1
Guinea	1 100	950	650	37	44	103	44	23
Guinea-Bissau	930	840	560	<77	136	95	28	29
Guyana	210	240	250	<27	<13	15	13	15
Haiti	670	510	380	174	73	3.9	40	25
Honduras	290	150	120	57	22	0.0	5.0	2.9
Hungary	23	10	14	…	…	…	3.5	0.7
Iceland	7	6	4	0.7[a]	0.1[a]	…	0.4	0.3
India	560	370	190	13	11	2.3	39	22
Indonesia	430	310	190	0.6	11	3.8	55	27
Iran (Islamic Republic of)	83	44	23	<1	6.0	0.0	3.8	2.9
Iraq	110	71	67	…	…	0.0	4.7	2.9
Ireland	6	6	9	…	…	…	1.5	0.4
Israel	12	9	2	…	…	…	0.6	0.2
Italy	10	4	4	2.8[a]	1.4[a]	…	0.9	0.4
Jamaica	98	88	80	105	46	…	0.6	0.2
Japan	14	10	6	…	…	…	2.2	1.7
Jordan	86	65	50	…	…	…	0.8	0.5
Kazakhstan	91	71	26	…	…	…	33	7.8
Kenya	490	570	400	412	133	28	19	22
Kiribati	250	200	130	…	…	…	15	17
Kuwait	12	8	14	0.0[a]	0.1[a]	…	0.8	0.9
Kyrgyzstan	85	100	75	<2	<9	0.0	25	9.5
Lao People's Democratic Republic	1 100	600	220	<2	<8	4.5	21	11
Latvia	57	42	13	…	…	…	13	2.6
Lebanon	64	37	16	…	…	…	1.2	1.5
Lesotho	720	680	490	858	755	…	16	17
Liberia	1 200	1 100	640	67	40	69	54	46
Libya	31	21	15	…	…	…	5.3	6.8

Morbidity									Member State
MDG 6									
Incidence rate (per 100 000 population)					Prevalence (per 100 000 population)				
HIV/AIDS[d]		Malaria[e]	Tuberculosis[g]		HIV/AIDS[d]		Tuberculosis[g]		
2001	2012	2012	2000	2012	2001	2012	2000	2012	
237	<58	2 386	619	620	1 323	892	775	897	Djibouti
...	...	...	14	13	...	...	28	25	Dominica
67	<5	13	100	62	728	438	159	98	Dominican Republic
...	...	4.1	107	59	314	338	187	98	Ecuador
...	...	...	26	17	2.9	8.1	42	29	Egypt
...	...	0.2	37	25	434	396	56	34	El Salvador
...	...	24 767	101	139	2 276	4 259	130	164	Equatorial Guinea
45	<8	1 282	157	93	738	290	194	152	Eritrea
...	...	...	67	23	...	...	97	29	Estonia
185	22	4 563	421	247	1 912	827	429	224	Ethiopia
...	...	...	54	24	<61	<114	112	30	Fiji
...	...	...	12	5.5	...	...	16	7.2	Finland
...	...	...	13	8.2	...	...	19	12	France
468	62	24 892	527	428	3 348	2 490	898	563	Gabon
122	<56	29 095	225	284	569	798	373	490	Gambia
<11	<23	0.0	256	116	32	152	516	158	Georgia
...	...	...	12	5.6	...	...	18	7.8	Germany
144	31	27 337	152	72	1 385	930	257	92	Ghana
...	...	...	7.4	4.5	...	...	9.5	6.3	Greece
...	...	...	4.4	4.1	...	...	8.6	6.8	Grenada
...	...	58	68	60	424	383	129	110	Guatemala
...	...	38 333	234	178	716	1 031	429	274	Guinea
320	219	28 120	192	242	1 584	2 480	290	312	Guinea-Bissau
...	...	7 910	104	109	435	902	139	131	Guyana
160	84	1 299	271	213	1 818	1 435	400	296	Haiti
...	...	164	114	54	682	323	169	82	Honduras
...	...	...	37	18	...	...	51	29	Hungary
...	...	...	5.3	3.5	...	...	8.1	4.3	Iceland
25	11	1 523	216	176	222	169	438	230	India
14	31	2 278	204	185	39	245	474	297	Indonesia
...	...	1.2	26	21	22	93	41	33	Iran (Islamic Republic of)
...	...	0.0	50	45	...	...	61	73	Iraq
...	...	...	12	8.6	...	...	16	11	Ireland
...	...	...	10	7.6	...	...	14	11	Israel
...	...	...	7.1	6.7	...	...	9.0	9.4	Italy
111	50	...	6.5	6.6	1 288	1 024	8.1	9.5	Jamaica
...	...	...	36	19	...	...	51	26	Japan
...	...	...	8.1	5.8	...	...	10	8.5	Jordan
...	...	...	351	137	...	...	668	189	Kazakhstan
426	228	8 200	286	272	5 024	3 812	273	299	Kenya
...	...	...	372	429	...	...	487	628	Kiribati
...	...	...	31	26	...	...	41	33	Kuwait
<10	31	0.0	249	141	20	159	449	217	Kyrgyzstan
...	...	1 698	330	204	60	173	961	514	Lao People's Democratic Republic
...	...	...	121	53	...	...	194	76	Latvia
...	...	...	17	16	...	...	20	20	Lebanon
1 759	1 284	...	553	630	14 822	17 482	387	424	Lesotho
142	<12	27 793	242	304	1 110	521	482	495	Liberia
...	...	...	40	40	...	...	57	66	Libya

Member State	Age-standardized mortality rates by cause[a] (per 100 000 population)			Years of life lost[a] (per 100 000 population)				MDG 4 — Number of deaths among children aged <5 years[a] (000s)		Mortality — Distribution of causes of death among children aged <5 years[a,b] (%)							
	Communicable	Non-communicable	Injuries	All causes	Communicable	Non-communicable	Injuries			HIV		Diarrhoea		Measles		Malaria	
	2012			2012				2000	2012	2000	2012	2000	2012	2000	2012	2000	201
Lithuania	27	580	76	27 354	1 281	22 141	3 932	0	0	0	0	0	1	0	0	0	0
Luxembourg	21	317	31	12 889	750	10 773	1 367	0	0	0	0	0	0	0	0	0	0
Madagascar	430	649	89	39 785	24 877	10 233	4 675	71	44	1	1	15	10	8	1	5	7
Malawi	778	655	98	54 730	41 453	9 228	4 049	81	43	13	12	13	8	0	1	20	15
Malaysia	117	563	63	15 325	3 134	9 740	2 450	6	4	1	1	3	2	0	0	0	0
Maldives	59	487	35	11 070	2 173	7 691	1 205	0	0	0	0	6	2	0	0	0	0
Mali	588	866	120	76 206	55 170	14 432	6 603	102	82	1	1	14	12	3	1	25	14
Malta	24	364	19	14 285	767	12 632	886	0	0	0	0	0	0	0	0	0	0
Marshall Islands	…	…	…	…	…	…	…	0	0	…	…	…	…	…	…	…	…
Mauritania	619	555	83	45 160	31 786	9 373	4 001	11	11	1	0	13	10	5	1	9	10
Mauritius	62	577	44	21 106	2 399	16 472	2 235	0	0	0	0	2	1	0	0	0	0
Mexico	58	468	63	16 308	2 578	10 391	3 339	64	37	0	0	8	3	0	0	0	0
Micronesia (Federated States of)	…	…	…	…	…	…	…	0	0	0	0	13	8	1	0	0	0
Monaco	…	…	…	…	…	…	…	0	0	…	…	…	…	…	…	…	…
Mongolia	83	966	69	26 275	5 357	17 033	3 885	3	2	0	0	15	8	1	0	0	0
Montenegro	19	572	41	21 165	883	18 336	1 946	0	0	0	0	1	0	0	0	0	0
Morocco	…	708	47	…	…	…	…	31	23	0	0	10	6	0	0	0	0
Mozambique	998	594	175	73 589	53 997	11 531	8 061	122	84	5	6	12	9	4	0	25	18
Myanmar	316	709	102	32 620	13 566	14 286	4 767	80	49	0	0	12	7	3	4	2	2
Namibia	357	580	76	29 801	18 018	8 027	3 755	4	2	29	9	8	6	1	3	3	0
Nauru	…	…	…	…	…	…	…	0	0	…	…	…	…	…	…	…	…
Nepal	252	678	89	26 981	11 880	11 404	3 697	63	27	0	0	10	6	14	9	0	0
Netherlands	26	355	22	15 078	941	13 172	966	1	1	0	0	0	0	0	0	0	0
New Zealand	18	314	33	12 635	742	10 295	1 597	0	0	0	0	0	2	0	0	0	0
Nicaragua	75	547	64	18 896	4 947	10 740	3 209	6	3	0	1	14	7	0	0	0	0
Niger	740	649	98	70 633	54 270	10 726	5 637	121	90	0	0	16	12	5	0	27	19
Nigeria	866	674	146	81 624	59 843	13 237	8 544	1 035	827	2	3	11	10	15	1	23	20
Niue	…	…	…	…	…	…	…	0	0	…	…	…	…	…	…	…	…
Norway	25	336	26	14 003	894	11 991	1 117	0	0	0	0	0	1	0	0	0	0
Oman	84	478	53	10 812	2 583	5 787	2 443	1	1	0	0	2	1	0	0	0	0
Pakistan	296	669	99	37 478	20 789	11 796	4 893	518	408	0	0	15	11	1	1	0	0
Palau	…	…	…	…	…	…	…	0	0	…	…	…	…	…	…	…	…
Panama	82	375	69	16 459	3 975	8 760	3 724	2	1	1	0	6	10	0	0	0	0
Papua New Guinea	554	693	100	39 380	22 709	12 277	4 394	15	13	1	1	10	9	5	1	16	11
Paraguay	77	486	68	17 545	4 427	9 696	3 421	5	3	0	0	9	5	0	0	0	0
Peru	121	364	48	14 429	4 193	8 048	2 189	25	11	1	1	7	4	0	0	0	0
Philippines	227	720	54	23 711	8 000	13 013	2 698	91	69	0	0	11	7	0	0	0	0
Poland	23	494	49	21 595	940	18 222	2 433	3	2	0	0	0	0	0	0	0	0
Portugal	40	343	25	16 975	1 632	14 128	1 215	1	0	0	0	0	0	0	0	0	0
Qatar	28	407	41	5 736	635	3 410	1 690	0	0	0	0	1	0	0	0	0	0
Republic of Korea	34	302	53	12 080	944	8 755	2 381	3	2	0	0	1	1	0	0	0	0
Republic of Moldova	60	776	72	31 406	3 150	24 614	3 642	2	1	0	0	2	1	0	0	0	0
Romania	39	612	41	26 317	1 841	22 427	2 049	8	3	0	0	2	1	0	0	0	0
Russian Federation	74	790	103	37 717	3 877	28 356	5 483	34	17	2	1	2	1	0	0	0	0
Rwanda	402	585	106	40 122	24 964	9 517	5 642	79	24	3	1	19	10	1	1	6	4
Saint Kitts and Nevis	…	…	…	…	…	…	…	0	0	…	…	…	…	…	…	…	…
Saint Lucia	…	…	…	…	…	…	…	0	0	3	0	2	0	0	0	0	0
Saint Vincent and the Grenadines	…	…	…	…	…	…	…	0	0	3	1	3	0	0	0	0	0
Samoa	…	…	…	…	…	…	…	0	0	0	0	6	4	0	0	0	0

Mortality

Distribution of causes of death among children aged < 5 years[a,b]
(%)

Member State

Acute respiratory infections		Prematurity		Intrapartum-related complications		Neonatal sepsis		Congenital anomalies		Other diseases		Injuries		Member State
2000	2012	2000	2012	2000	2012	2000	2012	2000	2012	2000	2012	2000	2012	
9	4	15	12	8	7	2	8	38	33	12	19	16	15	Lithuania
0	1	18	14	20	4	2	4	12	11	32	50	16	16	Luxembourg
19	18	11	12	9	13	5	7	2	6	19	18	5	7	Madagascar
14	13	8	12	7	11	4	7	2	5	15	13	3	5	Malawi
9	7	23	24	9	9	3	3	26	26	19	21	7	7	Malaysia
17	8	22	24	8	8	5	4	15	30	23	19	4	5	Maldives
14	16	10	13	6	10	3	6	2	3	17	18	3	5	Mali
2	0	37	27	7	5	3	2	21	45	26	19	5	1	Malta
…	…	…	…	…	…	…	…	…	…	…	…	…	…	Marshall Islands
17	16	17	18	9	11	5	8	3	6	16	16	4	5	Mauritania
4	10	40	27	10	5	4	7	22	29	12	13	7	7	Mauritius
16	11	17	18	7	6	5	6	19	25	19	23	9	7	Mexico
18	18	15	18	14	11	5	6	9	11	18	18	7	8	Micronesia (Federated States of)
…	…	…	…	…	…	…	…	…	…	…	…	…	…	Monaco
22	18	14	14	8	10	3	4	8	16	21	19	8	11	Mongolia
3	5	28	30	29	40	1	2	14	8	21	13	2	1	Montenegro
17	13	19	23	14	14	8	9	9	13	18	16	6	7	Morocco
13	14	9	12	8	11	5	6	2	4	14	14	3	5	Mozambique
18	17	18	20	11	12	6	7	4	6	18	18	6	8	Myanmar
13	13	12	20	10	13	5	7	4	10	11	13	4	6	Namibia
…	…	…	…	…	…	…	…	…	…	…	…	…	…	Nauru
15	13	12	18	15	13	10	9	4	7	16	17	4	6	Nepal
2	2	21	20	12	12	3	5	36	33	20	24	6	4	Netherlands
6	5	21	25	6	8	1	2	29	22	24	18	13	17	New Zealand
18	15	20	21	9	9	3	4	11	19	22	20	3	3	Nicaragua
15	18	6	10	6	7	2	5	2	3	18	19	3	6	Niger
12	16	8	12	8	11	3	5	2	3	13	16	3	4	Nigeria
…	…	…	…	…	…	…	…	…	…	…	…	…	…	Niue
3	2	12	19	10	10	1	1	37	34	29	31	6	2	Norway
10	6	23	28	11	11	4	3	27	28	16	15	7	6	Oman
19	17	13	19	14	13	9	10	4	5	20	18	5	7	Pakistan
…	…	…	…	…	…	…	…	…	…	…	…	…	…	Palau
11	14	15	16	6	5	5	7	27	24	25	18	4	6	Panama
15	17	13	13	11	13	5	7	4	5	15	17	5	7	Papua New Guinea
16	12	24	24	8	8	5	7	14	21	20	18	4	5	Paraguay
15	11	19	20	8	8	4	5	13	23	27	22	4	7	Peru
20	18	17	18	11	12	7	7	9	12	18	17	7	8	Philippines
5	4	25	34	9	6	6	3	36	37	12	11	6	4	Poland
4	3	18	20	6	7	3	4	34	29	25	28	9	9	Portugal
5	4	29	30	10	9	4	2	24	27	17	18	9	8	Qatar
6	3	23	32	6	6	4	2	24	23	21	23	16	10	Republic of Korea
29	18	4	12	9	4	6	4	23	36	13	12	15	13	Republic of Moldova
30	26	21	26	6	5	1	1	20	24	13	10	8	6	Romania
14	8	23	22	7	7	5	4	23	30	16	19	9	9	Russian Federation
21	18	7	12	10	13	5	7	2	7	21	18	5	8	Rwanda
…	…	…	…	…	…	…	…	…	…	…	…	…	…	Saint Kitts and Nevis
4	18	34	0	16	0	1	0	11	32	23	46	6	5	Saint Lucia
3	2	37	37	11	12	4	2	16	11	16	29	6	6	Saint Vincent and the Grenadines
15	11	16	20	5	7	4	4	24	24	18	23	12	7	Samoa

Member State	Mortality							
	MDG 5			MDG 6				
	Maternal mortality ratio[c] (per 100 000 live births)			Cause-specific mortality rate (per 100 000 population)				
				HIV/AIDS[d]		Malaria[e]	Tuberculosis among HIV-negative people[f]	
	1990	2000	2013	2001	2012	2012	2000	2012
Lithuania	34	20	11	...	...	...	11	3.0
Luxembourg	6	11	11	...	...	...	0.2	0.4
Madagascar	740	550	440	29	28	27	69	46
Malawi	1 100	750	510	743	287	64	28	9.0
Malaysia	56	40	29	18	18	0.0	6.9	5.4
Maldives	430	110	31	<36	<30	...	5.4	2.0
Mali	1 100	860	550	74	33	87	12	9.0
Malta	12	11	9	...	...	...	0.3	0.4
Marshall Islands	...	...	...	...	...	...	62	111
Mauritania	630	480	320	<18	<26	50	57	93
Mauritius	70	28	73	1.3 [a]	5.5 [a]	...	0.7	1.0
Mexico	88	67	49	...	...	0.0	3.3	1.8
Micronesia (Federated States of)	170	130	96	...	...	...	65	24
Monaco	...	...	...	...	...	...	0.1	0.1
Mongolia	100	120	68	0.7	1.7	...	13	7.2
Montenegro	8	10	7	...	...	...	...	0.2
Morocco	310	200	120	<2	3.7	...	15	9.2
Mozambique	1 300	870	480	210	305	70	75	53
Myanmar	580	360	200	20	22	5.4	106	48
Namibia	320	270	130	483	219	0.1	24	14
Nauru	...	...	...	...	...	...	7.2	9.5
Nepal	790	430	190	6.7	15	0.1	21	20
Netherlands	11	15	6	...	...	...	0.2	0.2
New Zealand	18	12	8	0.1 [a]	0.1 [a]	...	0.3	0.1
Nicaragua	170	140	100	<2	<3	0.0	6.4	3.1
Niger	1 000	850	630	28	20	110	46	16
Nigeria	1 200	950	560	120	142	108	38	16
Niue	...	...	...	...	...	...	3.1	3.1
Norway	9	8	4	...	...	...	0.2	0.1
Oman	48	22	11	...	...	...	1.8	0.9
Pakistan	400	280	170	<1	2.0	1.1	69	34
Palau	...	...	...	...	...	...	26	4.4
Panama	98	79	85	53	<26	0.0	6.6	4.9
Papua New Guinea	470	340	220	23	<14	39	52	54
Paraguay	130	120	110	<9	<7	0.0	4.3	3.0
Peru	250	160	89	35	14	0.1	14	5.1
Philippines	110	120	120	<1	<1	0.0	40	24
Poland	17	8	3	...	...	...	2.9	1.8
Portugal	15	11	8	11 [a]	6.6 [a]	...	2.8	1.3
Qatar	11	9	6	...	...	...	0.7	0.2
Republic of Korea	18	19	27	...	...	0.0	2.7	5.4
Republic of Moldova	61	39	21	<25	37	...	17	18
Romania	170	53	33	2.3 [a]	0.9 [a]	...	9.5	5.6
Russian Federation	74	57	24	15 [a]	43 [a]	...	21	13
Rwanda	1 400	1 000	320	267	49	33	49	10
Saint Kitts and Nevis	...	...	...	...	...	...	2.4	2.5
Saint Lucia	60	44	34	...	...	...	0.8	1.2
Saint Vincent and the Grenadines	48	75	45	...	...	...	3.3	2.6
Samoa	150	89	58	...	...	...	3.1	3.2

	Morbidity								Member State
Incidence rate (per 100 000 population)					**Prevalence (per 100 000 population)**				
HIV/AIDS[d]		Malaria[e]	Tuberculosis[g]		HIV/AIDS[d]		Tuberculosis[g]		
2001	2012	2012	2000	2012	2001	2012	2000	2012	
...	...	...	103	66	...	...	157	93	Lithuania
...	...	...	12	6.5	...	...	17	10	Luxembourg
...	...	6 020	293	234	337	264	609	442	Madagascar
956	414	27 462	467	163	9 206	7 103	365	140	Malawi
26	25	34	95	80	227	280	148	101	Malaysia
...	...	...	60	41	<36	<30	81	65	Maldives
106	28	20 399	77	60	1 021	675	117	92	Mali
...	...	...	4.5	11	...	...	6.2	16	Malta
...	...	...	263	572	...	...	532	1 079	Marshall Islands
...	...	17 591	277	350	327	276	536	794	Mauritania
...	...	...	24	21	615	850	46	39	Mauritius
10	7.7	0.8	31	23	183	144	51	33	Mexico
...	...	...	279	194	...	...	560	270	Micronesia (Federated States of)
...	...	...	0.0	2.1	...	...	1.7	2.7	Monaco
...	...	...	254	223	8.7	38	431	380	Mongolia
...	...	...	...	18	...	...	...	25	Montenegro
...	...	...	117	103	30	92	161	140	Morocco
870	467	27 947	513	552	4 508	6 169	701	553	Mozambique
51	13	2 743	412	377	453	371	831	489	Myanmar
1 213	458	23	1 407	655	8 853	9 742	1 429	688	Namibia
...	...	...	46	54	...	...	72	91	Nauru
40	4.3	62	163	163	213	177	248	241	Nepal
...	...	...	9.0	6.3	...	...	11	8.2	Netherlands
...	...	...	10	7.6	...	...	13	10	New Zealand
<10	26	39	68	38	26	160	108	55	Nicaragua
69	6.6	27 726	191	104	500	270	396	166	Niger
320	153	28 710	172	108	2 044	2 030	326	161	Nigeria
...	...	...	0.0	37	...	...	47	46	Niue
...	...	...	5.7	7.5	...	...	7.1	10	Norway
...	...	...	17	13	...	...	26	18	Oman
1.6	10	1 945	231	231	6.8	48	573	376	Pakistan
...	...	...	156	24	...	...	256	65	Palau
...	...	26	47	48	682	439	52	64	Panama
63	<14	14 255	349	348	408	347	586	541	Papua New Guinea
...	...	0.0	49	45	66	196	72	63	Paraguay
...	...	189	184	95	358	252	268	121	Peru
<1	1.8	23	329	265	6.8	15	775	461	Philippines
...	...	...	33	21	...	...	44	28	Poland
...	...	...	47	26	...	...	57	34	Portugal
...	...	...	54	41	...	...	72	60	Qatar
...	...	2.7	54	108	...	...	184	146	Republic of Korea
41	52	...	147	160	345	533	254	249	Republic of Moldova
...	...	...	181	94	...	...	295	144	Romania
...	...	...	127	91	...	...	206	121	Russian Federation
198	68	5 714	325	86	2 761	1 806	417	114	Rwanda
...	...	...	0.0	4.3	...	...	7.3	5.1	Saint Kitts and Nevis
...	...	...	12	3.3	...	...	15	4.8	Saint Lucia
...	...	...	26	24	...	...	51	24	Saint Vincent and the Grenadines
...	...	...	23	18	...	...	34	30	Samoa

Member State	Age-standardized mortality rates by cause[a] (per 100 000 population)			Years of life lost[a] (per 100 000 population)				MDG 4 Number of deaths among children aged <5 years[a] (000s)		Mortality Distribution of causes of death among children aged <5 years[a,b] (%)							
	Communicable	Non-communicable	Injuries	All causes	Communicable	Non-communicable	Injuries			HIV		Diarrhoea		Measles		Malaria	
	2012			2012				2000	2012	2000	2012	2000	2012	2000	2012	2000	2012
San Marino	...	...	...	...	...	...	...	0	0	...	...	...	...	...	...	...	...
Sao Tome and Principe	...	...	...	...	...	...	...	0	0	2	1	14	9	0	1	9	8
Saudi Arabia	71	549	41	10 140	1 841	6 721	1 577	13	5	0	0	3	1	0	0	0	0
Senegal	588	558	89	39 510	26 368	9 505	3 637	53	30	0	1	11	7	5	1	24	17
Serbia	20	657	32	25 600	895	23 163	1 543	1	1	0	0	1	0	0	0	0	0
Seychelles	...	...	...	...	...	...	...	0	0	...	...	...	...	...	...	...	...
Sierra Leone	1 327	964	150	113 198	82 802	21 114	9 282	43	39	0	0	13	14	12	6	25	14
Singapore	68	264	17	9 884	1 527	7 562	794	0	0	0	0	0	1	0	0	0	0
Slovakia	35	533	39	21 026	1 313	17 777	1 936	1	0	0	0	1	0	0	0	0	0
Slovenia	15	369	44	17 324	589	14 708	2 027	0	0	0	0	0	0	0	0	0	0
Solomon Islands	231	710	75	24 215	9 927	11 096	3 192	0	1	0	0	7	8	0	0	16	2
Somalia	927	551	188	94 542	71 921	11 605	11 017	66	66	0	0	14	12	23	13	2	2
South Africa	612	711	104	50 128	30 989	14 121	5 017	74	49	36	17	9	7	1	1	0	0
South Sudan	827	623	143	70 179	50 404	12 108	7 667	49	40	2	3	18	11	3	2	7	6
Spain	19	323	18	14 511	823	12 838	851	2	2	0	0	0	0	0	0	0	0
Sri Lanka	75	501	89	18 190	2 592	11 909	3 689	6	4	0	0	5	2	0	0	2	0
Sudan	496	551	134	46 269	29 142	10 558	6 569	112	92	0	1	15	11	6	4	3	2
Suriname	89	372	68	16 418	4 516	8 530	3 373	0	0	1	5	6	1	0	0	8	0
Swaziland	884	702	119	66 341	48 011	11 412	6 918	4	3	35	15	10	9	0	0	0	0
Sweden	19	333	26	15 323	792	13 327	1 204	0	0	0	0	0	0	0	0	0	0
Switzerland	14	292	25	13 079	609	11 297	1 173	0	0	0	0	0	0	0	0	0	0
Syrian Arab Republic	41	573	308	28 718	2 807	7 685	18 227	12	8	0	0	10	9	0	0	0	0
Tajikistan	148	753	52	29 749	14 692	11 930	3 128	17	15	0	0	16	11	0	0	0	0
Thailand	123	449	73	20 794	4 570	12 846	3 379	21	9	2	1	6	3	0	1	0	0
The former Yugoslav Republic of Macedonia	17	637	24	20 504	823	18 585	1 096	0	0	0	0	9	0	0	0	0	0
Timor-Leste	344	671	69	34 299	21 132	9 304	3 862	4	2	0	0	15	9	0	0	13	4
Togo	682	679	93	61 629	43 673	12 507	5 449	22	22	4	1	10	9	6	1	24	18
Tonga	...	...	...	...	...	...	...	0	0	0	0	4	2	0	0	0	0
Trinidad and Tobago	80	705	98	27 577	3 611	18 921	5 045	1	0	3	1	1	0	0	0	0	0
Tunisia	65	509	39	15 707	2 762	11 153	1 792	5	3	0	0	6	3	0	0	0	0
Turkey	44	555	39	17 160	2 361	12 651	2 148	52	18	0	0	3	1	0	0	0	0
Turkmenistan	116	1 025	93	36 555	8 879	22 123	5 552	7	6	0	0	15	9	0	0	0	0
Tuvalu	...	...	...	...	...	...	...	0	0	...	...	...	...	...	...	...	...
Uganda	697	664	167	60 022	41 005	10 918	8 098	167	103	7	7	12	9	8	0	18	13
Ukraine	69	749	67	35 801	3 734	28 498	3 569	8	6	2	1	3	2	0	0	0	0
United Arab Emirates	36	547	32	5 551	918	3 086	1 546	1	1	0	0	1	1	0	0	0	0
United Kingdom	29	359	21	16 092	1 187	13 889	1 016	5	4	0	0	1	0	0	0	0	0
United Republic of Tanzania	584	570	129	48 220	32 565	9 699	5 956	177	98	10	6	12	8	2	0	19	10
United States of America	31	413	44	17 754	1 337	14 258	2 159	32	29	0	0	2	2	0	0	0	0
Uruguay	46	446	54	19 426	1 972	14 879	2 575	1	0	0	0	3	1	0	0	0	0
Uzbekistan	86	811	47	24 124	6 840	14 571	2 713	34	25	0	0	15	9	0	0	0	0
Vanuatu	...	...	...	...	...	...	...	0	0	0	0	7	6	0	0	9	2
Venezuela (Bolivarian Republic of)	63	408	100	17 784	3 209	8 639	5 936	12	9	0	0	11	5	0	0	0	0
Viet Nam	96	435	59	17 798	4 475	10 594	2 730	39	33	0	1	14	7	8	2	0	0
Yemen	515	627	84	36 832	21 708	10 259	4 865	67	43	0	0	16	10	5	1	1	1
Zambia	764	587	156	66 252	49 853	9 379	7 020	76	50	14	6	12	9	5	1	19	16
Zimbabwe	711	599	82	57 699	42 568	9 782	5 349	39	39	45	9	6	9	0	1	2	1

Mortality

Distribution of causes of death among children aged <5 years[a,b] (%)

Member State

Acute respiratory infections		Prematurity		Intrapartum-related complications		Neonatal sepsis		Congenital anomalies		Other diseases		Injuries		Member State
2000	2012	2000	2012	2000	2012	2000	2012	2000	2012	2000	2012	2000	2012	
...	...	...	...	...	...	...	...	...	...	...	...	...	...	San Marino
19	16	14	13	10	13	6	7	5	10	17	16	5	7	Sao Tome and Principe
11	5	25	31	12	12	4	3	22	27	13	15	9	6	Saudi Arabia
13	13	12	15	8	13	5	8	3	7	14	13	3	5	Senegal
5	6	30	39	16	11	5	2	27	22	11	15	5	4	Serbia
...	...	...	...	...	...	...	...	...	...	...	...	...	...	Seychelles
13	17	9	9	6	9	3	5	2	4	15	18	3	4	Sierra Leone
8	8	21	26	4	7	2	1	34	25	25	25	6	6	Singapore
12	8	30	32	5	6	1	1	28	31	17	14	5	6	Slovakia
0	1	28	49	8	4	5	6	39	12	13	22	7	5	Slovenia
14	17	14	14	12	13	7	7	10	12	13	18	6	9	Solomon Islands
15	19	10	10	7	11	3	4	2	3	18	21	4	5	Somalia
12	16	11	14	7	10	3	4	4	6	14	18	4	7	South Africa
19	20	11	14	7	10	3	6	2	4	21	19	4	5	South Sudan
2	2	22	21	8	10	5	7	35	31	22	25	6	4	Spain
11	6	22	25	8	9	5	4	26	29	17	20	5	4	Sri Lanka
19	18	14	14	10	12	6	8	3	6	19	18	5	7	Sudan
8	8	20	26	7	10	14	9	12	16	16	18	8	6	Suriname
13	15	10	14	10	12	5	7	3	6	12	16	3	6	Swaziland
2	4	16	14	9	10	4	5	45	30	20	34	4	4	Sweden
2	1	25	34	8	11	3	4	31	30	23	16	9	4	Switzerland
14	9	23	25	12	11	3	6	20	17	14	14	5	10	Syrian Arab Republic
22	19	13	14	10	13	6	7	5	8	21	19	7	8	Tajikistan
13	8	22	24	7	8	6	5	21	29	18	17	5	5	Thailand
8	4	36	62	11	8	2	2	17	12	15	10	3	1	The former Yugoslav Republic of Macedonia
18	21	10	11	10	15	5	8	2	5	21	20	6	7	Timor-Leste
12	15	12	12	9	12	5	7	3	5	12	15	3	5	Togo
11	9	22	24	7	8	6	5	24	26	17	17	10	8	Tonga
3	8	38	28	27	9	3	4	12	26	10	17	2	7	Trinidad and Tobago
15	9	20	25	10	12	4	5	18	24	21	18	6	6	Tunisia
16	8	23	26	10	9	2	5	15	25	24	20	5	5	Turkey
21	17	15	17	11	12	5	6	7	11	20	19	7	8	Turkmenistan
...	...	...	...	...	...	...	...	...	...	...	...	...	...	Tuvalu
14	15	9	12	7	11	4	6	2	5	15	16	4	6	Uganda
16	10	18	22	6	7	3	3	26	26	16	20	10	9	Ukraine
5	4	30	30	11	10	3	2	27	30	15	16	9	8	United Arab Emirates
4	4	34	40	6	7	3	1	24	27	23	19	5	3	United Kingdom
14	15	8	11	10	14	5	8	2	7	14	15	3	6	United Republic of Tanzania
3	3	27	28	5	5	3	2	25	25	23	23	11	12	United States of America
9	12	22	18	7	4	7	11	26	27	19	20	7	6	Uruguay
22	19	13	14	9	11	4	4	9	13	21	19	8	10	Uzbekistan
13	11	19	23	9	10	5	4	17	19	14	21	5	4	Vanuatu
8	10	24	25	9	9	9	9	15	22	17	9	7	11	Venezuela (Bolivarian Republic of)
15	13	19	21	7	7	3	5	16	22	15	18	2	4	Viet Nam
20	19	13	15	9	13	6	8	3	5	21	19	6	7	Yemen
13	15	7	11	8	12	4	6	2	4	14	15	3	5	Zambia
9	15	10	17	9	14	5	8	3	6	8	15	2	5	Zimbabwe

Member State	Mortality							
	MDG 5			MDG 6				
	Maternal mortality ratio[c] (per 100 000 live births)			Cause-specific mortality rate (per 100 000 population)				
				HIV/AIDS[d]		Malaria[e]	Tuberculosis among HIV-negative people[f]	
	1990	2000	2013	2001	2012	2012	2000	2012
San Marino	...	...	...	...	...	...	0.0	0.0
Sao Tome and Principe	410	300	210	<71	<53	43	13	16
Saudi Arabia	41	24	16	...	...	0.0	3.9	3.9
Senegal	530	480	320	13	14	59	26	20
Serbia	18	7	16	...	...	...	...	1.5
Seychelles	...	...	...	...	...	...	2.0	1.8
Sierra Leone	2 300	2 200	1 100	25	55	108	59	143
Singapore	8	19	6	...	...	...	3.2	1.7
Slovakia	15	12	7	0.1 [a]	0.0 [a]	...	1.0	0.6
Slovenia	11	12	7	0.4 [a]	0.1 [a]	...	0.9	1.0
Solomon Islands	320	210	130	...	...	5.4	42	15
Somalia	1 300	1 200	850	26	25	29	68	64
South Africa	150	150	140	438	449	0.1	44	59
South Sudan	1 800	1 200	730	100	119	56	...	30
Spain	7	5	4	...	...	...	1.0	0.6
Sri Lanka	49	55	29	<1	<1	0.0	10	1.1
Sudan	720	540	360	...	...	15	27	22
Suriname	84	120	130	<106	<37	0.1	1.2	2.6
Swaziland	550	520	310	713	443	0.2	34	63
Sweden	6	5	4	0.4 [a]	0.2 [a]	...	0.2	0.1
Switzerland	8	7	6	1.8 [a]	0.5 [a]	...	0.5	0.2
Syrian Arab Republic	130	75	49	...	...	...	3.4	2.1
Tajikistan	68	89	44	<2	<12	0.0	20	7.6
Thailand	42	40	26	97	31	0.3	31	14
The former Yugoslav Republic of Macedonia	15	15	7	0.0 [a]	0.0 [a]	...	10	0.8
Timor-Leste	1 200	680	270	...	...	14	...	74
Togo	660	580	450	158	108	83	12	8.7
Tonga	71	91	120	...	...	...	3.6	2.5
Trinidad and Tobago	89	59	84	41 [a]	16 [a]	...	1.9	2.1
Tunisia	91	65	46	<1	<1	...	2.7	2.9
Turkey	48	33	20	...	...	0.0	3.2	0.5
Turkmenistan	66	81	61	...	...	...	28	8.4
Tuvalu	...	...	...	...	...	...	68	37
Uganda	780	650	360	424	174	55	35	13
Ukraine	49	35	23	18 [a]	46 [a]	...	23	13
United Arab Emirates	16	11	8	...	...	...	1.0	0.1
United Kingdom	10	11	8	...	...	...	0.7	0.5
United Republic of Tanzania	910	770	410	339	167	44	17	13
United States of America	12	13	28	5.2 [a]	2.5 [a]	...	0.3	0.1
Uruguay	42	35	14	5.1 [a]	6.3 [a]	...	2.1	1.5
Uzbekistan	66	48	36	7.0	8.6	0.0	17	2.1
Vanuatu	170	120	86	...	...	3.6	16	7.9
Venezuela (Bolivarian Republic of)	93	91	110	28	13	0.2	2.7	2.4
Viet Nam	140	82	49	6.7	13	0.1	33	20
Yemen	460	370	270	<3	<4	5.3	19	5.6
Zambia	580	610	280	745	215	78	31	28
Zimbabwe	520	680	470	1 252	288	9.1	17	33

Morbidity   Member State

MDG 6									
Incidence rate (per 100 000 population)					Prevalence (per 100 000 population)				
HIV/AIDS[d]		Malaria[e]	Tuberculosis[g]		HIV/AIDS[d]		Tuberculosis[g]		
2001	2012	2012	2000	2012	2001	2012	2000	2012	Member State
...	...	...	4.3	1.5	...	...	8.5	2.0	San Marino
<353	<53	12 375	114	93	<705	731	159	159	Sao Tome and Principe
...	...	0.3	20	15	...	...	26	17	Saudi Arabia
47	14	27 925	155	137	264	312	273	219	Senegal
...	...	...	...	23	...	...	...	31	Serbia
...	...	...	37	30	...	...	57	39	Seychelles
141	51	19 027	264	674	618	965	537	1 304	Sierra Leone
...	...	...	51	50	...	...	68	73	Singapore
...	...	...	22	6.8	...	...	28	9.5	Slovakia
...	...	...	21	7.5	...	...	28	9.0	Slovenia
...	...	7 160	185	97	...	...	364	151	Solomon Islands
...	...	6 395	285	286	376	306	604	581	Somalia
1 399	700	33	576	1 003	9 512	11 589	568	857	South Africa
...	...	29 891	...	146	1 777	1 419	...	257	South Sudan
...	...	...	23	14	...	...	30	17	Spain
<3	<2	0.4	66	66	10	14	115	109	Sri Lanka
...	...	13 535	144	114	...	...	262	207	Sudan
<106	<94	79	86	41	732	740	128	58	Suriname
1 618	966	43	803	1 349	13 614	17 291	573	907	Swaziland
...	...	...	5.4	7.2	...	...	7.5	9.6	Sweden
...	...	...	9.3	6.0	...	...	12	7.1	Switzerland
...	...	...	35	18	...	...	43	24	Syrian Arab Republic
<16	27	0.3	220	108	22	149	493	160	Tajikistan
38	13	205	171	119	1 050	663	286	159	Thailand
...	...	...	41	18	...	...	61	26	The former Yugoslav Republic of Macedonia
...	...	8 320	...	498	...	...	...	758	Timor-Leste
353	73	23 543	72	73	2 635	1 929	114	104	Togo
...	...	...	28	14	...	...	39	26	Tonga
106	<75	...	18	24	815	1 070	23	28	Trinidad and Tobago
...	...	...	25	31	<5	21	35	41	Tunisia
...	...	0.0	33	22	...	...	45	23	Turkey
...	...	...	209	75	...	...	400	99	Turkmenistan
...	...	...	357	241	...	...	626	377	Tuvalu
374	380	24 597	427	179	4 094	4 262	380	175	Uganda
71	24	...	108	93	475	506	164	137	Ukraine
...	...	...	12	1.7	...	...	22	2.4	United Arab Emirates
...	...	...	12	15	...	...	16	20	United Kingdom
381	174	17 318	236	165	4 340	3 082	234	176	United Republic of Tanzania
...	...	...	6.6	3.6	...	...	8.6	4.7	United States of America
...	...	...	22	27	253	389	29	34	Uruguay
...	...	0.0	287	78	147	104	647	135	Uzbekistan
...	...	3 742	110	65	...	...	166	89	Vanuatu
...	...	288	34	33	339	360	50	52	Venezuela (Bolivarian Republic of)
37	15	29	197	147	195	285	353	218	Viet Nam
...	...	1 812	116	49	23	79	198	70	Yemen
984	396	26 087	713	427	9 082	7 861	524	388	Zambia
1 063	501	7 844	726	562	14 679	9 969	389	433	Zimbabwe

	Age-standardized mortality rates by cause[a] (per 100 000 population)			Years of life lost[a] (per 100 000 population)				MDG 4 — Number of deaths among children aged <5 years[a] (000s)		Mortality — Distribution of causes of death among children aged <5 years[a,b] (%)							
	Communicable	Non-communicable	Injuries	All causes	Communicable	Non-communicable	Injuries			HIV		Diarrhoea		Measles		Malaria	
	2012			2012				2000	2012	2000	2012	2000	2012	2000	2012	2000	201
Ranges of country values																	
Minimum	9	244	17	5 551	413	3 086	794	0	0	0	0	0	0	0	0	0	0
Median	83	570	65	23 080	4 427	12 108	3 339	4	3	0	0	7	4	0	0	0	0
Maximum	1 327	1 025	308	113 198	82 802	28 498	18 227	2 417	1 407	46	19	19	15	24	16	29	27
WHO region																	
African Region	683	652	116	63 153	44 628	12 045	6 480	4 014	3 070	5	3	13	10	8	1	18	15
Region of the Americas	63	437	62	18 202	2 955	12 048	3 198	417	237	1	0	8	4	0	0	0	0
South-East Asia Region	232	656	99	29 553	11 937	13 451	4 165	3 156	1 787	0	0	14	10	4	2	0	1
European Region	45	496	49	22 738	2 191	18 126	2 421	228	136	0	0	7	4	0	0	0	0
Eastern Mediterranean Region	214	654	91	30 396	14 426	11 173	4 796	1 180	905	0	0	14	10	4	2	1	1
Western Pacific Region	56	499	50	17 716	2 518	12 929	2 268	847	415	0	0	8	5	1	0	0	0
Income group																	
Low income	502	625	104	49 141	32 289	11 333	5 520	3 135	2 170	4	2	14	10	6	2	12	10
Lower middle income	272	673	99	34 806	16 641	13 554	4 611	5 204	3 533	1	1	13	10	6	1	7	7
Upper middle income	75	558	59	19 610	3 778	13 004	2 829	1 375	756	2	2	8	6	1	0	2	3
High income	34	397	44	18 559	1 474	14 943	2 142	129	90	1	0	2	1	0	0	0	0
Global	178	539	73	28 311	11 315	13 343	3 654	9 848	6 554	2	2	13	9	5	2	8	7

Mortality

Distribution of causes of death among children aged <5 years[a,b]
(%)

Acute respiratory infections		Prematurity		Intrapartum-related complications		Neonatal sepsis		Congenital anomalies		Other diseases		Injuries		
2000	2012	2000	2012	2000	2012	2000	2012	2000	2012	2000	2012	2000	2012	
0	0	4	0	3	0	0	0	2	3	6	9	2	1	Minimum
13	12	18	19	9	10	4	6	13	19	18	18	6	6	Median
30	32	43	62	29	40	14	11	45	45	32	50	23	20	Maximum
14	16	9	12	8	11	4	6	2	4	15	17	3	5	African Region
13	11	21	21	9	9	6	6	15	21	20	20	7	7	Region of the Americas
18	14	16	26	12	11	8	8	5	7	17	16	5	5	South-East Asia Region
16	12	20	21	9	10	4	5	17	21	20	19	7	8	European Region
18	17	14	18	12	12	7	8[c]	5	7	19	18	5	7	Eastern Mediterranean Region
26	15	14	17	16	14	4	4	7	13	12	21	11	11	Western Pacific Region
16	16	10	13	9	11	5	6	2	5	17	17	4	6	Low income
17	15	14	20	11	11	6	7	5	6	16	16	4	5	Lower middle income
21	13	16	17	13	12	4	5	9	14	15	20	9	9	Upper middle income
7	4	24	26	7	7	4	3	27	29	19	21	9	9	High income
17	15	13	17	11	11	6	7	5	7	16	17	5	6	Global

	Mortality							
	MDG 5 Maternal mortality ratio[c] (per 100 000 live births)			MDG 6 Cause-specific mortality rate (per 100 000 population)				
				HIV/AIDS[d]		Malaria[e]	Tuberculosis among HIV-negative people[f]	
	1990	2000	2013	2001	2012	2012	2000	2012
Ranges of country values								
Minimum	6	4	1	0.0	0.0	0.0	0.0	0.0
Median	98	82	68	23	17	3.7	7.3	4.1
Maximum	2 300	2 200	1 100	1 252	755	136	143	143
WHO region								
African Region	960	820	500	221	377	63	38	26
Region of the Americas	110	81	68	15	20	0.1	3.5	1.9
South-East Asia Region	520	340	190	13	22	2.3	43	25
European Region	42	29	17	5.1	20	...	8.1	3.9
Eastern Mediterranean Region	340	300	170	2.0	5.5	4.1	29	16
Western Pacific Region	110	78	45	2.1	6.8	0.2	12	5.8
Income group								
Low income	900	740	450	141	178	36	49	32
Lower middle income	500	380	240	25	54	13	38	21
Upper middle income	120	93	57	19	42	1.0	9.4	5.1
High income	24	18	17	4.8	15	...	3.7	2.3
Global	380	330	210	32	56	11	22	13

a. Mortality Data [online database]. Geneva: World Health Organization; 2014 (http://www.who.int/gho/mortality_burden_disease/life_tables/en/index.html). The column in Table 2 labelled "Communicable" shows the rates for communicable diseases, maternal causes, conditions arising during the neonatal period and nutritional deficiencies. Rates are age-standardized to WHO's world standard population. Ahmad OB, Boschi-Pinto C, Lopez AD, Murray CJL, Lozano R, Inoue M. Age standardization of rates: a new WHO standard. Geneva: World Health Organization; 2001 (GPE Discussion Paper Series No. 31) (http://www.who.int/healthinfo/paper31.pdf, accessed 14 March 2014). WHO regional, income-group and global aggregates include country figures not shown. For regional groupings refer to WHO methods and data sources for global causes of death 2000-2012 (Global Health Estimates Technical Paper WHO/HIS/HSI/GHE/2014.7).

b. Individual percentages may not add up to 100% due to rounding.

c. WHO, UNICEF, UNFPA, United Nations Population Division and The World Bank. Trends in Maternal Mortality: 1990–2013. Geneva: World Health Organization; 2014. In preparation at the time of printing of this report. See report for the regional groupings used.

d. Global Report. UNAIDS report on the global AIDS epidemic 2013. Geneva: UNAIDS; 2013 (http://www.unaids.org/en/media/unaids/contentassets/documents/epidemiology/2013/gr2013/UNAIDS_Global_Report_2013_en.pdf, accessed 14 March 2014). WHO regional, income-group and global aggregates may include country estimates not available for reporting. For uncertainty ranges see the report.

e. World Malaria Report 2013. Geneva: World Health Organization; 2013 (http://www.who.int/malaria/publications/world_malaria_report_2013/en/).

f. These are classified as deaths from tuberculosis (A15–A19, B90) according to the International Statistical Classification of Diseases and Related Health Problems, 10th Revision. Geneva: World Health Organization; 2008 (http://apps.who.int/classifications/icd10/browse/2010/en/). Global Tuberculosis Report 2013. Geneva: World Health Organization; 2013 (http://www.who.int/tb/publications/global_report/). WHO regional, income-group and global aggregates include territories. For uncertainty ranges see the full report.

g. Data are for all forms of tuberculosis including tuberculosis in people with HIV infection. Global Tuberculosis Report 2013. Geneva: World Health Organization; 2013 (http://www.who.int/tb/publications/global_report/). WHO regional, income-group and global aggregates include territories. For uncertainty ranges see the full report.

Table 2

Morbidity

MDG 6									
Incidence rate (per 100 000 population)					Prevalence (per 100 000 population)				
HIV/AIDS[d]		Malaria[e]	Tuberculosis[g]		HIV/AIDS[d]		Tuberculosis[g]		
2001	2012	2012	2000	2012	2001	2012	2000	2012	
<1	<1	0	0	2	0.1	5.2	2	2	Minimum
106	46	1 698	72	54	453	438	123	82	Median
1 759	1 284	38 333	1 407	1 349	16 694	17 482	1 693	1 304	Maximum
377	176	18 579	310	255	3 203	2 774	397	303	African Region
20	15	139	41	29	303	315	60	40	Region of the Americas
22	12	1 462	220	187	213	185	449	264	South-East Asia Region
20	18	...	73	40	170	244	129	56	European Region
5.5	9.9	3 083	118	109	36	68	256	180	Eastern Mediterranean Region
6.8	5.9	84	119	87	43	75	210	128	Western Pacific Region
178	89	11 165	309	246	1 788	1 428	485	352	Low income
54	29	4 648	205	165	411	411	416	237	Lower middle income
42	26	215	109	86	340	416	166	107	Upper middle income
15	16	...	32	23	190	265	52	31	High income
56	33	3 752	148	122	494	511	263	169	Global

3. Selected infectious diseases

Table 3 has been compiled from official national reports of case numbers for selected infectious diseases. Decisions on which diseases to include have primarily been made on the basis of data availability. Where possible, a distinction is made between zero cases reported and no information available for a country. In isolation, the numbers shown provide no indication of the relative risk of disease, nor of the quality of disease reporting in different countries. However, the table does provide an indication of the current status of officially reported infectious disease data at the global level, and of the major reporting gaps. Given the variations in the methods used by countries to obtain these numbers, no attempt has been made to calculate incidence or prevalence.

To meaningfully interpret the figures provided, both epidemiological patterns and data-collection efforts in specific countries must be considered. Some diseases (for example, malaria and yellow fever) are endemic to certain geographical regions, but are extremely rare elsewhere. Diseases such as cholera are liable to cause outbreaks that can cause case numbers to fluctuate widely over time. Because some diseases are best tackled with preventive measures such as mass drug treatment, reporting the number of cases is a lower priority than estimating the population at risk. For vaccine-preventable diseases, case numbers are affected by immunization rates. Diseases such as Japanese encephalitis and malaria are difficult to identify without specialized laboratory tests that are often not available in developing countries. In many settings, cases of some diseases are identified through clinical signs and symptoms alone.

Despite ongoing efforts to enhance disease surveillance and response, many countries face challenges in accurately identifying, diagnosing and reporting infectious diseases due to the remoteness of communities, lack of transport and communication infrastructures, and a shortage of skilled health care workers and laboratory facilities to ensure accurate diagnosis. No inferences can be drawn from the figures shown concerning the efforts or progress that countries are making in controlling particular diseases. Case numbers are also a poor indication of the burden of disease. Diseases such as poliomyelitis and leprosy have low mortality rates but result in a heavy loss of healthy years of life. Some diseases with very small initial case numbers can potentially cause devastating epidemics, and so mandatory reporting is essential. For diseases that are considered eradicable, such as poliomyelitis, case reporting is essential to ensure that eradication efforts are targeted to the affected areas.

Some diseases are reported under the International Health Regulations, while others are monitored by countries or by WHO in the context of specific control programmes. Further information on disease incidence and prevalence, as well as on immunization coverage rates for vaccine-preventable diseases, can be obtained from the relevant WHO programme.

Member State	Number of reported cases								
	Cholera[a]	Diphtheria[b]	Human African trypanosomiasis[c]	Japanese encephalitis[b]	Leishmaniasis[c]	Leprosy[d]	Malaria[e]	Measles[b]	Meningitis[f]
	2012	2012	2012	2012	2012	2012	2012	2012	2013
Afghanistan	12	0	…	…	33 918	37	391 365	2 787	…
Albania	…	0	…	0	…	…	…	9	…
Algeria	…	0	…	0	9 127	…	887	18	…
Andorra	…	0	…	…	…	…	…	0	…
Angola	1 215	15	70	…	…	431	1 496 834	4 458	…
Antigua and Barbuda	…	0	…	…	…	0	…	0	…
Argentina	…	0	…	…	7	310	4	2	…
Armenia	…	0	…	…	…	…	…	0	…
Australia	5 [j]	0	…	1	…	4	…	199	…
Austria	…	0	…	0	…	…	…	36	…
Azerbaijan	…	0	…	0	…	…	4	0	…
Bahamas	1 [j]	0	…	…	…	…	…	0	…
Bahrain	…	0	…	0	…	…	…	0	…
Bangladesh	…	16	…	52	1 902	3 688	29 518	1 986	…
Barbados	…	0	…	…	…	…	…	0	…
Belarus	…	0	…	0	…	…	…	10	…
Belgium	…	1	…	0	…	…	…	109	…
Belize	…	0	…	…	…	0	37	0	…
Benin	625	0	0	…	…	243	1 151 038	288	833
Bhutan	…	0	…	27	…	18	82	1	…
Bolivia (Plurinational State of)	…	0	…	…	…	…	7 415	0	…
Bosnia and Herzegovina	…	0	…	…	…	…	…	22	…
Botswana	…	0	…	…	…	1	308	7	…
Brazil	…	0	…	…	26 911	33 303	242 758	2	…
Brunei Darussalam	…	0	…	0	…	2	…	1	…
Bulgaria	…	0	…	0	2	…	…	1	…
Burkina Faso	143	0	0	…	…	313	6 089 101	7 362	2 917
Burundi	214	…	…	…	…	…	2 151 076	49	…
Cabo Verde	…	0	…	0	…	…	8 751	0	…
Cambodia	…	…	…	55	…	475	45 553	15	…
Cameroon	363	…	7	…	…	502	313 315	609	1 010
Canada	…	1	…	…	…	…	…	10	…
Central African Republic	21	0	381	…	…	152	451 012	141	210 [k]
Chad	…	…	197	…	…	…	590 786	120	371
Chile	…	0	…	…	…	…	…	0	…
China	77 [l]	0	…	1 763	218	1 210	2 718	6 183	…
Colombia	…	0	…	…	9 766	392	60 179	1	…
Comoros	…	…	…	…	…	…	49 840	1	…
Congo	1 181	1	39	0	…	…	117 640	260	…
Cook Islands	…	0	…	0	…	…	…	0	…
Costa Rica	…	0	…	…	1 722	6	8	0	…
Côte d'Ivoire	424	…	9	…	0	1 030	2 168 215	137	255
Croatia	…	0	…	0	…	…	…	2	…
Cuba	417	0	…	…	…	258	…	0	…
Cyprus	…	0	…	…	…	…	…	1	…
Czech Republic	…	0	…	0	…	…	…	22	…
Democratic People's Republic of Korea	…	0	…	0	…	0	21 850	0	…
Democratic Republic of the Congo	33 661	…	5 983	…	…	3 607	6 263 607	72 029	9 339 [m]
Denmark	…	0	…	…	…	…	…	2	…

Mumps[b]	Pertussis[b]	Poliomyelitis[g]	Congenital rubella syndrome[b]	Rubella[b]	Neonatal tetanus[b]	Total tetanus[b]	Tuberculosis[h]	Yellow fever[b]	Member State
2012	2012	2013	2012	2012	2012	2012	2012	2012	
...	1 497	17 i	...	...	21	37	29 381	...	Afghanistan
18	16	0	0	1	0	0	408	0	Albania
0	104	0	0	420	0	0	21 880	0	Algeria
1	3	0	0	0	0	0	9	0	Andorra
...	1 259	0	...	65	6	543	51 819	0	Angola
0	0	0	0	0	0	0	3	0	Antigua and Barbuda
4 619	1 239	0	0	1	0	10	8 758	0	Argentina
6	8	0	0	1	0	1	1 213	...	Armenia
195	23 855	0	1	35	0	7	1 305	0	Australia
...	571	0	...	23	...	0	620	0	Austria
126	18	0	0	0	0	7	6 363	0	Azerbaijan
0	0	0	0	0	0	0	32	0	Bahamas
29	3	0	0	4	0	0	225	0	Bahrain
...	13	0	...	3 245	109	614	168 683	...	Bangladesh
0	0	0	0	7	0	0	4	0	Barbados
61	576	0	0	10	0	0	4 783	0	Belarus
2 687	548	0	1	0	0	0	909	0	Belgium
2	44	0	0	0	0	0	84	0	Belize
...	0	0	0	41	4	7	3 966	0	Benin
198	0	0	0	2	0	0	1 130	0	Bhutan
0	0	0	0	0	0	0	8 257	3	Bolivia (Plurinational State of)
7 881	19	0	0	17	0	0	1 409	...	Bosnia and Herzegovina
...	0	0	...	163	0	0	6 161	...	Botswana
0	5 400	0	0	0	2	314	75 122	0	Brazil
14	3	0	0	1	0	0	243	0	Brunei Darussalam
58	102	0	0	18	0	2	2 081	0	Bulgaria
...	0	0	...	677	1	1	5 210	0	Burkina Faso
...	0	0	...	11	1	1	6 921	...	Burundi
40	0	0	0	18	0	2	420	0	Cabo Verde
17	54	0	32	185	15	15	40 185	0	Cambodia
...	...	8 i	...	147	23	23	24 802	31	Cameroon
54	4 845	0	0	2	...	4	1 653	3	Canada
...	124	0	...	11	65	74	8 084	0	Central African Republic
...	...	4 i	...	...	225	225	10 585	48	Chad
876	5 762	0	0	0	0	6	2 394	0	Chile
479 518	2 183	0	...	40 156	674	...	890 645	...	China
9 397	3 289	0	0	2	2	50	11 424	0	Colombia
...	...	0	...	0	...	...	120	...	Comoros
0	12	0	0	22	2	2	11 303	1	Congo
0	0	0	0	0	0	0	1	0	Cook Islands
30	130	0	0	0	0	1	475	0	Costa Rica
...	...	0	...	298	9	9	23 762	4	Côte d'Ivoire
95	61	0	0	1	0	1	...	0	Croatia
0	0	0	0	0	0	0	734	0	Cuba
3	16	0	0	0	0	0	63	0	Cyprus
3 902	738	0	1	6	0	0	565	0	Czech Republic
11	8	0	0	1	0	0	91 885	0	Democratic People's Republic of Korea
...	3 407	0	...	1 860	1 252	1 296	108 984	1	Democratic Republic of the Congo
15	980	0	0	0	0	0	...	...	Denmark

3. Selected infectious diseases

Member State	Cholera[a] 2012	Diphtheria[b] 2012	Human African trypanosomiasis[c] 2012	Japanese encephalitis[b] 2012	Leishmaniasis[c] 2012	Leprosy[d] 2012	Malaria[e] 2012	Measles[b] 2012	Meningitis[f] 2013
Djibouti	...	0	...	...	...	2	25	709	...
Dominica	...	0	...	...	...	0	...	0	...
Dominican Republic	7 919	0	...	...	...	124	952	0	...
Ecuador	...	0	...	...	...	86	558	72	...
Egypt	...	0	...	...	1 260	644	...	245	...
El Salvador	...	0	...	...	21	3	19	0	...
Equatorial Guinea	...	0	2	...	...	4	15 169	1 190	...
Eritrea	...	8	...	...	...	...	42 178	194	...
Estonia	...	0	...	0	...	...	...	4	...
Ethiopia	...	...	...	...	2 500	3 776	3 876 745	4 347	...
Fiji	...	...	...	...	...	3	...	0	...
Finland	...	...	...	...	...	...	...	...	...
France	...	...	...	...	...	...	...	...	...
Gabon	...	...	9	...	...	30	137 695	2	...
Gambia	...	0	...	0	...	33	271 038	0	248 [n]
Georgia	...	0	...	0	...	...	5	31	...
Germany	...	9	...	...	...	...	...	166	...
Ghana	9 548	0	0	...	...	...	8 774 516	1 613	454
Greece	...	0	...	0	51	...	...	3	...
Grenada	...	0	...	...	...	2	...	0	...
Guatemala	...	0	...	...	607	0	5 346	0	...
Guinea	7 350	0	70	...	...	438	1 220 574	6	480
Guinea-Bissau	3 068	0	...	0	...	...	50 381	0	...
Guyana	...	0	...	...	7	19	31 601	0	...
Haiti	112 076	0	...	...	...	...	25 423	0	...
Honduras	...	0	...	...	1 927	4	6 434	0	...
Hungary	...	0	...	...	...	...	...	2	...
Iceland	...	0	...	0	...	...	...	0	...
India	...	2 525	...	...	20 571	134 752	1 067 824	18 668	...
Indonesia	...	1 192	...	...	...	18 994	2 051 425	15 489	...
Iran (Islamic Republic of)	53	150	...	...	21 014	21	1 629	332	...
Iraq	4 693	3	...	...	3 531	1	8	15	...
Ireland	...	0	...	0	...	...	...	107	...
Israel	...	0	...	...	...	...	...	211	...
Italy	...	0	...	...	81	...	...	376	...
Jamaica	...	0	...	...	...	...	...	0	...
Japan	3 [j]	0	...	2	...	3	...	228	...
Jordan	...	0	...	...	103	0	...	3	...
Kazakhstan	...	0	...	0	...	...	...	55	...
Kenya	...	...	2	0	457	...	5 788 381	...	...
Kiribati	...	0	...	0	...	94	...	0	...
Kuwait	...	0	...	0	0	16	...	27	...
Kyrgyzstan	...	0	...	...	...	...	3	0	...
Lao People's Democratic Republic	...	130	...	23	...	88	46 819	32	...
Latvia	...	8	...	0	...	...	...	3	...
Lebanon	...	0	...	0	2	1	...	9	...
Lesotho	...	0	...	0	...	...	...	179	...
Liberia	219	0	...	0	...	...	1 407 455	43	...
Libya	...	...	...	0	...	4	...	320	...

Mumps[b] 2012	Pertussis[b] 2012	Poliomyelitis[g] 2013	Congenital rubella syndrome[b] 2012	Rubella[b] 2012	Neonatal tetanus[b] 2012	Total tetanus[b] 2012	Tuberculosis[h] 2012	Yellow fever[b] 2012	Member State
...	...	0	...	0	0	...	3 474	...	Djibouti
0	0	0	0	0	0	0	7	0	Dominica
0	11	0	0	0	1	40	4 262	0	Dominican Republic
799	54	0	0	0	1	1	5 456	1	Ecuador
...	0	0	...	35	6	...	8 453	...	Egypt
351	37	0	0	0	0	7	2 053	0	El Salvador
...	0	0	0	...	0	0	...	0	Equatorial Guinea
2 350	208	0	...	18	0	19	3 143	0	Eritrea
4	149	0	0	0	0	0	259	0	Estonia
...	...	9	...	795	40	...	145 323	0	Ethiopia
...	...	0	...	25	...	...	210	...	Fiji
...	...	0	...	...	...	...	261	...	Finland
...	...	0	...	...	...	...	...	...	France
...	...	0	...	2	2	2	4 929	0	Gabon
0	0	0	0	39	0	0	2 333	1	Gambia
50	346	0	0	75	0	6	3 940	0	Georgia
...	...	0	1	...	...	...	4 043	0	Germany
...	...	0	0	272	0	456	14 753	3	Ghana
2	56	0	0	0	0	7	...	0	Greece
2	0	0	0	0	0	0	1	0	Grenada
143	273	0	0	0	0	0	3 442	0	Guatemala
...	...	0	...	55	8	...	11 407	0	Guinea
0	0	0	0	23	0	0	1 939	0	Guinea-Bissau
0	0	0	0	0	0	0	748	0	Guyana
0	0	0	0	0	0	0	16 568	0	Haiti
138	48	0	0	0	2	17	3 014	0	Honduras
4	5	0	0	7	0	5	1 159	0	Hungary
0	36	0	0	2	0	0	10	0	Iceland
...	44 154	0	...	1 025	588	2 404	1 289 836	...	India
...	...	0	...	1 020	106	106	328 824	...	Indonesia
...	1 329	0	0	30	2	13	11 042	...	Iran (Islamic Republic of)
1 482	2 314	0	...	22	11	34	8 664	...	Iraq
170	458	0	0	10	0	1	341	0	Ireland
93	2 730	0	0	1	0	0	506	0	Israel
322	225	0	...	85	0	64	...	...	Italy
0	2	0	0	0	0	4	91	0	Jamaica
71 549	4 087	0	5	2 353	0	116	20 857	0	Japan
194	4	0	0	0	0	0	331	...	Jordan
67	43	0	0	13	0	1	18 006	0	Kazakhstan
0	...	14	0	...	2	2	92 987	0	Kenya
0	0	0	0	0	0	0	346	0	Kiribati
61	83	0	1	13	0	0	737	0	Kuwait
350	62	0	0	6	0	0	6 195	...	Kyrgyzstan
...	412	0	...	78	11	36	4 118	0	Lao People's Democratic Republic
41	257	0	0	8	0	0	959	0	Latvia
12	53	0	0	3	0	2	630	0	Lebanon
0	0	0	0	68	0	0	10 776	0	Lesotho
0	0	0	0	39	12	12	8 093	17	Liberia
111	197	0	...	1	0	0	1 549	0	Libya

Number of reported cases

Member State	Number of reported cases								
	Cholera[a]	Diphtheria[b]	Human African trypanosomiasis[c]	Japanese encephalitis[b]	Leishmaniasis[c]	Leprosy[d]	Malaria[e]	Measles[b]	Meningitis[f]
	2012	2012	2012	2012	2012	2012	2012	2012	2013
Lithuania	...	0	...	0	...	...	...	0	...
Luxembourg	...	0	...	...	...	...	...	2	...
Madagascar	...	1	...	...	...	1 474	359 420	2	...
Malawi	187	...	18	...	...	...	3 659 565	11	...
Malaysia	282 [o]	0	...	22	...	325	4 725	1 868	...
Maldives	...	0	...	0	...	7	...	0	...
Mali	219	...	0	...	...	228	2 171 739	341	358
Malta	...	...	...	...	...	...	...	...	...
Marshall Islands	...	0	...	0	...	137	...	0	...
Mauritania	...	0	...	...	...	...	165 834	35	14
Mauritius	...	0	...	0	...	...	...	0	...
Mexico	2	0	...	...	571	216	833	0	...
Micronesia (Federated States of)	...	...	...	...	...	252	...	0	...
Monaco	...	...	...	...	...	...	...	5	...
Mongolia	...	0	...	0	...	0	...	0	...
Montenegro	...	0	...	0	...	...	...	0	...
Morocco	...	0	...	...	2 990	38	...	...	...
Mozambique	647	...	...	...	...	758	1 813 984	145	...
Myanmar	174	19	...	14	...	3 013	480 586	2 175	...
Namibia	...	2	...	...	...	...	3 163	86	...
Nauru	...	...	...	...	...	2	...	11	...
Nepal	34	138	...	75	575	3 492	70 272	3 362	...
Netherlands	...	1	...	...	...	...	...	10	...
New Zealand	...	0	...	0	...	1	...	68	...
Nicaragua	...	0	...	...	1 884	8	1 235	0	...
Niger	5 284	0	...	0	...	464	3 525 112	272	311
Nigeria	597	...	2	...	0	3 805	2 087 068	6 447	871
Niue	...	0	...	0	...	...	...	0	...
Norway	...	0	...	0	...	...	...	4	...
Oman	...	0	...	0	3	7	...	13	...
Pakistan	144 [p]	98	...	...	6 598	377	4 285 449	8 046	...
Palau	...	0	...	0	...	2	...	0	...
Panama	...	0	...	...	1 811	3	844	0	...
Papua New Guinea	...	0	...	0	...	283	643 214	0	...
Paraguay	...	0	...	...	253	515	15	0	...
Peru	...	0	...	...	7 527	32	31 436	0	...
Philippines	1 864	...	...	...	...	2 150	7 133	1 536	...
Poland	...	0	...	0	...	...	...	71	...
Portugal	...	0	...	...	...	...	...	23	...
Qatar	...	0	...	0	...	24	...	160	...
Republic of Korea	...	0	...	20	...	5	555	2	...
Republic of Moldova	...	0	...	0	...	...	...	11	...
Romania	...	0	...	0	...	...	...	7 450	...
Russian Federation	1 [j]	5	...	...	...	...	...	2 123	...
Rwanda	9	0	...	...	...	41	483 470	75	...
Saint Kitts and Nevis	...	0	...	...	...	...	...	0	...
Saint Lucia	...	0	...	...	...	5	...	0	...
Saint Vincent and the Grenadines	...	0	...	...	...	0	...	0	...
Samoa	...	0	...	0	...	8	...	1	...

Number of reported cases									Member State
Mumps[b]	Pertussis[b]	Poliomyelitis[g]	Congenital rubella syndrome[b]	Rubella[b]	Neonatal tetanus[b]	Total tetanus[b]	Tuberculosis[h]	Yellow fever[b]	
2012	2012	2013	2012	2012	2012	2012	2012	2012	
62	154	0	0	0	0	2	1 635	0	Lithuania
0	10	0	0	1	...	0	45	0	Luxembourg
...	33	0	...	110	9	490	25 782	...	Madagascar
...	...	0	...	56	1	1	20 335	...	Malawi
...	217	0	1	789	9	34	21 851	...	Malaysia
14	0	0	0	0	0	0	110	0	Maldives
...	...	0	...	19	10	108	5 446	0	Mali
...	...	0	...	...	...	...	42	...	Malta
3	0	0	0	0	0	0	145	0	Marshall Islands
...	30	0	0	...	0	0	2 616	0	Mauritania
11	0	0	1	9	0	0	128	0	Mauritius
5 683	978	0	0	0	0	28	20 470	0	Mexico
...	...	0	...	...	...	...	144	...	Micronesia (Federated States of)
...	...	0	...	...	...	1	...	...	Monaco
9 060	0	0	0	240	0	0	4 128	0	Mongolia
104	2	0	...	0	0	0	98	0	Montenegro
...	...	0	...	...	...	...	28 635	...	Morocco
...	...	0	...	428	...	110	47 741	...	Mozambique
...	2	0	...	21	29	75	141 170	...	Myanmar
0	2	0	...	42	3	3	10 003	...	Namibia
...	...	0	...	...	...	...	...	...	Nauru
35 874	1 595	0	...	801	32	359	35 195	...	Nepal
398	13 552	0	0	1	0	1	920	0	Netherlands
26	5 598	0	0	4	0	2	293	0	New Zealand
4	68	0	0	0	0	1	2 790	0	Nicaragua
0	0	1 [i]	0	77	3	75	10 989	0	Niger
...	11 628	56 [i]	...	239	110	112	92 818	0	Nigeria
0	0	0	0	0	0	0	0	0	Niue
30	4 231	0	0	1	0	1	...	0	Norway
679	165	0	0	13	0	1	382	0	Oman
...	60	138 [i]	...	483	320	320	267 475	...	Pakistan
0	0	0	0	0	0	0	4	0	Palau
134	47	0	0	0	0	10	1 520	0	Panama
...	6 472	0	...	33	32	32	20 557	...	Papua New Guinea
247	44	0	0	0	1	5	2 416	0	Paraguay
...	1 173	0	0	0	0	17	29 760	9	Peru
...	0	0	...	100	131	...	216 627	...	Philippines
2 779	4 682	0	0	6 263	0	19	7 054	0	Poland
158	224	0	1	3	0	3	2 490	0	Portugal
382	0	0	1	20	0	0	728	0	Qatar
7 147	230	0	1	27	0	17	43 702	0	Republic of Korea
131	92	0	0	3	0	0	4 409	0	Republic of Moldova
163	82	0	55	20 812	0	7	16 036	0	Romania
394	7 220	0	0	1 003	0	21	105 753	...	Russian Federation
...	0	0	5	172	0	0	6 091	0	Rwanda
0	0	0	0	0	0	0	2	0	Saint Kitts and Nevis
0	0	0	0	0	0	0	11	0	Saint Lucia
0	0	0	0	0	0	0	30	0	Saint Vincent and the Grenadines
0	0	0	...	0	0	0	22	0	Samoa

Member State	Number of reported cases								
	Cholera[a]	Diphtheria[b]	Human African trypanosomiasis[c]	Japanese encephalitis[b]	Leishmaniasis[c]	Leprosy[d]	Malaria[e]	Measles[b]	Meningitis[f]
	2012	2012	2012	2012	2012	2012	2012	2012	2013
San Marino	...	0	...	0	...	...	...	1	...
Sao Tome and Principe	...	0	...	...	...	2	12 550	0	...
Saudi Arabia	...	0	...	...	1 472	4	3 406	294	...
Senegal	1	...	...	...	...	224	366 912	46	379
Serbia	...	0	...	...	...	...	...	0	...
Seychelles	...	0	...	0	...	...	...	0	...
Sierra Leone	23 124	...	...	...	...	236	1 537 322	678	...
Singapore	2[j]	0	...	0	...	15	...	42	...
Slovakia	...	0	...	0	...	...	...	0	...
Slovenia	...	0	...	0	...	...	...	2	...
Solomon Islands	...	0	...	0	...	13	57 296	0	...
Somalia	22 576	65	...	...	410	139	59 709	9 983	...
South Africa	...	...	...	...	...	15	6 846	32	...
South Sudan	...	...	317	...	5 012	1 801	1 125 039	1 952	259[q]
Spain	...	0	...	0	...	...	...	1 204	...
Sri Lanka	...	0	...	60	...	2 191	93	51	...
Sudan	...	18	...	...	3 165	727	964 698	8 523	1 110
Suriname	...	0	...	...	260	27	569	0	...
Swaziland	...	0	...	0	...	...	626	0	...
Sweden	...	2	...	0	...	...	...	30	...
Switzerland	...	...	...	...	...	...	...	61	...
Syrian Arab Republic	...	0	...	0	53 000	...	...	13	...
Tajikistan	...	0	...	...	...	...	33	16	...
Thailand	29	63	...	54	...	220	32 569	5 197	...
The former Yugoslav Republic of Macedonia	...	0	...	...	...	...	...	7	...
Timor-Leste	...	0	...	0	...	70	6 148	16	...
Togo	61	0	0	...	...	...	697 374	238	266
Tonga	...	0	...	0	...	...	...	0	...
Trinidad and Tobago	...	0	...	...	...	...	...	0	...
Tunisia	...	0	...	0	5 416	0	...	48	...
Turkey	...	...	...	...	...	...	376	...	...
Turkmenistan	...	1	...	...	...	...	...	0	...
Tuvalu	...	0	...	...	...	3	...	0	...
Uganda	6 326	...	91	...	87	264	10 338 093	2 027	...
Ukraine	...	5	...	...	...	...	...	12 746	...
United Arab Emirates	...	0	...	...	...	...	...	132	...
United Kingdom	17[j]	0	...	0	...	19	...	2 092	...
United Republic of Tanzania	286	0	4	0	...	2 528	2 441 750	1 668	...
United States of America	18[r]	1	...	...	...	168	...	55	...
Uruguay	...	0	...	...	...	5	...	0	...
Uzbekistan	...	...	...	...	...	...	1	...	...
Vanuatu	...	0	...	...	...	...	36 708	0	...
Venezuela (Bolivarian Republic of)	...	0	...	...	...	692	52 803	1	...
Viet Nam	...	12	...	183	...	296	43 717	578	...
Yemen	...	0	...	...	3 671	392	165 678	2 177	...
Zambia	198	0	6	0	...	...	4 695 400	896	...
Zimbabwe	23	0	9	0	...	...	276 963	0	...

Table 3

Mumps[b]	Pertussis[b]	Poliomyelitis[g]	Congenital rubella syndrome[b]	Rubella[b]	Neonatal tetanus[b]	Total tetanus[b]	Tuberculosis[h]	Yellow fever[b]	Member State
2012	2012	2013	2012	2012	2012	2012	2012	2012	
2	0	0	0	0	0	0	…	0	San Marino
…	0	0	…	…	0	0	115	0	Sao Tome and Principe
64	6	0	…	18	14	21	3 690	…	Saudi Arabia
…	…	0	…	44	14	118	12 265	1	Senegal
584	51	0	0	14	0	3	1 872	…	Serbia
0	0	0	0	0	0	0	20	0	Seychelles
…	…	0	…	…	23	…	13 074	94	Sierra Leone
521	24	0	2	64	0	0	2 301	0	Singapore
5	950	0	0	0	0	0	321	0	Slovakia
8	178	0	0	0	0	1	134	0	Slovenia
0	0	0	…	…	0	0	361	0	Solomon Islands
…	3 784	191 [i]	…	…	224	…	11 975	…	Somalia
…	…	0	…	2 298	1	1	323 664	…	South Africa
…	…	0	…	20	48	…	8 403	0	South Sudan
9 539	3 439	0	1	64	0	12	5 677	0	Spain
3 558	61	0	12	54	0	8	9 155	0	Sri Lanka
…	109	0	…	191	128	137	18 775	…	Sudan
0	1	0	0	0	0	1	128	0	Suriname
0	0	0	0	23	0	0	7 165	0	Swaziland
33	289	0	0	50	0	0	593	0	Sweden
…	…	0	0	10	…	…	416	…	Switzerland
52	4	23	0	1	1	13	3 003	0	Syrian Arab Republic
1 518	5	0	0	1	0	0	6 508	…	Tajikistan
7 431	14	0	2	493	4	105	60 304	0	Thailand
97	9	0	…	4	0	2	346	0	The former Yugoslav Republic of Macedonia
0	0	0	0	8	4	10	3 828	0	Timor-Leste
…	32	0	0	33	20	20	2 843	12	Togo
0	4	0	0	0	0	0	11	0	Tonga
0	0	0	0	0	0	0	274	0	Trinidad and Tobago
…	0	0	18	615	0	2	3 239	0	Tunisia
…	…	0	…	…	…	…	14 139	…	Turkey
…	0	0	0	0	…	0	…	…	Turkmenistan
0	0	0	0	0	0	0	19	…	Tuvalu
…	…	0	…	2 027	149	1 019	44 663	32	Uganda
799	2 286	0	…	1 952	…	23	40 990	…	Ukraine
377	61	0	…	30	0	3	79	…	United Arab Emirates
3 178	11 980	0	0	70	0	6	8 269	0	United Kingdom
…	0	0	…	55	0	…	62 178	0	United Republic of Tanzania
229	47 693	0	3	9	1	37	9 945	0	United States of America
113	598	0	0	0	0	0	808	0	Uruguay
2 300	62	0	…	…	…	…	14 832	…	Uzbekistan
…	…	0	…	…	…	…	125	…	Vanuatu
0	8	0	0	0	1	14	6 495	0	Venezuela (Bolivarian Republic of)
…	98	0	92	185	39	253	102 112	…	Viet Nam
5 081	4 699	0	…	199	80	115	9 867	0	Yemen
…	0	0	0	134	0	0	40 726	0	Zambia
0	0	0	63	20	6	6	35 760	0	Zimbabwe

Number of reported cases

	Cholera[a]	Diphtheria[b]	Human African trypanosomiasis[c]	Japanese encephalitis[b]	Leishmaniasis[c]	Leprosy[d]	Malaria[e]	Measles[b]	Meningitis[f]
	2012	2012	2012	2012	2012	2012	2012	2012	2013

Ranges of country values

Minimum	1	0	0	0	0	0	1	0	14
Median	217	0	9	0	1 767	41	46 819	10	375
Maximum	112 076	2 525	5 983	1 763	53 000	134 752	10 338 093	72 029	9 339

WHO region

African Region	94 994	...	6 899	...	...	20 599	77 079 733	106 052	...
Region of the Americas	...	2	...	...	53 274	36 178	468 469	143	...
South-East Asia Region	...	3 953	...	...	23 048	166 445	3 760 367	46 945	...
European Region	...	32	...	...	...	...	...	27 030	...
Eastern Mediterranean Region	27 478	334	...	...	141 565	4 235	6 997 006	35 788	...
Western Pacific Region	2 233	142	...	2 069	218	5 371	888 438	10 764	...

Income group

Low income	216 339	247	...	...	...	27 200	58 957 355	112 313	...
Lower middle income	...	3 981	...	...	95 954	167 501	28 139 207	79 095	...
Upper middle income	14 687	234	...	1 839	87 988	37 869	2 078 743	26 223	...
High income	47	28	...	...	...	...	...	9 091	...

Global

Global	...	4 490	...	...	230 410	232 847	89 194 435	226 722	...

a. Cholera, 2012. Weekly Epidemiological Record. 2013;88(31):321–36 (www.who.int/wer).

b. Data provided by Member States through WHO/UNICEF Joint Reporting Form and WHO regional offices. Geneva: World Health Organization; 2013 (www.who.int/immunization_monitoring/data/en/, October 2013 update).

c. Neglected tropical diseases on the Global Health Observatory [online database]. Geneva: World Health Organization (http://apps.who.int/gho/data/node.main.A1629).

d. Global leprosy: update on the 2012 situation. Weekly Epidemiological Record. 2013;88(35):365–80 (www.who.int/wer).

e. World Malaria Report 2013. Annex 6A Reported malaria cases and deaths, 2012, . Geneva: World Health Organization; 2013 (http://www.who.int/malaria/publications/world_malaria_report_2013/en/).

f. Suspected meningitis cases reported to WHO Global Alert and Response (GAR) in African countries under enhanced surveillance up to 29 December 2013.

g. Data from World Health Organization, Polio Eradication Initiative, as of 15 January 2014. (Updated information can be found at: http://www.who.int/immunization_monitoring_surveillance/data/en/). Confirmed polio cases refer to any circulating polioviruses from AFP (Wild poliovirus and circulating Vaccine Derived Poliovirus – cVDPV). Afghanistan, Nigeria and Pakistan are currently endemic countries. For non-endemic countries, cases are the result of importation.

h. The number of new and relapse tuberculosis cases diagnosed and treated in national tuberculosis control programmes and notified to WHO. Global Tuberculosis Report 2013. Geneva: World Health Organization; 2013 (www.who.int/tb/publications/global_report/). WHO regional and global figures include territories.

i. Figures include 3 cVDPV in Afghanistan; 4 cVDPV in Cameroon; 4 cVDPV in Chad; 1 cVDPV in Niger; 3 cVDPV in Nigeria; 45 cVDPV in Pakistan; 1 cVDPV in Somalia; 1 cVDPV in Yemen.

j. All cases are imported.

k. Number of cases reported up to 1 December 2013.

l. 2 of 77 reported cases are imported.

m. Number of cases reported up to 24 November 2013.

n. Number of cases reported up to 8 December 2013.

o. 81 of 282 reported cases are imported.

p. Laboratory-confirmed cases only.

q. Number of cases reported up to 13 October 2013.

r. 17 of 18 reported cases are imported.

Number of reported cases

Mumps[b]	Pertussis[b]	Poliomyelitis[g]	Congenital rubella syndrome[b]	Rubella[b]	Neonatal tetanus[b]	Total tetanus[b]	Tuberculosis[h]	Yellow fever[b]	
2012	2012	2013	2012	2012	2012	2012	2012	2012	
0	0	0	0	0	0	0	0	0	Minimum
32	36	0	0	9	0	1	3 690	0	Median
479 518	47 693	191	92	40 156	1 252	2 404	1 289 836	94	Maximum
...	16 839	92	...	10 830	2 001	4 737	1 344 122	245	African Region
22 821	71 744	0	3	21	11	567	219 349	16	Region of the Americas
...	45 847	0	...	6 670	872	3 681	2 130 120	...	South-East Asia Region
38 238	57 521	0	60	30 536	0	197	286 765	...	European Region
...	14 368	369	...	1 698	855	698	420 769	...	Eastern Mediterranean Region
568 050	43 237	0	...	44 275	911	...	1 375 713	...	Western Pacific Region
...	10 824	236	...	10 846	2 309	4 566	1 240 145	205	Low income
...	71 003	225	...	6 950	1 607	4 216	2 650 652	...	Lower middle income
518 605	20 979	0	...	66 032	719	...	1 648 886	...	Upper middle income
106 237	146 750	0	19	10 202	15	354	237 154	3	High income
687 120	249 556	461	...	94 030	4 650	10 392	5 776 838	...	Global

4. Health service coverage

Health service coverage indicators reflect the extent to which people in need actually receive important health interventions. Such interventions include: reproductive-health services; the provision of skilled care to women during pregnancy and childbirth; immunization to prevent common childhood infections; vitamin A supplementation in children; and the prevention and treatment of disease in children, adolescents and adults. Table 4 presents data on the following related MDG indicators: unmet need for family planning; contraceptive prevalence; antenatal care coverage; births attended by skilled health personnel; measles immunization coverage among 1-year-olds; children aged < 5 years sleeping under insecticide-treated nets; children aged < 5 years with fever who received treatment with any antimalarial; antiretroviral therapy coverage among people eligible for treatment; case-detection rate for all forms of tuberculosis; and treatment-success rate for smear-positive tuberculosis.

Data are also presented on births by caesarean section; postnatal care coverage; neonates protected at birth against neonatal tetanus; 1-year-olds immunized against diphtheria, tetanus and pertussis, hepatitis B and *Haemophilus influenzae* type B; children aged 6–59 months who received vitamin A supplementation; children aged < 5 years with acute respiratory infection (ARI) symptoms taken to a health facility; children aged < 5 years with suspected pneumonia receiving antibiotics; children aged < 5 years with diarrhoea receiving oral rehydration therapy (ORT); and coverage of antiretroviral therapy among pregnant women with HIV to prevent mother-to-child transmission (MTCT).

Coverage indicators are typically calculated by dividing the number of people receiving a defined intervention by the population eligible for – or in need of – the intervention. For example, immunization coverage among 1-year-old children can be calculated from the number of children having received a specific vaccine divided by the total population of 1-year-old children in each country. For indicators on antenatal care, births attended by skilled health personnel and births by caesarean section, the denominator is the total number of live births in the defined population.

The main sources of data on health service coverage are household surveys and completed questionnaires on health service use. The principal types of surveys used are the UNICEF Multiple Indicator Cluster Survey (MICS), the Demographic and Health Survey (DHS) and country health and economic surveys. Other sources of data include the administrative records of routine service provision, which provide data on the numerator. The denominator is estimated on the basis of census projections. It should be borne in mind that administrative records tend to overestimate coverage as a result of double counting in the numerator and uncertainty in the denominator. Although household surveys are generally considered to be more reliable, these are subject to respondent reporting errors as well as to margins of uncertainty due to sampling errors. In generating global estimates, it is good practice to reconcile data from multiple sources in order to maximize the accuracy of all estimates.

Unavoidable terminology differences also exist between countries, making standardization difficult. For example, there are significant variations across countries in the precise skills and training of health workers classified as "skilled birth attendants". Indicator definitions may also change over time. As a result of these and other issues, there may be limitations in the comparability of results across countries and over time. WHO regional aggregates are not available for several coverage indicators, reflecting both the limited availability of data for several indicators, and the fact that some conditions (such as malaria) are not of public health significance in all countries.

Table 4

Member State	Unmet need for family planning[a] (%)	Contraceptive prevalence[a] (%)	Antenatal care coverage[b] (%)		Births attended by skilled health personnel[b] (%)	Births by caesarean section[b] (%)	Postnatal care visit within two days of childbirth[b] (%)	Neonates protected at birth against neonatal tetanus[c] (%)	Immunization coverage among 1-year-olds[d] (%)					
									Measles			DTP3	HepB3	Hib3
			At least 1 visit	At least 4 visits										
	2006 –2012	2006 –2012	2006–2013		2006 –2013	2006 –2012	2006 –2012	2012	1990	2000	2012	2012	2012	2012
Afghanistan	...	22	46	15	36	4	23	60	20	27	68	71	71	71
Albania	13	69	97	67	99	19	83	87	88	95	99	99	99	99
Algeria	...	61	89	...	95	...	...	90	83	80	95	95	95	95
Andorra	...	...	...	...	...	...	...	...	...	97	98	99	97	98
Angola	...	18	68 k	47	49 k	...	...	72	38	41	97	91	91	91
Antigua and Barbuda	...	...	100 k	100	100 k	...	...	...	89	95	98	98	98	98
Argentina	...	...	91 l	25	99	23	...	...	93	91	94	91	91	91
Armenia	14	55	99	93	100	13	92	...	...	92	97	95	95	95
Australia	...	...	96 m	90 m,n	99 o	32	...	...	86	91	94	92	92	92
Austria	...	70	...	...	99 o	29	...	...	60	75	76	83	83	83
Azerbaijan	15	51	77	45	100 k	21	66	...	...	67	66	75	46	91
Bahamas	...	...	98 k	86	99 k	...	...	92	86	93	91	98	96	98
Bahrain	...	...	100 k	100	100 k	30	...	94	87	98	99	99	99	99
Bangladesh	14	61	50	26	31	17	27	94	65	72	96	96	96	96
Barbados	...	...	100 k	81	100 k	...	...	...	87	94	90	87	88	88
Belarus	...	...	100	100	100 k	24	...	...	...	98	98	98	97	22
Belgium	...	70	...	...	100 q	20	...	...	85	82	96	99	98	98
Belize	16	55	96	83	95	28	95	88	86	96	96	98	98	98
Benin	27	13	86	61	84	4	66	93	79	70	72	85	85	85
Bhutan	12	66	74	77	58	12	70	89	93	78	95	97	97	97
Bolivia (Plurinational State of)	20	61	86	72	71	19	28	76	53	84	84	80	80	80
Bosnia and Herzegovina	9	46	87	84	100	14	...	...	...	80	94	92	92	87
Botswana	...	53	94	73	99 k	...	...	92	87	91	94	96	96	96
Brazil	6	80	97 l	89	99 o	54	...	93	78	99	99	94	97	95
Brunei Darussalam	...	...	100 l	100	100 k	...	...	95	99	99	99	90	99	90
Bulgaria	...	69	...	...	100 k	33	...	...	99	89	94	95	95	95
Burkina Faso	25	16	95	34	67	2	72	88	79	48	87	90	90	90
Burundi	32	22	99	33	60	4	30	85	74	72	93	96	96	96
Cabo Verde	...	...	91 l	...	99	...	...	92	79	86	96	90	90	90
Cambodia	17	51	89	59	71	3	70	91	34	65	93	95	95	95
Cameroon	24	23	85 k	62	64 k	4	37	85	56	49	82	85	85	85
Canada	...	...	100 l	99	98 o	27	...	...	89	96	98	95	70	95
Central African Republic	...	19	55	38	40	5	...	66	82	36	49	47	47	47
Chad	28	5	43	23	17	2	...	43	32	28	64	45	45	45
Chile	...	64	...	...	100 o	37 r	...	...	97	97	90	90	90	90
China	...	85	94 l	...	96 o	27	...	...	98	84	99	99	99	...
Colombia	8	79	97	89	99	43	3 s	79	82	88	94	92	92	91
Comoros	...	...	92	...	82	...	...	85	87	70	85	86	86	86
Congo	...	45	90	79	90	6	64	83	75	34	80	85	85	85
Cook Islands	...	...	...	...	100 k	...	...	...	67	76	97	98	98	98
Costa Rica	...	82	95 l	97	99	22 t	...	...	90	82	90	91	91	90
Côte d'Ivoire	...	18	89	44	57	3	70	82	56	68	85	94	94	94
Croatia	...	...	96 l	95 u	100	19	...	...	...	93	95	96	98	96
Cuba	9	74	100 k	100	100 o	...	...	...	94	94	99	96	96	96
Cyprus	...	...	99 l	...	97 o	51	...	...	77	86	86	99	96	96
Czech Republic	4	86	98 l	95 u	100 o	25	...	...	...	98	98	99	99	99
Democratic People's Republic of Korea	...	...	100	94	100	13	...	93	98	78	99	96	96	32
Democratic Republic of the Congo	24	18	89	44	80	7	80	70	38	46	73	72	72	72
Denmark	...	...	...	...	98 o	21	...	...	84	99	90	94	...	94

Children aged 6–59 months who received vitamin A supplementation[e] (%)	Children aged < 5 years (%)					Pregnant women with HIV receiving antiretrovirals to prevent MTCT[h] (%)	Anti-retroviral therapy coverage among people eligible for treatment[h] (%)	Case-detection rate for all forms of tuberculosis[i] (%)		Smear-positive tuberculosis treatment-success rate[j] (%)		Member State
	With ARI symptoms taken to a health facility[e]	With suspected pneumonia receiving antibiotics[e]	With diarrhoea receiving ORT (ORS and/or RHF)[e]	MDG 6 Sleeping under insecticide-treated nets[f]	With fever who received treatment with any antimalarial[g]							
2006–2013	2006–2013			2006–2012		2012	2012	2000	2012	2000	2011	
51	61	64	70	4	...	...	8	18	52	85	91	Afghanistan
...	70	60	68	...	...	...	...	81	81	...	93	Albania
...	53	59	27	...	...	...	...	67	64	87	92	Algeria
...	...	...	...	...	...	...	...	87	87	50	100	Andorra
...	...	...	...	26	28	17	42	46	79	68	55	Angola
...	...	...	...	...	...	...	...	87	87	100	17	Antigua and Barbuda
...	...	...	...	...	...	...	81	79	84	47	52	Argentina
...	57	...	90	...	...	...	35	71	79	87	63	Armenia
...	...	...	...	...	...	...	...	87	87	72	77	Australia
...	...	...	...	...	...	...	...	87	93	73	71	Austria
9	33	...	31	...	...	...	24	9	72	90	78	Azerbaijan
...	...	...	...	...	...	...	...	87	87	...	70	Bahamas
...	...	...	...	...	...	...	...	87	87	73	34	Bahrain
60 p	35	71	81	...	1	...	27	25	49	81	92	Bangladesh
...	...	...	...	...	...	...	...	87	87	...	...	Barbados
...	...	...	...	...	...	...	45	81	72	...	60	Belarus
...	...	...	...	...	...	...	...	87	85	66	77	Belgium
65	82	71	55	...	...	...	71	110	65	78	...	Belize
49	31	29	54	...	38	40	67	45	57	78	90	Benin
...	74	49	81	...	...	...	12	50	85	90	91	Bhutan
25	51	64	44	...	...	...	35	65	62	79	86	Bolivia (Plurinational State of)
...	87	76	55	...	...	...	...	100	76	94	70	Bosnia and Herzegovina
...	...	...	...	...	...	>95	>95	58	75	77	81	Botswana
...	50	...	51	...	...	...	...	74	82	71	76	Brazil
...	...	...	...	...	...	...	...	87	87	63	66	Brunei Darussalam
...	...	...	...	...	...	...	...	72	90	...	86	Bulgaria
63	56	47	24	47	35	66	62	28	58	60	78	Burkina Faso
81	55	43	41	44	17	54	58	33	54	80	92	Burundi
...	...	...	...	...	...	...	>95	...	59	64	77	Cabo Verde
71	64	39	34	...	0	...	84	27	66	91	93	Cambodia
...	30	45	22	11	23	64	45	11	48	77	80	Cameroon
...	...	...	...	...	...	...	...	87	100	35	62	Canada
78	22	31	38	...	34	...	...	...	49	58	68	Central African Republic
98	26	31	48	...	43	14	40	...	56	...	68	Chad
...	...	...	...	...	...	...	86	87	87	82	71	Chile
...	...	...	...	...	...	...	...	33	89	93	95	China
...	65	...	74	...	...	...	55	68	73	80	77	Colombia
...	...	...	...	...	28	...	...	58	49	93	25	Comoros
65	52	59	37	31	25	19	39	84	68	69	71	Congo
...	...	...	...	...	...	...	...	87	87	...	0	Cook Islands
...	77	72	78	...	...	...	74	43	93	57	88	Costa Rica
61	38	29	22	37	18	68	49	25	69	57	78	Côte d'Ivoire
...	...	...	...	...	...	...	...	87	...	...	...	Croatia
...	97	70	53	...	...	...	>95	82	70	93	88	Cuba
...	...	...	...	...	...	...	...	87	100	...	64	Cyprus
...	...	...	...	...	...	...	...	87	99	70	69	Czech Republic
98	80	88	92	...	...	...	...	39	91	82	90	Democratic People's Republic of Korea
82	40	42	53 v	6	39	13	31	40	51	78	87	Democratic Republic of the Congo
...	...	...	...	...	...	...	...	87	...	86	...	Denmark

4. Health service coverage

Member State	MDG 5								Immunization coverage among 1-year-olds[d] (%)					
	Unmet need for family planning[a] (%)	Contraceptive prevalence[a] (%)	Antenatal care coverage[b] (%)		Births attended by skilled health personnel[b] (%)	Births by caesarean section[b] (%)	Postnatal care visit within two days of childbirth[b] (%)	Neonates protected at birth against neonatal tetanus[c] (%)			MDG 4			
			At least 1 visit	At least 4 visits					Measles			DTP3	HepB3	Hib3
	2006–2012	2006–2012	2006–2013		2006–2013	2006–2012	2006–2012	2012	1990	2000	2012	2012	2012	2012
Djibouti	…	18	81	…	78	…	…	79	85	50	83	81	81	81
Dominica	…	…	100 [k]	…	100 [k]	…	…	…	88	99	99	97	97	97
Dominican Republic	11	73	96	95	95	44	82	90	70	85	79	85	74	70
Ecuador	…	…	84 [k]	…	91	…	…	85	60	99	94	99	98	99
Egypt	12	60	74	66	79	28	65	86	86	98	93	93	93	…
El Salvador	…	72	94 [l]	78 [n]	85 [o]	28 [w]	…	90	98	97	93	92	92	92
Equatorial Guinea	…	…	91	67	68	…	44	75	88	51	51	33	…	…
Eritrea	…	…	…	…	…	…	…	94	…	76	99	99	99	99
Estonia	…	…	100 [l]	97 [n]	99 [o]	20	…	…	…	93	94	94	94	94
Ethiopia	26	29	34	19	10	2	7	68	38	33	66	61	61	61
Fiji	…	…	…	…	100 [k]	…	…	94	84	81	99	99	99	99
Finland	…	…	…	…	100 [o]	16	…	…	97	96	97	99	…	99
France	…	76	100 [l]	99	97 [o]	21	…	…	71	84	89	99	74	98
Gabon	…	31	95 [k]	78	89 [k]	10	59	75	76	55	71	82	82	82
Gambia	22	13	86	72	57	3	…	92	86	89	95	98	98	98
Georgia	12	53	98 [k]	82	100	35	73	…	…	73	93	92	92	92
Germany	…	…	…	…	98 [o]	32	…	…	75	92	97	93	86	94
Ghana	36	24	96	87	67	11	68	88	61	90	88	92	92	92
Greece	…	…	…	…	…	…	…	…	76	89	99	99	98	94
Grenada	…	…	100 [k]	…	100 [k]	…	…	…	85	92	94	97	97	97
Guatemala	…	…	93 [l]	…	51	16	26 [x]	85	68	86	93	96	96	96
Guinea	…	6	85 [k]	50	45 [k]	2	41 [x]	80	35	42	58	59	59	59
Guinea-Bissau	6	14	93	68	43	2	…	80	53	71	69	80	76	76
Guyana	29	43	86	79	87	13	79	90	73	86	99	97	97	97
Haiti	37	35	90	67	37	6	32	76	31	55	58	60	…	…
Honduras	17	65	94	89	83	19	85	94	90	98	93	88	88	88
Hungary	…	…	…	…	99 [k]	32	…	…	99	99	99	99	…	99
Iceland	…	…	…	…	…	17	…	…	99	91	90	89	…	89
India	21	55	75 [l]	50 [u]	67 [o]	8	48	87	56	59	74	72	70	…
Indonesia	11	62	96 [k]	88	83 [k]	12	80	85	58	76	80	64	64	…
Iran (Islamic Republic of)	…	…	…	…	…	48	…	95	85	99	98	99	98	…
Iraq	8	53	78	50	91	22	…	85	75	86	69	69	77	46
Ireland	…	…	100	…	100 [o]	28	…	…	78	79	92	95	95	95
Israel	…	…	…	…	…	20	…	…	91	97	96	94	97	93
Italy	…	…	98 [l]	85	100 [o]	38	…	…	43	74	90	97	97	96
Jamaica	…	…	99 [l]	87	96 [k]	15	…	80	74	88	93	99	99	99
Japan	…	…	…	…	100 [o]	19	…	…	73	96	96	98	…	…
Jordan	13	59	99	94	100	19	82	90	87	94	98	98	98	98
Kazakhstan	12	51	98	87	100	16	…	…	…	99	96	99	95	97
Kenya	26	46	92	47	44	6	42	73	78	78	93	83	83	83
Kiribati	28	22	…	…	98 [k]	…	…	…	75	80	91	94	94	94
Kuwait	…	…	100 [l]	…	99 [o]	…	…	95	66	99	99	98	98	98
Kyrgyzstan	…	48	97	…	99	7	…	…	…	98	98	96	96	96
Lao People's Democratic Republic	…	…	53	37	40	4	…	80	32	42	72	79	79	79
Latvia	…	…	98 [l]	… [y]	99 [o]	24	…	…	…	97	90	92	91	91
Lebanon	…	…	…	…	…	…	…	…	61	71	80	82	84	82
Lesotho	23	47	92	70	62	7	48	83	80	74	85	83	83	83
Liberia	36	11	96	66	61	4	60	91	0	63	80	77	77	77
Libya	…	…	93	…	100 [o]	…	…	…	89	93	98	98	98	98

Children aged 6–59 months who received vitamin A supplementation (%)	Children aged <5 years (%)					Pregnant women with HIV receiving antiretrovirals to prevent MTCT[h] (%)	Anti-retroviral therapy coverage among people eligible for treatment[h] (%)	Case-detection rate for all forms of tuberculosis[i] (%)		Smear-positive tuberculosis treatment-success rate[j] (%)		Member State
	With ARI symptoms taken to a health facility[e]	With suspected pneumonia receiving antibiotics[e]	With diarrhoea receiving ORT (ORS and/or RHF)[e]	Sleeping under insecticide-treated nets[f] (MDG 6)	With fever who received treatment with any antimalarial[g]							
2006–2013	2006–2013			2006–2012		2012	2012	2000	2012	2000	2011	
18	...	43	71	...	1	20	31	89	65	62	82	Djibouti
...	...	...	...	...	...	...	...	...	75	...	100	Dominica
29	67	...	45	...	...	...	77	61	67	70	83	Dominican Republic
...	...	...	...	...	...	...	55	52	60	...	78	Ecuador
12	73	58	28	...	...	...	37	63	62	87	88	Egypt
52	59	...	58	...	...	...	47	68	130	79	93	El Salvador
30	54	27	44	42	...	...	...	...	...	...	...	Equatorial Guinea
50	45	...	58	...	13	46	73	110	55	76	87	Eritrea
...	...	...	...	...	...	...	...	87	87	70	59	Estonia
53	27	7	31	33	26	41	61	33	64	80	90	Ethiopia
...	...	...	...	...	...	...	43	33	99	85	93	Fiji
...	...	...	...	...	...	...	...	87	87	...	67	Finland
...	...	...	...	...	...	...	...	80	...	...	...	France
54	68	50	37	39	26	70	62	...	71	...	51	Gabon
73	68	70	65	...	30	...	55	56	46	...	88	Gambia
...	...	...	...	...	...	...	72	36	78	63	76	Georgia
...	...	...	...	...	...	...	...	87	87	77	70	Germany
74	41	56	59	38	53	95	58	38	81	50	86	Ghana
...	...	...	...	...	...	...	...	87	...	...	...	Greece
...	...	...	...	...	...	...	...	0	23	...	100	Grenada
...	60	...	44	...	...	...	51	38	38	86	86	Guatemala
41	37	38	37	...	28	44	50	27	56	68	82	Guinea
79	52	35	81	...	51	33	37	52	48	...	73	Guinea-Bissau
55	65	18	59	24	6	...	93	54	86	55	72	Guyana
44	38	46	58	12	3	>95	60	45	76	71	84	Haiti
73	64	60	71	...	0	...	58	90	70	86	88	Honduras
...	...	...	...	...	...	...	...	81	65	64	...	Hungary
...	...	...	...	...	...	...	...	87	87	100	...	Iceland
16	67	13	26	...	8	...	50	49	59	34	88	India
61	75	39	47	3	1	...	17	20	72	87	90	Indonesia
...	...	...	...	...	...	...	13	70	70	85	85	Iran (Islamic Republic of)
28	74	67	34	...	...	...	...	81	59	92	89	Iraq
...	...	...	...	...	...	...	...	87	87	84	64	Ireland
...	...	...	...	...	...	...	...	87	87	83	77	Israel
...	...	...	...	...	...	...	...	87	...	74	...	Italy
...	...	...	...	...	...	...	69	75	50	45	47	Jamaica
...	...	...	...	...	...	...	...	87	86	45	...	Japan
11	77	87	28	...	...	...	...	80	82	90	92	Jordan
...	81	87	65	...	...	...	...	50	81	79	61	Kazakhstan
30	56	50	72	46	23	53	73	72	79	80	88	Kenya
...	...	...	...	...	...	...	...	82	80	91	94	Kiribati
...	...	...	...	...	...	...	...	87	87	69	93	Kuwait
...	...	...	68	...	...	...	23	50	80	82	78	Kyrgyzstan
59	54	57	61	...	2	...	51	13	30	77	92	Lao People's Democratic Republic
...	...	...	...	...	...	...	...	69	87	72	73	Latvia
...	...	...	...	...	...	...	...	100	86	92	80	Lebanon
34	67	...	71	...	...	58	54	95	83	...	74	Lesotho
43	51	49	62	26	57	87	43	21	64	80	86	Liberia
...	...	...	...	...	...	...	...	65	63	...	59	Libya

Table 4

Member State	MDG 5								Immunization coverage among 1-year-olds[d] (%)					
	Unmet need for family planning[a] (%)	Contra-ceptive preva-lence[a] (%)	Antenatal care coverage[b] (%)		Births attended by skilled health person-nel[b] (%)	Births by cae-sarean section[b] (%)	Postnatal care visit within two days of child-birth[b] (%)	Neonates protected at birth against neonatal tetanus[c] (%)			MDG 4			
											Measles		DTP3	HepB3	Hib3
			At least 1 visit	At least 4 visits											
	2006 –2012	2006 –2012	2006–2013		2006 –2013	2006 –2012	2006 –2012	2012	1990	2000	2012	2012	2012	2012
Lithuania	…	63	…	…	…	25	…	…	…	97	93	93	93	93
Luxembourg	…	…	100	97 z	100 o	31	…	…	80	91	96	99	95	99
Madagascar	19	40	86	49	44	2	46	78	47	57	69	86	86	86
Malawi	26	46	95	46	71	5	43	89	81	73	90	96	96	96
Malaysia	…	…	97 l	…	99 k	16 aa	…	90	70	88	95	99	98	99
Maldives	29	35	99	85	99	41	67	95	96	99	98	99	99	…
Mali	28	8	74	35	58	2	22 s	89	43	49	59	74	74	74
Malta	…	…	…	…	100 o	34	…	…	80	74	93	99	93	99
Marshall Islands	8	45	92 l	77	90	9	64	…	52	94	78	80	80	67
Mauritania	…	9	72	…	57	…	…	80	38	46	75	80	80	80
Mauritius	…	…	…	…	100 o	44 ab	…	95	76	84	99	98	98	98
Mexico	12	71	96 k	… y	95 k	39	55 ac	88	75	96	99	99	99	99
Micronesia (Federated States of)	…	…	…	…	100 k	11	…	…	81	85	91	81	82	66
Monaco	…	…	…	…	…	…	…	…	99	99	99	99	99	99
Mongolia	22	55	99 k	81	99 k	21	…	…	92	92	99	99	99	99
Montenegro	…	39	…	…	100 o	24	…	…	…	…	90	94	90	94
Morocco	12	67	77	55	74 k	16	…	89	79	93	99	99	99	99
Mozambique	…	12	60	51	19	4	…	83	59	71	82	76	76	76
Myanmar	…	46	83 k	43 z	71 k	…	…	93	68	84	84	85	38	…
Namibia	21	55	95	70	81	13	65	83	…	69	76	84	84	84
Nauru	24	36	94 k	40	97 k	8	66	…	0	8	96	79	79	79
Nepal	28	50	58	50	36	5	45	82	57	71	86	90	90	90
Netherlands	…	69	…	…	…	17	…	…	94	96	96	97	…	97
New Zealand	…	…	…	…	96 o	24	…	…	90	85	92	93	93	93
Nicaragua	11	72	95	88	88 k	30	7 ae	81	82	86	99	98	98	98
Niger	16	14	83	15	29	1	12 s	84	25	37	73	74	74	74
Nigeria	19	14	61	57	38 k	5	38	60	54	33	42	41	41	10
Niue	…	…	…	…	100 k	…	…	…	99	99	99	98	98	99
Norway	…	…	…	…	99 o	17	…	…	87	88	94	95	…	95
Oman	…	…	99 l	83	99 k	17 af	…	91	98	99	99	98	97	98
Pakistan	25	27	73 k	28	52 k	7	39	75	50	59	83	81	81	81
Palau	…	…	90 l	81	100 k	…	…	…	98	83	91	89	89	89
Panama	…	52	94 l	…	94	20	72 ae	…	73	97	98	85	85	85
Papua New Guinea	27	32	65 l	29	43 o	…	…	70	67	62	67	63	63	63
Paraguay	5	79	96 l	91	95 o	33	77 ag	85	69	92	91	87	87	87
Peru	6	69	96	94	87	25	93	85	64	97	94	95	95	95
Philippines	22	49	95	78	72	11	77	76	85	78	85	86	70	23
Poland	…	…	…	…	100 o	35	…	…	95	97	98	99	98	99
Portugal	…	87	…	…	…	35	…	…	85	87	97	98	98	98
Qatar	…	…	91 k	85	100 k	…	…	…	79	91	97	92	92	92
Republic of Korea	…	80	100 l	… y	100 o	37	…	…	93	95	99	99	99	…
Republic of Moldova	…	…	…	…	99 k	16	…	…	…	89	91	92	94	90
Romania	…	…	…	…	99 k	37	…	…	92	98	94	89	96	92
Russian Federation	…	80	…	…	100 k	22	…	…	…	97	98	97	97	18
Rwanda	21	52	98	35	69	7	18	85	83	74	97	98	98	98
Saint Kitts and Nevis	…	…	100 k	…	100 k	…	…	…	99	99	95	97	98	98
Saint Lucia	…	…	99 k	99	99 k	…	…	…	82	88	99	98	98	98
Saint Vincent and the Grenadines	…	…	100 k	…	99 k	…	…	…	96	96	94	96	96	97
Samoa	48	29	93 k	58	81 k	13	66	…	89	93	85	92	99	99

Children aged 6–59 months who received vitamin A supplementation[e] (%)	Children aged <5 years (%)					Pregnant women with HIV receiving antiretrovirals to prevent MTCT[h] (%)	Anti-retroviral therapy coverage among people eligible for treatment[h] (%)	MDG 6				Member State
	With ARI symptoms taken to a health facility[e]	With suspected pneumonia receiving antibiotics[e]	With diarrhoea receiving ORT (ORS and/or RHF)[e]	MDG 6 Sleeping under insecticide-treated nets[f]	With fever who received treatment with any antimalarial[g]			Case-detection rate for all forms of tuberculosis[i] (%)		Smear-positive tuberculosis treatment-success rate[j] (%)		
2006–2013	2006–2013			2006–2012		2012	2012	2000	2012	2000	2011	
...	...	...	...	...	...	...	...	74	82	73	73	Lithuania
...	...	...	...	...	...	...	...	87	130	...	0	Luxembourg
72	42	...	29	45	20	...	1	...	49	70	83	Madagascar
86	70	...	69	39	33	60	69	45	78	73	85	Malawi
...	...	...	...	...	...	...	42	68	93	78	79	Malaysia
48	74	...	63	...	...	...	26	80	80	97	81	Maldives
72	30	...	40	70	32	...	52	53	61	...	68	Mali
...	...	...	...	...	...	...	...	87	87	100	58	Malta
...	...	...	...	...	...	...	...	25	48	91	88	Marshall Islands
56	45	24	31	...	20	...	35	41	20	...	73	Mauritania
...	...	...	...	...	...	...	36	55	49	93	90	Mauritius
...	...	...	...	...	...	...	82	58	75	76	86	Mexico
...	...	...	...	...	...	...	...	30	72	93	96	Micronesia (Federated States of)
...	...	...	...	...	...	...	...	...	...	...	...	Monaco
61	87	72	56 v,ad	...	...	...	...	51	66	87	86	Mongolia
...	89	57	98	...	...	...	...	...	87	...	86	Montenegro
21	50	49	40	...	...	...	49	86	86	89	80	Morocco
75	50	12	62	7	30	86	45	23	34	75	...	Mozambique
56	69	34	66 v	...	...	...	48	15	71	82	86	Myanmar
52	72	...	69	10	20	94	90	40	68	56	84	Namibia
...	...	...	...	...	...	...	...	87	...	25	...	Nauru
87	50	...	31	...	1	...	32	78	78	84	90	Nepal
...	...	...	...	...	...	...	...	87	87	76	81	Netherlands
...	...	...	...	...	...	...	...	87	87	30	56	New Zealand
62	64	...	68	...	...	...	72	70	120	82	86	Nicaragua
60	53	11	47	...	19	...	46	22	62	65	80	Niger
65	35	45	38	5	45	17	32	12	51	79	85	Nigeria
...	...	...	...	...	...	...	...	...	0	...	...	Niue
...	...	...	...	...	...	...	...	87	...	70	...	Norway
...	...	...	...	...	...	...	...	87	87	93	97	Oman
72	64	42	42	...	3	...	14	3	65	74	92	Pakistan
...	...	...	...	...	...	...	...	...	80	...	57	Palau
...	...	...	...	...	...	...	76	81	84	60	84	Panama
...	...	...	...	...	...	39	79	56	82	63	69	Papua New Guinea
...	...	...	...	...	...	...	73	74	81	66	78	Paraguay
15	59	48	67	...	...	...	59	81	100	90	74	Peru
76	50	42	59	...	0	...	73	47	84	88	90	Philippines
...	...	...	...	...	...	...	...	87	87	72	60	Poland
...	...	...	...	...	...	...	...	87	89	79	80	Portugal
...	...	...	...	...	...	...	...	87	87	66	49	Qatar
98	80	88	92 ah	...	...	...	...	87	82	83	80	Republic of Korea
...	...	...	...	...	...	...	29	49	79	63	62	Republic of Moldova
...	...	...	...	...	...	...	...	68	79	70	85	Romania
...	...	...	...	...	...	...	...	75	81	68	54	Russian Federation
93	50	...	35	56	11	87	87	22	62	61	89	Rwanda
...	...	...	...	...	...	...	...	...	87	...	100	Saint Kitts and Nevis
...	...	...	...	...	...	...	...	49	180	100	57	Saint Lucia
...	...	...	...	...	...	...	...	57	110	100	56	Saint Vincent and the Grenadines
...	87	54	87	...	...	...	...	110	66	92	83	Samoa

Member State	Unmet need for family planning[a] (%) 2006–2012	Contra-ceptive preva-lence[a] (%) 2006–2012	Antenatal care coverage[b] (%) At least 1 visit 2006–2013	Antenatal care coverage[b] (%) At least 4 visits 2006–2013	Births attended by skilled health person-nel[b] (%) 2006–2013	Births by cae-sarean section[b] (%) 2006–2012	Postnatal care visit within two days of child-birth[b] (%) 2006–2012	Neonates protected at birth against neonatal tetanus[c] (%) 2012	Immunization coverage among 1-year-olds[d] (%) Measles 1990	Measles 2000	Measles 2012	DTP3 2012	HepB3 2012	Hib3 2012
San Marino	...	...	...	...	...	34	...	...	0	74	87	96	96	96
Sao Tome and Principe	38	38	98	72	81	5	37	...	71	69	92	96	96	96
Saudi Arabia	...	24	98[l]	...	98[k]	22[af]	...	...	88	94	98	98	98	98
Senegal	30	13	95	50	51	6	68	91	51	48	84	92	92	92
Serbia	7	61	99	94	100	25	...	...	...	89	87	91	97	90
Seychelles	...	...	...	...	99[k]	23	...	...	86	97	98	98	99	98
Sierra Leone	27	11	91	75	61[k]	5	58	87	0	37	80	84	84	84
Singapore	...	...	100[l]	...	100[o]	...	...	...	84	96	95	96	96	...
Slovakia	...	...	...	...	100[k]	29	...	...	...	98	99	99	99	99
Slovenia	...	...	...	...	100[o]	18	...	...	...	95	95	96	...	96
Solomon Islands	11	35	74	65	70	6	51	85	70	85	85	90	90	90
Somalia	...	15	22	6	9	...	...	64	30	24	46	42	...	...
South Africa	...	...	...	...	...	...	...	77	79	72	79	68	73	68
South Sudan	...	4	40	17	17	<1	...	0	...	...	62	59	...	...
Spain	...	66	...	...	...	25	...	...	99	94	97	97	96	97
Sri Lanka	7	68	99	93	99	26	71	95	80	99	99	99	99	99
Sudan	29	9	69	47	20	7	...	74	...	...	85	92	92	92
Suriname	...	46	90	67	90	19	...	93	65	84	73	84	84	84
Swaziland	13	65	97	77	82	12	22	86	85	92	88	95	95	95
Sweden	...	...	...	...	...	17	...	...	96	91	97	98	...	98
Switzerland	...	...	...	...	...	33	...	...	90	81	92	95	...	95
Syrian Arab Republic	...	58	88[k]	...	96[k]	...	27	94	87	84	61	45	43	45
Tajikistan	...	28	79	53	87	4	80	...	...	88	94	94	94	94
Thailand	3	80	99[l]	80	99	...	...	91	80	94	98	99	98	...
The former Yugoslav Republic of Macedonia	...	...	99	94	89	25	...	...	...	97	97	96	96	96
Timor-Leste	32	22	84	55	29	2	25	81	...	...	62	67	67	...
Togo	37	15	51	55	44	9	...	81	73	58	72	84	84	84
Tonga	...	...	98[l]	86	99[k]	...	...	...	86	95	95	95	95	95
Trinidad and Tobago	...	43	95	100	100[k]	18	...	...	70	90	85	92	92	92
Tunisia	7	63	84	85	74[k]	27	...	96	93	95	96	97	97	97
Turkey	6	73	92	74	91	37	80	90	78	87	98	97	96	97
Turkmenistan	...	...	99[l]	...	100[k]	6	...	...	...	96	99	97	98	97
Tuvalu	24	31	93	67	93	7	51	...	95	81	98	97	97	97
Uganda	34	30	95	48	58	5	33	85	52	57	82	78	78	78
Ukraine	10	67	99	75[z]	99	10	87	...	...	99	79	76	46	83
United Arab Emirates	...	...	100[l]	...	100[k]	21	...	...	80	94	94	94	94	94
United Kingdom	...	84	...	...	...[ai]	...	...	...	87	88	93	97	...	97
United Republic of Tanzania	25	34	88	43	49	5	31	88	80	78	97	92	92	92
United States of America	8	76	...	97	99	33	...	...	90	91	92	95	92	90
Uruguay	...	...	96[l]	92	100	33	...	...	97	89	96	95	95	95
Uzbekistan	...	65	99	...	100	9	...	...	...	99	99	99	99	99
Vanuatu	...	38	84	...	74	...	...	75	66	61	52	68	59	68
Venezuela (Bolivarian Republic of)	...	...	...	61	96[k]	32[af]	...	50	61	84	87	81	81	81
Viet Nam	4	78	94	60	92	20	...	91	88	97	96	97	97	97
Yemen	...	28	65[k]	29	34	7	...	66	69	71	71	82	82	82
Zambia	27	41	94	60	47	3	39	81	90	85	83	78	78	78
Zimbabwe	15	59	90	65	66	5	27	66	87	75	90	89	89	89

Children aged 6–59 months who received vitamin A supplementation[e] (%)	Children aged <5 years (%)					Pregnant women with HIV receiving antiretrovirals to prevent MTCT[h] (%)	Anti-retroviral therapy coverage among people eligible for treatment[h] (%)	MDG 6 Case-detection rate for all forms of tuberculosis[i] (%)		Smear-positive tuberculosis treatment-success rate[j] (%)		Member State
	With ARI symptoms taken to a health facility[e]	With suspected pneumonia receiving antibiotics[e]	With diarrhoea receiving ORT (ORS and/or RHF)[e]	MDG 6 Sleeping under insecticide-treated nets[f]	With fever who received treatment with any antimalarial[g]							
2006–2013	2006–2013			2006–2012		2012	2012	2000	2012	2000	2011	
...	...	...	...	...	...	...	...	87	...	0	...	San Marino
48	75	60	57	56	8	...	44	61	66	78	72	Sao Tome and Principe
...	...	...	...	...	...	...	...	87	87	73	61	Saudi Arabia
78	50	...	27	29	8	...	62	56	65	52	85	Senegal
...	90	82	73	...	...	...	...	...	87	...	87	Serbia
...	...	...	...	...	...	...	...	69	73	82	67	Seychelles
91	74	58	84	25	62	93	33	34	32	77	88	Sierra Leone
...	...	...	...	...	...	...	...	87	87	71	83	Singapore
...	...	...	...	...	...	...	...	87	87	82	91	Slovakia
...	...	...	...	...	...	...	...	87	87	84	81	Slovenia
...	...	...	...	...	19	...	...	40	67	81	90	Solomon Islands
24	13	32	21	...	8	...	12	27	41	83	86	Somalia
...	...	...	...	...	...	83	80	59	62	63	79	South Africa
...	...	...	...	...	51	13	8	...	53	...	73	South Sudan
...	...	...	...	...	...	...	...	87	87	...	73	Spain
...	58	...	63	...	0	...	34	67	66	79	87	Sri Lanka
...	...	...	...	16	65	...	...	50	44	75	70	Sudan
...	76	71	72	...	0	...	66	22	58	68	76	Suriname
68	58	61	81	1	2	83	82	69	43	...	73	Swaziland
...	...	...	...	...	...	...	...	87	87	79	83	Sweden
...	...	...	...	...	...	...	...	87	87	...	...	Switzerland
3	77	71	68	...	...	...	...	89	77	78	84	Syrian Arab Republic
77	63	...	72	...	...	...	28	20	75	77	80	Tajikistan
...	84	65	68	...	...	...	76	32	76	69	85	Thailand
...	...	...	...	...	...	...	...	75	89	86	95	The former Yugoslav Republic of Macedonia
51	71	45	78	41	6	...	...	...	69	...	91	Timor-Leste
88	32	41	31 v,ad	35	34	86	46	40	59	...	85	Togo
...	...	...	...	...	...	...	...	88	73	93	100	Tonga
...	...	...	...	...	...	...	...	87	87	68	72	Trinidad and Tobago
...	59	...	74	...	...	...	55	86	96	91	87	Tunisia
...	...	...	...	...	...	...	...	87	87	73	90	Turkey
...	...	...	...	...	...	...	...	43	...	81	...	Turkmenistan
...	...	...	...	...	...	...	...	48	80	86	75	Tuvalu
57	79	47	48	32	65	72	64	29	69	63	77	Uganda
...	...	...	...	...	...	...	41	62	96	...	58	Ukraine
...	...	...	...	...	...	...	...	32	50	74	73	United Arab Emirates
...	...	...	...	...	...	...	...	89	88	...	80	United Kingdom
61	31	...	59	25	54	77	61	68	79	78	88	United Republic of Tanzania
...	...	...	...	...	...	...	...	87	87	83	78	United States of America
...	...	...	...	...	...	...	65	87	87	85	85	Uruguay
72	68	56	79	...	...	...	43	22	66	80	78	Uzbekistan
...	63	48	54	...	53	...	...	75	78	88	82	Vanuatu
...	...	...	...	...	...	...	71	77	65	76	80	Venezuela (Bolivarian Republic of)
83	73	68	66	...	1	...	58	56	76	92	93	Viet Nam
...	...	38	87	8	...	...	14	67	85	72	88	Yemen
63	68	47	67	28	34	>95	79	69	68	67	88	Zambia
66	48	31	63	91	2	82	79	56	46	69	81	Zimbabwe

		Antenatal care coverage[b] (%)		Births attended by skilled health personnel[b] (%)	Births by cae-sarean section[b] (%)	Postnatal care visit within two days of child-birth[b] (%)	Neonates protected at birth against neonatal tetanus[c] (%)	Immunization coverage among 1-year-olds[d] (%)					
Unmet need for family planning[a] (%)	Contra-ceptive preva-lence[a] (%)								Measles		DTP3	HepB3	Hib3
		At least 1 visit	At least 4 visits					1990	2000	2012	2012	2012	2012
2006 –2012	2006 –2012	2006–2013		2006 –2013	2006 –2012	2006 –2012	2012						

Ranges of country values

Minimum	3	4	22	6	9	<1	3	0	0	8	42	33	38	10
Median	19	49	94	72	96	17	58	85	80	88	93	94	94	94
Maximum	48	87	100	100	100	54	95	96	99	99	99	99	99	99

WHO region

African Region	25	27	75	47	48	4	41	75	58	53	73	72	72	65
Region of the Americas	9	74	95	86	94	36	...	85	80	93	94	93	91	91
South-East Asia Region	14	59	76	54	67	10	50	88	59	65	78	75	72	11
European Region	10	69	...	...	98	24	...	90	83	91	94	95	79	83
Eastern Mediterranean Region	20	46	71	39	58	16	43	77	67	72	83	83	81	58
Western Pacific Region	6	80	94	...	93	24	...	83	94	85	97	97	91	14

Income group

Low income	22	39	72	38	46	6	37	79	56	59	80	80	76	74
Lower middle income	16	54	78	56	64	9	51	81	61	64	75	73	71	27
Upper middle income	6	79	93	...	95	32	...	86	90	87	96	95	95	40
High income	10	70	...	...	99	28	...	91	84	91	94	96	76	74

Global

Global	12	63	81	56	72	16	48	81	73	73	84	83	79	45

[a.] 2013 Update for the MDG Database. New York: United Nations, Department of Economic and Social Affairs, Population Division; 2013 (http://www.un.org/en/development/desa/population/publications/dataset/fertility/). WHO regional and income-group aggregates are population-weighted averages of model-based country estimates for the reference year (2011) from Model-based Estimates and Projections of Family Planning Indicators: 2013 Revision (http://www.un.org/en/development/desa/population/theme/family-planning/cp_model.shtml)

[b.] WHO global database on maternal health indicators, 2014 update. Geneva: World Health Organization (http://www.who.int/gho). Antenatal care coverage only includes visits to a skilled provider (doctor, nurse and/or midwife). Contraceptive prevalence refers to any method. Births attended by skilled health personnel refer to doctor, nurse and/or midwife. Postnatal care was surveyed only for the mother.

[c.] Proportion of neonates protected at birth against neonatal tetanus through maternal immunization with tetanus toxoid, based on a mathematical model taking into account the mother's immunization in infancy, during pregnancy and in tetanus campaigns. WHO/UNICEF estimates of national immunization coverage. Geneva: World Health Organization; 2013 (http://www.who.int/immunization_monitoring/routine/immunization_coverage/en/index4.html). Estimates based on data available up to July 2013. This indicator applies only to countries where tetanus is recommended for girls and women and therefore WHO regional, income-group and global aggregates relate only to these same Member States.

[d.] Measles = measles-containing vaccine (MCV); DTP3 = 3 doses of diphtheria-tetanus pertussis vaccine; HepB3 = 3 doses of hepatitis B vaccine; Hib3 = 3 doses of Haemophilus influenzae type B vaccine. WHO/UNICEF estimates of national immunization coverage. Geneva: World Health Organization; 2013 (http://www.who.int/immunization_monitoring/routine/immunization_coverage/en/index4.html).

Estimates based on data available up to July 2013. For countries recommending the first dose of measles vaccine in children older than 12 months of age, the indicator is calculated as the proportion of children less than 24 months of age receiving one dose of measles-containing vaccine. Complete coverage estimates available online at the above website.

[e.] Data compiled by WHO from Demographic and Health Surveys (DHS) and Multiple Indicator Cluster Surveys (MICS), January 2014 (http://dhsprogram.com and http://www.unicef.org/statistics/index_24302.html). Vitamin A supplementation data refer to the six months preceding the survey; data on children receiving oral rehydration salts (ORS) and/or recommended home fluids (RHF) refer to the two weeks preceding the survey; and data on children who were ill with a cough accompanied by rapid breathing (ARI symptoms) and who were taken to a health facility and/or received antibiotics refer to the two weeks preceding the survey. The WHO regional, income-group and global aggregates are population and prevalence weighted from available survey data and may differ from previously reported aggregates.

[f.] World Malaria Report 2013. Annex 5: Household surveys, 2008–2012. Geneva: World Health Organization; 2013 (http://www.who.int/malaria/publications/world_malaria_report_2013/en/).

[g.] The State of the World's Children. 2014 in Numbers: Every Child Counts. New York: UNICEF; 2014. See Table 3: Health (http://www.unicef.org/sowc2014/numbers/).

[h.] Global Aids response progress reporting 2013. Geneva: UNAIDS, 2013 (http://apps.who.int/iris/bitstream/10665/78126/1/9789292530068_eng.pdf?ua=1, accessed 14 March 2014). WHO regional and global aggregates include low- and middle-income countries only. Income groups were derived using the 2012 World Bank list of economies. For uncertainty ranges see the report or visit http://www.who.int/gho/hiv/en/.

Children aged 6–59 months who received vitamin A supplementation[e] (%)	Children aged <5 years (%)					Pregnant women with HIV receiving antiretrovirals to prevent MTCT[h] (%)	Anti-retroviral therapy coverage among people eligible for treatment[h] (%)	Case-detection rate for all forms of tuberculosis[i] (%)		Smear-positive tuberculosis treatment-success rate[j] (%)		
	With ARI symptoms taken to a health facility[e]	With suspected pneumonia receiving antibiotics[e]	With diarrhoea receiving ORT (ORS and/or RHF)[e]	Sleeping under insecticide-treated nets[f]	With fever who received treatment with any antimalarial[g]							
2006–2013	2006–2013			2006–2012		2012	2012	2000	2012	2000	2011	
3	13	7	21	1	0	13	1	0	0	0	0	Minimum
61	60	49	58	30	20	65	52	69	78	78	81	Median
98	97	88	98	91	65	>95	>95	110	180	100	100	Maximum
65	49	...	44	25	...	64	63	39	59	71	82	African Region
...	...	...	...	...	...	88	75	70	79	76	78	Region of the Americas
29	66	...	37	...	...	15	55	41	62	50	89	South-East Asia Region
...	...	...	...	...	...	>95	38	59	79	75	66	European Region
45	61[v]	...	48	...	...	10	15	25	63	81	88	Eastern Mediterranean Region
...	...	...	...	...	...	36	53	39	85	90	94	Western Pacific Region
64	49	...	51	30	...	76	62	34	60	78	87	Low income
39	63	...	39	...	...	49	49	41	64	56	88	Lower middle income
...	...	...	...	...	...	93	73	43	79	81	87	Upper middle income
...	...	...	...	...	...	...	...	81	80	67	63	High income
46	59	...	44	...	...	62	61	42	67	69	87	Global

Table 4

i. The case-detection rate for all forms of tuberculosis is the estimated number of new and relapse tuberculosis cases diagnosed and treated in national tuberculosis control programmes and notified to WHO, divided by WHO's estimate of the number of incident tuberculosis cases for the same year, expressed as a percentage. Global Tuberculosis Report 2013. Geneva: World Health Organization; 2013 (http://www.who.int/tb/publications/global_report/). For uncertainty ranges see the full report. WHO regional, income-group and global aggregates include territories.

j. The treatment-success rate for new pulmonary smear-positive tuberculosis cases is the proportion of new smear-positive tuberculosis cases registered under a national tuberculosis control programme in a given year that successfully completed treatment – with or without bacteriological evidence of success ("cured" and "treatment completed" respectively). Global Tuberculosis Report 2013. Geneva: World Health Organization; 2013 (http://www.who.int/tb/publications/global_report/). WHO regional, income-group and global aggregates include territories.

k. Definition of skilled personnel differs from standard definition.

l. Skilled personnel not defined.

m. Data only include information from Queensland, South Australia, Tasmania, Australian Capital Territory and the Northern Territory.

n. Five or more visits.

o. Institutional births.

p. Data refer to children aged 9–59 months.

q. Separate surveys for Wallonie, Brussels and the Flemish region all report institutional births above 99%.

r. Data from the public system only.

s. Only women who gave birth outside of a health facility.

t. Caesarean section covered by the Costa Rican Social Security Fund (Caja Costarricense del Seguro Social – CCSS).

u. Three or more visits.

v. ORT and/or RHF and/or increased fluids.

w. Data from national health institutions only.

x. No timing of postnatal visit was provided.

y. Mean number of visits reported is more than seven.

z. Six or more visits.

aa. Data from public hospitals only.

ab. The figure includes data from government and private hospitals.

ac. Postnatal care visit occurred 1 to 15 days postpartum.

ad. Continued feeding.

ae. Postnatal care visit occurred 0 to 7 days postpartum.

af. Deliveries in Ministry of Health institutions only.

ag. Postnatal care visit occurred 0 to 15 days postpartum.

ah. ORS or any other fluid.

ai. Separate datasets for England, Wales, Scotland and Northern Ireland report figures of 25, 26, 29 and 30 respectively.

5. Risk factors

Table 5 presents information on indicators for certain risk factors that are associated with increased mortality and morbidity. These preventable risk factors include: unsafe water and lack of sanitation; use of solid fuels in households; low birth weight; poor infant-feeding practices; childhood under-nutrition and overnutrition; diabetes; hypertension; obesity; harmful consumption of alcohol; use of tobacco; and unsafe sex.

Unsafe water supplies and inadequate levels of sanitation and hygiene increase the transmission of diarrhoeal diseases (including cholera); trachoma; and hepatitis. The use of solid fuels in households is a proxy indicator for household air pollution. Using solid fuels such as wood, charcoal and crops is associated with increased mortality from pneumonia and other acute lower respiratory diseases among children, as well as increased mortality from chronic obstructive pulmonary disease, lung cancer (where coal is used) and other diseases among adults.

More than one in 10 babies are born preterm (born alive before 37 weeks of pregnancy) and one million die from the complications of such births each year. More than three quarters of premature babies can be saved with feasible and cost-effective care.

Child growth is the most widely used measure of children's nutritional status. Included in the estimates presented in Table 5 are the four indicators: "wasted"; "stunted"; "underweight" (which is an MDG indicator); and "overweight". Stunting (i.e. low height-for-age) reflects the cumulative effects of under-nutrition and infections since birth – and even before birth. Evidence of this condition indicates chronic malnutrition, which is likely to have serious and long-lasting impacts on health. Being underweight may reflect wasting (i.e. low weight-for-height) which indicates acute weight loss and/or stunting. Thus, it is a composite indicator that is more difficult to interpret. Fewer data are available on the number of overweight children, although it is known that many countries face a double burden of malnutrition (with high numbers of underweight or stunted children) in some population groups coupled with high numbers of overweight children in other groups.

In adults, diabetes, hypertension and being overweight or obese increase the risk of cardiovascular disease and several types of cancer. These risks also contribute to non-fatal diseases such as arthritis and loss of vision due to diabetic retinopathy. Once considered a problem only in high-income countries, obesity is on the rise in low- and middle-income countries. The prevalence of hyperten-sion is highest in some low-income countries, whereas public health interventions have reduced its prevalence in many high-income countries.

The prevalence of current tobacco smoking is an important predictor of the future burden of tobacco-related diseases. Harmful use of alcohol can cause alcohol dependence, hepatic cirrhosis, cancer and injuries.

Data on risk factors and health-related behaviours are generally drawn from household surveys. It is important to note that the reliability of these estimates depends upon the overall quality of the sampling frames and methods used; on interviewer training, data-quality assurance procedures, and statistical data analyses; and on the ability and willingness of respondents to provide accurate responses. Where data from household surveys are not available, statistical techniques may be used to develop estimates.

Table 5

Member State	MDG 7 Population using improved drinking-water sources[a] (%)			Population using improved sanitation[a] (%)			Population using solid fuels[b] (%)	Preterm birth rate[c] (per 100 live births)	Infants exclusively breastfed for the first 6 months of life[d] (%)	Children aged <5 years[e] (%)				
										Wasted	Stunted	Underweight (MDG 1)		Overweight
	1990	2000	2012	1990	2000	2012	2012	2010	2006–2012	2006–2012		1990–1995	2006–2012	2006–2012
Afghanistan	...	22	64	...	23	29	81	12	54	...	...	...	...	...
Albania	...	96	96	79	84	91	38	9	3	9.4	23.1	...	6.3	23.4
Algeria	94	89	84	89	92	95	<5	7	7	...	...	9.2	...	...
Andorra	100	100	100	100	100	100	<5	...	...	...	...	...	...	...
Angola	42	46	54	29	42	60	56	13	...	8.2	29.2	...	15.6	...
Antigua and Barbuda	97	98	98	75	85	...	<5	6	...	...	...	...	...	...
Argentina	94	96	99	86	92	97	<5	8	55	...	...	1.7	...	...
Armenia	...	93	100	...	89	91	7	11	35	4.2	20.8	...	5.3	16.8
Australia	100	100	100	100	100	100	<5	8	...	0.0	1.8	...	0.2	8.0
Austria	100	100	100	100	100	100	<5	11	10	...	...	...	...	...
Azerbaijan	70	74	80	...	62	82	11	9	12	6.8	26.8	...	8.4	13.9
Bahamas	...	97	98	...	89	92	<5	10	...	...	...	...	...	...
Bahrain	95	99	100	99	99	99	<5	14	...	...	...	7.6	...	...
Bangladesh	68	76	85	33	45	57	89	14	64	15.7	41.4	61.5	36.8	1.9
Barbados	95	99	100	82	90	...	<5	9	...	...	...	...	...	...
Belarus	100	100	100	95	95	94	<5	4	19	...	...	...	...	...
Belgium	100	100	100	100	100	100	<5	8	...	...	...	...	...	...
Belize	73	85	99	76	83	91	14	10	15	3.3	19.3	5.4	6.2	7.9
Benin	57	66	76	5	9	14	94	11	33	16.0	44.6	...	21.3	17.9
Bhutan	...	86	98	...	35	47	37	10	49	5.9	33.6	...	12.8	7.6
Bolivia (Plurinational State of)	69	79	88	28	37	46	25	9	60	1.4	27.2	9.7	4.5	8.7
Bosnia and Herzegovina	97	98	100	...	95	95	58	8	22	2.3	8.9	...	1.5	17.4
Botswana	92	95	97	39	52	64	37	15	...	7.2	31.4	...	11.2	11.2
Brazil	88	93	98	67	75	81	6	9	40	1.6	7.1	...	2.2	7.3
Brunei Darussalam	...	...	...	...	...	...	<5	12	...	...	...	...	...	...
Bulgaria	100	100	99	99	100	100	12	8	...	...	...	...	...	...
Burkina Faso	44	60	82	8	12	19	95	11	25	10.9	32.9	29.6	24.4	2.8
Burundi	69	72	75	42	44	47	>95	11	69	6.1	57.5	...	29.1	2.9
Cabo Verde	...	83	89	...	44	65	31	11	...	...	...	11.8	...	...
Cambodia	22	42	71	3	16	37	89	11	74	10.8	40.9	...	29.0	1.9
Cameroon	51	62	74	40	42	45	78	13	20	5.8	32.6	18.0	15.1	6.5
Canada	100	100	100	100	100	100	<5	8	26	...	...	...	...	...
Central African Republic	59	62	68	15	17	22	>95	13	34	7.4	40.7	23.3	23.5	1.8
Chad	40	45	51	8	10	12	93	13	3	15.6	38.8	...	30.3	2.8
Chile	90	95	99	85	92	99	7	7	44	0.3	2.0	0.8	0.5	9.5
China	67	80	92	24	45	65	45	7	28	2.3	9.4	12.6	3.4	6.6
Colombia	88	90	91	69	75	80	15	9	43	0.9	12.7	6.3	3.4	4.8
Comoros	87	92	...	18	28	...	71	17	...	11.1	30.1	16.2	15.3	9.3
Congo	...	69	75	...	13	15	76	17	21	5.9	24.4	...	11.6	3.3
Cook Islands	100	100	100	...	92	97	17	...	...	...	...	...	...	...
Costa Rica	93	95	97	88	91	94	6	14	19	1.0	5.6	2.5	1.1	8.1
Côte d'Ivoire	76	78	80	15	18	22	79	14	12	7.1	28.0	20.9	14.1	2.8
Croatia	98	98	99	98	98	98	7	6	...	...	...	0.6	...	...
Cuba	...	91	94	81	87	93	7	6	49	...	...	...	...	...
Cyprus	100	100	100	100	100	100	<5	15	...	...	...	...	...	...
Czech Republic	100	100	100	100	100	100	<5	7	...	...	...	0.9	...	...
Democratic People's Republic of Korea	100	100	98	...	61	82	92	11	89	4.0	27.9	...	15.2	0.0
Democratic Republic of the Congo	43	44	46	17	23	31	93	12	37	8.5	43.5	30.7	24.2	4.9

118

Prevalence of raised fasting blood glucose[f] (≥ 25 years) (%)		Prevalence of raised blood pressure[g] (≥ 25 years) (%)		Adults aged ≥20 years who are obese[h] (%)		Alcohol consumption among adults aged ≥15 years[i] (litres of pure alcohol per person per year)	Prevalence of smoking any tobacco product among adults aged ≥15 years[j] (%)		Prevalence of current tobacco use among adolescents aged 13–15 years[k] (%)		Prevalence of condom use by adults aged 15–49 years during higher-risk sex[l] (%)		Population aged 15–24 years with comprehensive correct knowledge of HIV/AIDS[m] (%)		Member State
Male	Female	Male	Female	Male	Female		Male	Female	Male	Female	Male	Female	Male	Female	
2008		2008		2008		2010	2011		2006–2012		2006–2010		2006–2010		
8.9[n]	9.5[n]	27.2[n]	27.9[n]	1.5[n]	3.3[n]	0.7	...	...	...	...	...	...	...	...	Afghanistan
10.3[n]	9.0[n]	39.3	31.7	21.7	20.5	7.0	48	5	18	7	37	...	22	36	Albania
9.0	9.3	33.9	33.2	10.7	24.3	1.0	28	2	...	...	...	...	...	...	Algeria
10.4[n]	7.0[n]	29.2[n]	17.5[n]	25.7[n]	22.6[n]	13.8	...	...	...	...	...	...	...	...	Andorra
8.2[n]	8.7[n]	39.6[n]	33.8[n]	3.8[n]	10.2[n]	7.5	...	...	...	...	...	...	...	...	Angola
11.3[n]	12.0[n]	38.5[n]	27.5[n]	18.1[n]	33.1[n]	5.4	...	...	24	16	...	...	...	...	Antigua and Barbuda
11.0	10.3	31.0	17.9	27.4	31.0	9.3	30	16	23	25	...	...	...	...	Argentina
11.5[n]	11.5[n]	42.1	37.0	14.4	30.2	5.3	47	2	11	4	72	...	...	...	Armenia
9.6	6.7	22.8	13.7	25.2	24.9	12.2	21	19	...	...	...	...	...	...	Australia
7.1	4.6	28.7	19.8	19.2	17.1	10.3	46	47	...	...	...	...	...	...	Austria
12.1[n]	12.3[n]	36.6	30.9	15.8	32.1	2.3	34	<1	11	2	26	0	5	5	Azerbaijan
12.7[n]	13.7[n]	37.6[n]	25.6[n]	26.7[n]	42.6[n]	6.9	...	...	18	15	...	...	...	...	Bahamas
13.5	12.1	34.5	32.9	28.9	38.2	2.1	35	8	...	...	...	...	...	...	Bahrain
9.2	9.9	27.4[n]	27.9[n]	1.0	1.3	0.2	48	2	9	5	...	...	...	...	Bangladesh
12.8	15.2	35.4	29.1	21.6	44.2	6.8	13	2	35	23	...	...	...	...	Barbados
10.4[n]	10.0[n]	44.3	32.9	19.7[n]	26.4[n]	17.5	50	11	...	...	...	...	...	...	Belarus
9.3[n]	6.4[n]	24.6	16.8	21.2	16.9	11.0	31	23	...	...	...	...	...	...	Belgium
8.7	12.7	30.2	22.4	24.4	45.4	8.5	22	2	22	15	...	...	0	43	Belize
6.7	6.5	38.1	34.1	3.5	9.5	2.1	21	3	...	...	22	30	14	8	Benin
12.0	12.6	29.0	26.9	4.7	6.6	0.7	...	...	28	12	...	...	...	...	Bhutan
8.9[n]	10.2[n]	30.7[n]	23.5[n]	10.0	27.1	5.9	42	18	21	16	35	...	28	22	Bolivia (Plurinational State of)
11.4[n]	10.4[n]	38.7	38.4	22.7	25.3	7.1	44	27	16	11	44	17	47	48	Bosnia and Herzegovina
8.0[n]	10.0[n]	39.1	37.9	3.0	22.8	8.4	36	7	27	21	...	...	...	...	Botswana
10.4	10.0	39.4	26.6	16.5	22.1	8.7	22	13	...	...	...	...	...	...	Brazil
8.7[n]	5.9[n]	23.6[n]	16.9[n]	8.5[n]	7.2[n]	0.9	32	4	...	...	...	...	...	...	Brunei Darussalam
10.4[n]	8.9[n]	40.0	31.2	22.0	20.4	11.4	48	31	26	32	...	...	...	...	Bulgaria
8.9[n]	8.7[n]	36.7[n]	35.2[n]	1.7	3.0	6.8	...	...	...	...	27	62	36	31	Burkina Faso
6.2[n]	5.9[n]	42.2[n]	39.5[n]	2.8[n]	3.7[n]	9.3	...	...	21	17	14	14	47	45	Burundi
15.6	14.7	47.7	38.4	6.3	15.3	6.9	14	3	15	12	73	51	89	90	Cabo Verde
4.7	5.2	22.5	16.8	1.6	2.8	5.5	42	3	8	5	40	...	44	44	Cambodia
9.5	10.4	35.6	29.8	7.0	15.1	8.4	...	...	...	...	43	37	34	29	Cameroon
10.9[n]	8.3[n]	17.4	13.2	24.6	23.9	10.2	20	15	...	...	...	...	...	...	Canada
7.3[n]	8.0[n]	39.1	34.5[n]	2.0	5.3	3.8	...	...	...	...	...	...	27	17	Central African Republic
8.8[n]	8.7[n]	35.5	31.3	2.4	3.8	4.4	20	4	21	14	...	...	...	...	Chad
11.2	9.5	39.4	27.4	24.5	33.6	9.6	44	38	...	...	...	...	...	...	Chile
9.6	9.4	29.8	25.6	4.6	6.5	6.7	47	2	...	...	...	...	...	...	China
6.7	6.1	34.3	26.5	11.9	23.7	6.2	31	5	...	...	...	34	0	24	Colombia
7.9[n]	7.6[n]	40.8[n]	36.5[n]	3.5	5.3	0.2	25	2	22	15	...	...	...	...	Comoros
7.8[n]	8.5[n]	40.3	36.1	2.8	7.5	3.9	9	3	28	20	28	29	22	8	Congo
20.5	21.1	40.1	28.1	59.7	68.5	6.4	41	27	34	36	...	...	...	...	Cook Islands
10.1	10.2	31.6	22.5	20.9	28.3	5.4	24	8	16	13	...	...	...	...	Costa Rica
9.2[n]	9.7[n]	41.6	35.7	3.9	9.7	6.0	16	9	26	11	...	...	...	...	Côte d'Ivoire
10.2[n]	8.4[n]	42.4	34.2	22.8	19.4	12.2	36	30	29	28	...	...	...	...	Croatia
11.3	12.0	33.2[n]	28.7[n]	13.3	27.5	5.2	...	...	20	15	...	...	...	...	Cuba
10.2[n]	6.8[n]	28.9	18.5	24.8	21.9	9.2	41	18	29	11	...	...	...	...	Cyprus
11.5	9.1	39.3	27.7	30.5	26.5	13.0	40	32	35	38	...	...	...	...	Czech Republic
7.7[n]	7.5[n]	26.7[n]	23.7[n]	3.7[n]	3.9[n]	3.7	...	...	...	...	...	...	...	8	Democratic People's Republic of Korea
6.6[n]	7.8[n]	38.5	33.3	0.7	3.0	3.6	16	5	...	...	16	9	21	15	Democratic Republic of the Congo

119

5. Risk factors

Member State	Population using improved drinking-water sources[a] (%)			Population using improved sanitation[a] (%)			Population using solid fuels[b] (%)	Preterm birth rate[c] (per 100 live births)	Infants exclusively breastfed for the first 6 months of life[d] (%)	Children aged <5 years[e] (%)				
										Wasted	Stunted	Underweight		Overweight
	1990	2000	2012	1990	2000	2012	2012	2010	2006–2012	2006–2012		1990 –1995	2006 –2012	2006 –2012
Denmark	100	100	100	100	100	100	<5	7	...	...	...	...	...	...
Djibouti	77	82	92	62	62	61	14	12	1	21.5	33.5	...	29.8	8.1
Dominica	...	94	...	...	81	...	7	12	...	...	...	...	...	...
Dominican Republic	89	86	81	73	77	82	8	11	8	2.3	10.1	8.4	3.4	8.3
Ecuador	74	80	86	57	70	83	<5	5	44	...	...	...	...	...
Egypt	93	96	99	72	86	96	<5	7	53	7.9	30.7	10.5	6.8	20.5
El Salvador	75	84	90	50	61	70	21	13	31	1.6	20.6	7.2	6.6	5.7
Equatorial Guinea	...	51	...	...	89	...	78	17	...	...	...	...	...	...
Eritrea	43	54	...	9	11	...	63	12	...	...	...	36.9	...	...
Estonia	99	99	99	95	95	95	12	6	...	...	...	...	...	...
Ethiopia	13	29	52	2	8	24	>95	10	52	10.1	44.2	43.3	29.2	1.8
Fiji	85	91	96	57	74	87	40	10	...	...	...	6.9	...	...
Finland	100	100	100	100	100	100	<5	6	...	...	...	...	...	...
France	100	100	100	100	100	100	<5	7	...	...	...	...	...	...
Gabon	...	84	92	...	39	41	21	16	6	3.4	17.5	...	6.5	7.7
Gambia	76	83	90	...	61	60	>95	14	36	9.5	23.4	...	17.4	1.9
Georgia	85	89	99	96	95	93	46	9	...	1.6	11.3	...	1.1	19.9
Germany	100	100	100	100	100	100	<5	9	...	...	...	...	...	...
Ghana	54	71	87	7	10	14	84	15	46	6.2	22.7	25.1	13.4	1.4
Greece	96	99	100	97	98	99	<5	7	...	...	...	...	...	...
Grenada	97	97	97	98	98	98	<5	10	...	...	...	...	...	...
Guatemala	81	87	94	62	71	80	64	8	50	1.1	48.0	21.7	13.0	4.9
Guinea	52	63	75	8	13	19	>95	14	21	5.6	35.8	21.2	16.3	3.1
Guinea-Bissau	36	52	74	...	12	20	>95	11	38	5.8	32.2	...	18.1	3.2
Guyana	77	86	98	76	79	84	7	13	33	5.3	19.5	16.1	11.1	6.7
Haiti	61	61	62	19	21	24	93	14	40	5.2	21.9	23.7	11.6	3.6
Honduras	73	81	90	48	63	80	51	12	31	1.4	22.7	15.8	7.1	5.2
Hungary	96	99	100	100	100	100	12	9	...	...	...	...	...	...
Iceland	100	100	100	100	100	100	<5	7	...	...	...	...	...	...
India	70	81	93	18	25	36	63	13	46	20.0	47.9	56.6	43.5	1.9
Indonesia	70	78	85	35	47	59	47	16	42	12.3	39.2	29.8	18.6	12.3
Iran (Islamic Republic of)	92	94	96	71	79	89	<5	13	28	4.0	6.8	13.8	4.1	...
Iraq	78	80	85	...	75	85	<5	7	20	7.4	22.6	10.4	8.5	11.8
Ireland	100	100	100	99	99	99	<5	6	15	...	...	...	...	...
Israel	100	100	100	100	100	100	<5	8	...	...	...	...	...	...
Italy	100	100	100	...	...	...	<5	7	...	...	...	...	...	...
Jamaica	93	93	93	79	80	80	13	10	...	3.5	4.8	4.0	3.2	4.0
Japan	100	100	100	100	100	100	<5	6	...	...	...	...	...	...
Jordan	97	97	96	97	98	98	<5	14	23	2.4	7.8	4.8	3.0	4.7
Kazakhstan	94	94	93	96	97	97	9	9	32	4.1	13.1	6.7	3.7	13.3
Kenya	43	52	62	25	27	30	84	12	32	7.0	35.2	20.1	16.4	5.0
Kiribati	50	59	67	28	34	40	45	10	69	...	...	...	14.2	...
Kuwait	99	99	99	100	100	100	<5	11	...	2.4	4.3	9.2	2.2	9.5
Kyrgyzstan	73	79	88	91	91	92	34	10	56	2.7	17.7	...	3.4	8.5
Lao People's Democratic Republic	...	45	72	...	28	65	>95	11	40	7.3	47.6	39.8	31.6	1.3
Latvia	98	98	98	...	79	...	6	5	29	...	...	...	...	...
Lebanon	100	100	100	...	98	...	<5	8	15	...	...	...	...	...
Lesotho	78	79	81	...	24	30	62	12	54	3.9	39.0	13.8	13.5	7.3

120

Table 5

Prevalence of raised fasting blood glucose[f] (≥ 25 years) (%)		Prevalence of raised blood pressure[g] (≥ 25 years) (%)		Adults aged ≥20 years who are obese[h] (%)		Alcohol consumption among adults aged ≥15 years[i] (litres of pure alcohol per person per year)	Prevalence of smoking any tobacco product among adults aged ≥15 years[j] (%)		Prevalence of current tobacco use among adolescents aged 13–15 years[k] (%)		MDG 6 Prevalence of condom use by adults aged 15–49 years during higher-risk sex[l] (%)		Population aged 15–24 years with comprehensive correct knowledge of HIV/AIDS[m] (%)		Member State
Male	Female	Male	Female	Male	Female		Male	Female	Male	Female	Male	Female	Male	Female	
2008		2008		2008		2010	2011		2006–2012		2006–2010		2006–2010		
8.8[n]	5.9[n]	26.5	15.6	17.1	15.4	11.4	30	27	...	...	...	...	...	...	Denmark
9.7[n]	9.4[n]	38.8[n]	32.5[n]	6.7[n]	13.8[n]	1.3	...	...	23	14	...	...	...	...	Djibouti
15.6	20.7	41.9	35.3	10.1	39.1	7.1	11	4	30	20	...	...	...	...	Dominica
8.0	9.0	35.6	29.5	14.4	29.3	6.9	17	16	24	14	45	35	34	41	Dominican Republic
9.2[n]	9.8[n]	32.3[n]	23.9[n]	15.7	28.2	7.2	...	...	...	...	...	...	...	...	Ecuador
7.0	7.4	27.1	27.0	22.5	46.3	0.4	46	<1	20	4	...	...	...	...	Egypt
11.3	10.7	27.8	20.7	20.2	32.9	3.2	24	3	18	11	...	...	...	...	El Salvador
8.7[n]	8.7[n]	43.5[n]	35.8[n]	7.9[n]	14.8[n]	6.6	...	...	25	17	...	...	...	...	Equatorial Guinea
7.8[n]	7.3[n]	32.2	28.1	1.3	2.3	1.1	13	<1	8	5	18	2	34	25	Eritrea
9.0	7.8	47.3	33.2	20.2	17.6	10.3	43	21	34	28	...	...	...	...	Estonia
7.3[n]	7.0[n]	33.0	28.3	0.9	1.6	4.2	...	...	...	...	16	47	34	24	Ethiopia
13.2	16.4	32.5	29.7	21.3	42.2	3.0	...	...	18	10	...	...	...	...	Fiji
10.3	6.3	34.9	22.7	21.0	18.6	12.3	27	20	...	...	...	...	...	...	Finland
7.2	4.3	29.1	16.2	16.8	14.6	12.2	39	32	...	...	...	...	...	...	France
9.1[n]	9.9[n]	40.0	33.0	8.4	21.5	10.9	19	3	...	...	51	44	36	29	Gabon
9.9	11.3	39.7	34.2	2.3	14.4	3.4	32	3	...	...	...	...	...	...	Gambia
11.9[n]	11.1[n]	42.6	34.3	15.9[n]	25.7[n]	7.7	55	3	15	3	...	...	...	...	Georgia
9.8	6.3	31.1	20.7	23.1	19.2	11.8	35	25	...	...	...	...	...	...	Germany
9.9	10.3	32.7	31.6	4.4	11.7	4.8	14	7	14	11	26	18	34	28	Ghana
9.5	7.9	25.1	19.8	18.8	16.1	10.3	46	34	...	...	...	...	...	...	Greece
11.1[n]	12.4[n]	35.9[n]	28.1[n]	14.9[n]	32.1[n]	12.5	...	...	25	17	...	...	...	...	Grenada
11.5	14.0	28.5	22.2	13.8	26.7	3.8	20	2	20	13	...	...	...	...	Guatemala
8.8[n]	8.6[n]	38.4[n]	36.8[n]	4.3	5.1	0.7	23	2	31	20	...	...	...	...	Guinea
8.6[n]	9.1[n]	37.6[n]	35.3[n]	2.6[n]	8.1[n]	4.0	...	...	...	...	...	...	...	...	Guinea-Bissau
10.8[n]	13.1[n]	32.1[n]	28.0[n]	8.3[n]	27.1[n]	8.1	27	6	25	16	65	48	47	54	Guyana
9.6[n]	9.6[n]	33.6[n]	28.1[n]	8.4	8.4	6.4	...	...	...	...	43	43	40	34	Haiti
8.6	8.4	30.8	25.1	12.9	26.3	4.0	...	...	...	...	...	27	0	30	Honduras
10.6[n]	8.5[n]	42.7	31.3	26.2	22.9	13.3	35	27	41	30	...	...	...	...	Hungary
10.9[n]	6.9[n]	25.8	14.2	23.4	20.3	7.1	19	18	...	...	...	...	...	...	Iceland
11.1	10.8	23.1	22.6	1.3	2.5	4.3	25	4	19	8	23	12	36	20	India
6.6	7.1	32.5	29.3	2.5	6.9	0.6	67	3	41	6	...	...	...	...	Indonesia
9.3	10.5	30.9	26.9	13.6	29.5	1.0	26	<1	33	20	...	...	...	...	Iran (Islamic Republic of)
12.7	12.5	30.1[n]	28.7[n]	22.3	36.2	0.5	31	4	...	...	...	...	...	...	Iraq
8.4	5.6	34.9	20.7	25.7	23.3	11.9	...	...	...	...	...	...	...	...	Ireland
10.2	8.7	23.1	16.5	23.2	27.6	2.8	35	17	...	...	...	...	...	...	Israel
8.8	5.4	28.6	20.6	19.3	14.9	6.7	31	18	...	...	...	...	...	...	Italy
10.2	12.9	32.3	28.0	10.0	38.2	4.9	...	...	31	25	...	...	...	...	Jamaica
7.2	4.7	26.4	16.7	5.5	3.5	7.2	34	11	...	...	...	...	...	...	Japan
17.2	18.1	26.0	20.3	27.3	41.7	0.7	47	6	34	19	...	...	5	13	Jordan
12.5[n]	10.8[n]	40.4[n]	31.8[n]	20.2	27.4	10.3	40	9	12	8	...	...	...	...	Kazakhstan
7.6[n]	7.8[n]	37.1	33.0	2.5	6.8	4.3	26	<1	15	15	37	32	55	47	Kenya
23.6	24.9	31.2	21.6	37.7	53.6	3.0	67	37	43	32	...	...	...	...	Kiribati
17.0	14.8	29.0	23.7	37.2	52.4	0.1	35	4	25	11	...	...	...	...	Kuwait
11.1[n]	10.4[n]	38.5[n]	33.4[n]	11.7	21.6	4.3	45	2	10	4	...	...	...	...	Kyrgyzstan
7.1[n]	7.6[n]	28.1	24.0	1.7	4.1	7.3	48	4	19	6	...	...	...	...	Lao People's Democratic Republic
10.4[n]	9.0[n]	44.5[n]	32.7[n]	21.5	21.8	12.3	46	20	39	41	...	...	...	...	Latvia
13.0	11.0	33.9	26.1	26.4	29.7	2.4	...	...	...	...	...	...	...	...	Lebanon
9.0[n]	12.0[n]	36.4[n]	35.9[n]	3.1	26.6	6.5	...	...	26	22	52	39	29	39	Lesotho

Member State	Population using improved drinking-water sources[a] (%) MDG 7			Population using improved sanitation[a] (%)			Population using solid fuels[b] (%)	Preterm birth rate[c] (per 100 live births)	Infants exclusively breastfed for the first 6 months of life[d] (%)	Children aged <5 years[e] (%)				
										Wasted	Stunted	Underweight MDG 1		Overweight
												1990–1995	2006–2012	2006–2012
	1990	2000	2012	1990	2000	2012	2012	2010	2006–2012	2006–2012				
Liberia	...	61	75	...	14	17	>95	14	29	2.8	41.8	...	14.9	4.2
Libya	54	54	...	97	97	97	<5	8	...	6.5	21.0	4.3	5.6	22.4
Lithuania	87	91	96	84	89	94	<5	6	...	...	...	...	...	...
Luxembourg	100	100	100	100	100	100	<5	8	...	...	...	...	...	...
Madagascar	29	38	50	8	11	14	>95	14	51	...	49.2	35.5	...	...
Malawi	42	62	85	10	10	10	>95	18	71	4.1	47.8	24.4	13.8	9.2
Malaysia	88	96	100	84	92	96	<5	12	...	...	17.2	22.1	12.9	...
Maldives	93	95	99	68	79	99	7	8	48	10.2	20.3	32.5	17.8	6.5
Mali	28	45	67	15	18	22	>95	12	38	8.9	27.8	...	18.9	4.7
Malta	100	100	100	100	100	100	<5	6	...	...	...	...	...	...
Marshall Islands	92	93	95	65	70	76	32	12	27	...	...	...	...	...
Mauritania	30	40	50	16	21	27	56	15	19	11.6	22.0	43.3	19.5	1.2
Mauritius	99	99	100	89	89	91	<5	13	...	...	...	13.0	...	...
Mexico	82	89	95	66	75	85	14	7	15	1.6	13.6	...	2.8	9.0
Micronesia (Federated States of)	91	90	89	19	34	57	42	11	...	...	...	...	...	...
Monaco	100	100	100	100	100	100	<5	...	...	...	...	...	...	...
Mongolia	62	68	85	...	49	56	70	14	66	2.3	15.9	10.8	4.7	...
Montenegro	97	98	98	...	90	90	28	9	19	4.2	7.9	...	2.2	15.6
Morocco	73	78	84	52	64	75	<5	7	15	2.3	14.9	8.1	3.1	10.7
Mozambique	34	41	49	8	14	21	>95	16	43	6.1	43.1	23.9	15.6	7.9
Myanmar	56	67	86	...	61	77	93	12	24	7.9	35.1	28.8	22.6	2.6
Namibia	67	79	92	24	28	32	55	14	24	7.5	29.6	21.5	17.5	4.6
Nauru	...	93	96	66	66	66	<5	...	67	1.0	24.0	...	4.8	2.8
Nepal	66	77	88	6	21	37	80	14	70	11.2	40.5	44.1	29.1	1.5
Netherlands	100	100	100	100	100	100	<5	8	...	...	...	...	...	...
New Zealand	100	100	100	...	...	...	<5	8	...	...	...	...	...	...
Nicaragua	74	80	85	43	48	52	54	9	31	1.5	23.0	9.6	5.7	6.2
Niger	34	42	52	5	7	9	94	9	23	18.0	43.9	41.0	36.4	2.4
Nigeria	46	55	64	37	32	28	75	12	15	10.2	36.0	35.1	24.4	3.0
Niue	99	99	99	...	79	100	5	...	...	...	...	...	...	...
Norway	100	100	100	100	100	100	<5	6	...	...	...	...	...	...
Oman	79	84	93	82	89	97	<5	14	...	7.1	9.8	21.4	8.6	1.7
Pakistan	85	88	91	27	37	48	62	16	38	14.8	43.0	39.0	30.9	6.4
Palau	90	92	...	46	81	100	<5	...	...	...	...	...	...	...
Panama	84	90	94	60	67	73	17	8	14	1.2	19.1	...	3.9	...
Papua New Guinea	...	35	...	20	19	19	70	7	56	16.2	48.2	...	27.2	...
Paraguay	53	73	94	37	58	80	46	8	24	...	...	2.8	...	...
Peru	74	81	87	54	63	73	36	7	68	0.6	18.1	8.8	3.4	6.9
Philippines	84	88	92	57	66	74	49	15	34	7.3	33.6	29.9	20.2	4.3
Poland	...	...	...	...	89	...	<5	7	...	...	...	...	...	...
Portugal	96	98	100	94	98	100	<5	8	...	...	...	...	...	...
Qatar	100	100	100	100	100	100	<5	11	...	...	...	4.8	...	...
Republic of Korea	...	93	98	100	100	100	<5	9	89	...	...	...	...	...
Republic of Moldova	...	93	97	...	79	87	11	12	...	...	...	...	...	...
Romania	75	84	...	71	72	...	21	7	...	...	...	5.0	...	...
Russian Federation	93	95	97	74	72	70	<5	7	...	...	...	...	...	...
Rwanda	60	66	71	30	47	64	>95	10	85	3.0	44.3	24.3	11.7	7.1
Saint Kitts and Nevis	98	98	98	...	87	...	<5	...	...	...	...	...	...	...

Prevalence of raised fasting blood glucose[f] (≥ 25 years) (%)		Prevalence of raised blood pressure[g] (≥ 25 years) (%)		Adults aged ≥20 years who are obese[h] (%)		Alcohol consumption among adults aged ≥15 years[i] (litres of pure alcohol per person per year)	Prevalence of smoking any tobacco product among adults aged ≥15 years[j] (%)		Prevalence of current tobacco use among adolescents aged 13–15 years[k] (%)		MDG 6 Prevalence of condom use by adults aged 15–49 years during higher-risk sex[l] (%)		Population aged 15–24 years with comprehensive correct knowledge of HIV/AIDS[m] (%)		Member State
Male	Female	Male	Female	Male	Female		Male	Female	Male	Female	Male	Female	Male	Female	
2008		2008		2008		2010	2011		2006–2012		2006–2010		2006–2010		
8.4[n]	9.3[n]	38.5[n]	35.7[n]	3.1	7.7	4.7	18	2	...	...	22	14	27	21	Liberia
14.5	14.4	45.2	38.9	21.5	41.3	0.1	45	<1	11	5	...	...	...	...	Libya
11.2[n]	9.7[n]	45.5	34.3	23.9	24.7	15.4	43	25	38	29	...	...	...	...	Lithuania
9.9[n]	6.7[n]	28.5[n]	17.9[n]	24.5	22.2	11.9	...	...	...	...	...	...	...	...	Luxembourg
8.1[n]	7.0[n]	40.6	37.5	1.8	1.5	1.8	...	...	33	14	7	8	26	23	Madagascar
6.4	6.2	44.5	39.4	2.6	6.2	2.5	23	5	17	11	25	27	45	42	Malawi
11.6	11.2	28.8	24.6	10.4	17.9	1.3	43	1	35	9	...	...	...	...	Malaysia
7.8	7.5	30.6[n]	24.5[n]	6.5	26.1	1.2	42	7	15	7	...	...	...	35	Maldives
9.0[n]	9.5[n]	30.5	31.3	2.4	6.8	1.1	28	2	23	9	12	8	22	18	Mali
11.8	8.9	29.9	20.3	26.1	26.8	7.0	31	20	...	...	...	...	...	...	Malta
25.5	31.9	29.6	22.7	38.8	53.9	...	36	7	29	22	20	11	39	27	Marshall Islands
7.5	8.3	38.4[n]	33.9[n]	4.3	23.3	0.1	29	4	28	18	...	...	...	...	Mauritania
11.6	9.9	40.6[n]	34.5[n]	12.9	23.0	3.6	39	5	20	8	...	...	...	...	Mauritius
13.2	14.9	27.4	21.5	26.7	38.4	7.2	27	8	22	18	...	...	...	...	Mexico
14.0	19.8	36.9	27.0	30.9	53.4	3.3	...	...	52	40	...	...	...	...	Micronesia (Federated States of)
...	...	...	...	...	...	...	...	...	...	...	...	...	...	...	Monaco
10.9	8.9	44.8	32.9	11.9	20.7	6.9	48	6	26	16	...	...	...	...	Mongolia
9.8[n]	8.4[n]	42.0[n]	32.5[n]	22.8[n]	20.7[n]	8.7	...	...	7	6	...	...	22	22	Montenegro
10.6	10.9	34.0	37.6	11.1	23.1	0.9	32	2	11	7	...	...	...	...	Morocco
8.0[n]	8.2[n]	46.3	41.4	2.6	7.8	2.3	...	...	...	...	26	31	52	30	Mozambique
6.1	7.1	34.0	29.2	2.0	6.1	0.7	38	7	30	7	...	...	...	...	Myanmar
8.6[n]	9.6[n]	43.7	38.1	4.3	16.8	10.8	30	9	32	30	74	66	53	59	Namibia
12.8	15.2	40.3	29.9	67.5	74.7	3.5	52	50	...	...	...	...	...	...	Nauru
9.8	9.3	26.6[n]	28.6[n]	1.4	1.6	2.2	37	25	25	16	27	...	34	26	Nepal
6.1	4.1	28.9	17.6	16.1	16.1	9.9	29	23	...	...	...	...	...	...	Netherlands
11.1[n]	8.8[n]	22.8	15.1	26.2	27.7	10.9	21	19	19	22	...	...	...	...	New Zealand
8.6	9.4	31.9	24.7	16.8	31.3	5.0	...	...	...	...	...	...	...	...	Nicaragua
7.8[n]	8.3[n]	50.3	41.0	1.5	3.7	0.3	9	<1	12	6	7	8	16	13	Niger
7.9	12.0	38.6	41.2	5.1	9.0	10.1	10	2	...	...	33	23	33	22	Nigeria
...	...	...	...	...	...	8.0	...	...	14	19	...	...	...	...	Niue
10.6	7.7	33.7	22.2	21.6	17.9	7.7	28	26	...	...	...	...	...	...	Norway
12.0	12.3	32.4	27.5	19.4	25.9	0.9	13	<1	5	2	...	...	...	...	Oman
11.7	14.1	28.6	28.0	3.5	8.4	0.1	38	7	...	...	...	...	...	...	Pakistan
17.5[n]	19.0[n]	34.6[n]	25.5[n]	44.9[n]	56.3[n]	7.9	...	...	58	42	...	...	...	...	Palau
10.9[n]	11.2[n]	33.1[n]	23.3[n]	19.4	32.1	8.0	23	4	15	10	...	...	...	...	Panama
15.2	14.7	21.1	18.1	11.8	20.1	3.0	55	27	55	40	...	...	...	...	Papua New Guinea
10.6	10.1	34.6[n]	24.8[n]	16.2[n]	22.3[n]	8.8	30	8	21	13	...	...	...	...	Paraguay
5.8	6.1	26.0	19.6	11.1	21.7	8.1	...	...	22	17	...	31	...	19	Peru
6.5	6.6	28.7	23.6	4.5	8.3	5.4	44	10	19	9	...	...	...	21	Philippines
8.2	6.9	41.3	33.0	22.9	22.9	12.5	38	27	...	...	...	...	...	...	Poland
7.5	5.7	34.5	24.3	20.4	22.3	12.9	30	15	...	...	...	...	...	...	Portugal
12.4	11.0	34.4	27.6	30.8	39.3	1.5	...	...	25	13	...	...	...	...	Qatar
6.8	5.3	18.0	13.1	6.9	7.7	12.3	...	...	15	11	...	...	...	...	Republic of Korea
9.5[n]	11.1[n]	40.4[n]	34.0[n]	10.0	28.8	16.8	43	5	21	7	...	...	...	...	Republic of Moldova
10.0[n]	8.9[n]	39.0	32.9	16.3	19.0	14.4	38	18	18	10	...	...	...	...	Romania
10.5[n]	10.7[n]	37.2	31.8	18.4	29.8	15.1	59	25	...	...	...	...	...	...	Russian Federation
6.7[n]	6.1[n]	43.6[n]	40.2[n]	4.9	4.0	9.8	...	...	13	10	28	29	46	52	Rwanda
13.6[n]	14.6[n]	43.2	32.5	32.0	49.4	8.2	12	3	10	8	...	...	...	...	Saint Kitts and Nevis

5. Risk factors

Member State	Population using improved drinking-water sources[a] (%)			Population using improved sanitation[a] (%)			Population using solid fuels[b] (%)	Preterm birth rate[c] (per 100 live births)	Infants exclusively breastfed for the first 6 months of life[d] (%)	Children aged <5 years[e] (%)				
										Wasted	Stunted	Underweight (MDG 1)		Overweight
	1990	2000	2012	1990	2000	2012	2012	2010	2006–2012	2006–2012		1990–1995	2006–2012	2006–2012
Saint Lucia	93	94	94	58	62	...	<5	11	...	...	...	...	...	...
Saint Vincent and the Grenadines	88	93	95	63	73	...	<5	12	...	...	...	...	...	...
Samoa	89	93	99	93	92	92	61	6	51	...	...	...	...	...
San Marino	...	...	...	...	...	...	<5	...	...	...	...	...	...	...
Sao Tome and Principe	...	78	97	...	21	34	71	11	51	11.2	31.6	...	14.4	11.6
Saudi Arabia	92	95	97	92	97	100	<5	6	...	...	...	13.5	...	...
Senegal	60	66	74	35	43	52	56	10	38	8.7	15.5	19.0	14.4	0.7
Serbia	99	100	99	96	96	97	32	7	14	3.5	6.6	...	1.6	15.6
Seychelles	96	96	96	97	97	97	<5	12	...	...	...	...	...	...
Sierra Leone	37	47	60	11	12	13	>95	10	32	9.2	44.9	25.4	21.1	10.3
Singapore	100	100	100	99	100	100	<5	12	...	...	...	...	...	...
Slovakia	100	100	100	100	100	100	<5	6	...	...	...	...	...	...
Slovenia	100	100	100	100	100	100	<5	8	...	...	...	...	...	...
Solomon Islands	...	80	81	...	25	29	92	12	74	4.3	32.8	...	11.5	2.5
Somalia	...	23	...	...	22	...	>95	12	9	13.2	42.1	...	32.8	4.7
South Africa	81	87	95	58	65	74	13	8	...	4.7	23.9	8.0	8.7	...
South Sudan	...	...	57	...	...	9	>95	...	...	22.7	31.1	...	27.6	6.0
Spain	100	100	100	100	100	100	<5	7	...	...	...	...	...	...
Sri Lanka	68	79	94	68	79	92	74	11	76	11.8	19.2	33.8	21.6	0.8
Sudan	67	62	55	27	25	24	72	13 [o]	41	14.5	38.3	...	27.0	4.2
Suriname	...	89	95	...	81	80	11	9	3	5.0	8.8	...	5.8	4.0
Swaziland	39	52	74	49	52	57	62	14	44	0.8	31.0	...	5.8	10.7
Sweden	100	100	100	100	100	100	<5	6	...	...	...	...	...	...
Switzerland	100	100	100	100	100	100	<5	7	...	...	...	...	...	...
Syrian Arab Republic	86	88	90	85	89	96	<5	11	29	11.5	27.5	11.5	10.1	17.9
Tajikistan	...	60	72	...	90	94	37	11	34	9.9	26.2	...	12.1	5.9
Thailand	86	92	96	82	91	93	24	12	15	4.7	15.7	16.3	7.0	8.0
The former Yugoslav Republic of Macedonia	99	99	99	...	90	91	33	7	23	1.8	4.9	...	1.3	12.4
Timor-Leste	...	54	70	...	37	39	94	12	52	18.9	57.7	...	45.3	5.8
Togo	48	53	61	13	12	11	>95	13	62	4.8	29.8	...	16.5	1.6
Tonga	99	99	99	95	94	91	45	8	...	...	...	...	...	...
Trinidad and Tobago	90	92	...	93	92	92	<5	8	13	...	...	...	...	...
Tunisia	82	89	97	73	82	90	<5	9	9	3.0	10.0	8.1	2.0	14.0
Turkey	85	93	100	84	87	91	<5	12	42	0.8	12.3	8.7	1.7	...
Turkmenistan	...	83	71	98	98	99	<5	10	...	...	...	...	...	...
Tuvalu	90	94	98	73	78	83	17	...	35	3.3	10.0	...	1.6	6.3
Uganda	42	56	75	26	30	34	>95	14	63	4.8	33.7	21.5	14.1	3.8
Ukraine	...	97	98	...	95	94	<5	7	18	...	...	...	...	...
United Arab Emirates	100	100	100	97	97	98	<5	8	...	...	...	...	...	...
United Kingdom	100	100	100	100	100	100	<5	8	...	...	...	...	...	...
United Republic of Tanzania	55	54	53	7	9	12	>95	11	50	6.6	34.8	25.1	13.6	5.5
United States of America	98	99	99	100	100	100	<5	12	16 [p]	0.5	2.6	0.9	0.8	7.9
Uruguay	95	97	99	92	94	96	<5	10	57	1.1	11.7	...	4.5	7.7
Uzbekistan	90	89	87	84	91	100	11	9	26	4.5	19.6	...	4.4	12.8
Vanuatu	62	76	91	...	42	58	85	13	35	5.9	25.9	...	11.7	4.7
Venezuela (Bolivarian Republic of)	90	92	...	82	89	...	<5	8	28	4.1	13.4	6.7	2.9	6.4
Viet Nam	61	77	95	37	54	75	51	9	17	4.4	23.3	36.9	12.0	4.6
Yemen	66	60	55	24	39	53	33	13	...	3.6	...	29.6	46.6	13.0
Zambia	49	53	63	41	41	43	83	13	61	5.6	45.8	21.2	14.9	8.4
Zimbabwe	79	80	80	41	40	40	70	17	31	3.1	32.3	11.7	10.1	5.8

Prevalence of raised fasting blood glucose[f] (≥ 25 years) (%)		Prevalence of raised blood pressure[g] (≥ 25 years) (%)		Adults aged ≥20 years who are obese[h] (%)		Alcohol consumption among adults aged ≥15 years[i] (litres of pure alcohol per person per year)	Prevalence of smoking any tobacco product among adults aged ≥15 years[j] (%)		Prevalence of current tobacco use among adolescents aged 13–15 years[k] (%)		MDG 6				Member State
											Prevalence of condom use by adults aged 15–49 years during higher-risk sex[l] (%)		Population aged 15–24 years with comprehensive correct knowledge of HIV/AIDS[m] (%)		
Male	Female	Male	Female	Male	Female		Male	Female	Male	Female	Male	Female	Male	Female	
2008		2008		2008		2010	2011		2006–2012		2006–2010		2006–2010		
10.3[n]	11.8[n]	37.1[n]	27.4[n]	11.9	31.9	10.4	...	...	25	17	...	...	...	...	Saint Lucia
11.1[n]	12.5[n]	35.4[n]	27.5[n]	16.4[n]	33.5[n]	6.6	...	...	24	15	...	...	...	...	Saint Vincent and the Grenadines
21.2	23.7	37.2	28.3	45.3	66.7	3.6	...	...	26	20	...	...	6	3	Samoa
...	...	...	...	...	...	...	...	...	...	...	...	...	...	...	San Marino
9.3[n]	10.3[n]	46.3	42.4	6.4	15.4	7.1	8	3	31	23	33	28	43	43	Sao Tome and Principe
22.0	21.7	32.9	28.7	29.5	43.5	0.2	38	<1	21	9	...	...	...	...	Saudi Arabia
9.3[n]	10.6[n]	37.9[n]	34.4[n]	3.2	12.5	0.6	16	<1	20	10	21	22	31	29	Senegal
10.3[n]	8.2[n]	42.5	33.6	25.5	20.3	12.6	38	27	11	10	...	...	...	...	Serbia
13.7	13.2	43.2	31.9	15.1	33.7	5.6	31	8	27	25	...	...	...	...	Seychelles
9.2[n]	10.0[n]	41.9	40.5	3.6	10.1	8.7	48	20	...	...	15	7	28	17	Sierra Leone
7.5	5.4	24.3	18.5	6.6	6.2	2.0	...	...	...	...	...	...	...	...	Singapore
10.6[n]	9.2[n]	42.1[n]	32.5[n]	24.9[n]	24.3[n]	13.0	39	19	30	28	...	...	...	...	Slovakia
10.7[n]	8.8[n]	43.3[n]	32.8[n]	28.1[n]	25.9[n]	11.6	28	21	17	22	...	...	...	...	Slovenia
17.1	18.3	26.5	25.9	25.3	39.2	1.7	45	18	44	37	...	...	...	...	Solomon Islands
7.9[n]	7.7[n]	39.9[n]	35.7[n]	3.4[n]	7.1[n]	0.5	...	...	...	...	...	...	...	...	Somalia
11.9	11.7	39.9	34.9	23.2	42.8	11.0	28	8	24	19	...	...	...	...	South Africa
...	...	...	...	...	...	...	...	...	...	...	...	...	...	...	South Sudan
11.0	8.8	27.7	18.6	24.9	23.0	11.2	33	27	...	...	...	...	...	...	Spain
9.3	8.6	31.0	26.2	2.6	7.3	3.7	31	<1	16	5	...	...	...	...	Sri Lanka
8.6[n,o]	8.1[n,o]	39.9[n,o]	33.5[n,o]	4.1[n,o]	8.9[n,o]	2.7	...	...	10[o]	4[o]	...	...	...	...	Sudan
11.6[n]	13.5[n]	34.2[n]	26.7[n]	16.5[n]	34.6[n]	6.6	...	...	21	17	...	...	...	...	Suriname
9.0[n]	12.2[n]	40.5[n]	36.4[n]	6.1	37.1	5.7	16	2	16	9	56	55	52	52	Swaziland
8.1	6.0	29.7	19.3	18.2	15.0	9.2	25	24	...	...	...	...	...	...	Sweden
9.3	5.3	27.4	14.9	18.3	11.6	10.7	31	22	...	...	...	...	...	...	Switzerland
12.9[n]	12.8[n]	31.8[n]	29.6[n]	23.8	39.0	1.2	...	...	32	17	...	...	...	...	Syrian Arab Republic
10.7[n]	9.7[n]	37.4[n]	34.1[n]	8.0	11.6	2.8	...	...	...	...	...	...	...	...	Tajikistan
7.3	7.1	24.6	20.2	4.9	11.8	7.1	46	3	27	9	...	...	...	...	Thailand
10.4[n]	8.8[n]	39.8[n]	33.2[n]	21.6	18.9	6.7	...	...	12	12	...	...	...	...	The former Yugoslav Republic of Macedonia
6.4[n]	6.9[n]	28.2[n]	24.7[n]	1.5[n]	4.3[n]	0.6	...	...	40	24	19	...	20	12	Timor-Leste
8.7[n]	9.1[n]	38.8[n]	35.3[n]	3.0	6.1	2.3	14	2	18	8	...	...	...	...	Togo
17.0	19.3	34.1	27.0	49.1	70.3	1.6	43	12	45	28	...	...	...	...	Tonga
12.1[n]	13.0[n]	34.8	27.7	21.6	38.0	6.7	...	...	20	16	...	...	...	...	Trinidad and Tobago
12.0	12.7	32.4	31.6	13.9	33.4	1.5	52	11	20	4	...	...	...	...	Tunisia
10.1	9.8	24.0	24.9	22.8	35.6	2.0	42	13	20	13	...	...	...	...	Turkey
12.0[n]	10.1[n]	38.3[n]	32.8[n]	13.9	14.5	4.3	...	...	...	...	...	...	...	...	Turkmenistan
...	...	...	...	...	...	1.5	...	...	42	33	...	...	...	...	Tuvalu
6.8[n]	6.5[n]	42.9[n]	39.6[n]	4.3	4.9	9.8	16	3	19	16	13	16	38	32	Uganda
10.2[n]	10.2[n]	45.8	35.4	15.5	23.6	13.9	49	14	23	16	46	48	43	45	Ukraine
15.3	15.8	30.4	21.2	30.2	43.0	4.3	...	...	...	...	...	...	...	...	United Arab Emirates
7.8	5.7	27.7	19.1	24.4	25.2	11.6	22	22	...	...	...	...	...	...	United Kingdom
8.3	8.5	36.2	33.9	4.0	6.8	7.7	...	...	...	...	24	27	43	48	United Republic of Tanzania
12.6	9.1	17.0	14.2	30.2	33.2	9.2	...	...	15	11	...	...	...	...	United States of America
10.7	10.0	37.5	25.4	20.7	26.0	7.6	29	21	21	25	...	...	...	...	Uruguay
12.6	10.9	30.5	26.3	14.5	19.8	4.6	22	3	...	...	...	...	...	...	Uzbekistan
9.2	9.6	40.7	36.5	22.9	36.8	1.4	43	8	34	20	...	...	...	...	Vanuatu
11.1	10.9	37.1	25.4	26.6	34.8	8.9	...	...	11	7	...	...	...	...	Venezuela (Bolivarian Republic of)
7.5	7.9	29.1	23.3	1.2	2.0	6.6	46	2	7	2	...	...	...	...	Viet Nam
11.1[n]	11.0[n]	32.2[n]	29.3[n]	10.5[n]	22.7[n]	0.3	35	11	15	11	...	...	...	...	Yemen
7.2	7.5	41.0	37.9	1.2	7.0	4.0	24	4	25	26	28	33	37	34	Zambia
8.7[n]	9.9[n]	36.9	36.4	2.8	13.8	5.7	25	<1	...	...	33	48	47	52	Zimbabwe

Table 5

5. Risk factors

	MDG 7						Population using solid fuels[b] (%)	Preterm birth rate[c] (per 100 live births)	Infants exclusively breastfed for the first 6 months of life[d] (%)	Children aged <5 years[e] (%)				
	Population using improved drinking-water sources[a] (%)			Population using improved sanitation[a] (%)								MDG 1		
										Wasted	Stunted	Underweight		Overweight
	1990	2000	2012	1990	2000	2012	2012	2010	2006–2012	2006–2012		1990 –1995	2006 –2012	2006 –2012

Ranges of country values

Minimum	13	22	46	2	7	9	<5	4	1	0.0	1.8	0.6	0.2	0.0
Median	88	90	95	73	79	85	13	10	34	5.6	26.5	16.1	11.9	6.2
Maximum	100	100	100	100	100	100	>95	18	89	22.7	57.7	61.5	46.6	23.4

WHO region

African Region	50	57	66	27	29	33	78	12	35	9.8	39.9	34.3	24.6	6.4
Region of the Americas	90	93	96	80	84	88	9	10	31	1.0	7.8	4.8	2.0	7.6
South-East Asia Region	70	80	91	25	35	45	63	13	47	14.2	34.4	46.9	26.6	3.8
European Region	95	97	98	91	91	93	<5	8	...	1.3	7.5	9.8	1.5	12.1
Eastern Mediterranean Region	85	83	87	53	60	68	31	12	36	9.3	25.4	22.6	13.6	8.1
Western Pacific Region	71	82	93	36	53	70	40	8	30	2.8	9.7	17.5	3.9	5.3

Income group

Low income	52	58	69	19	30	37	91	12	47	9.1	37.2	39.9	21.8	4.6
Lower middle income	71	80	88	29	38	48	56	13	39	12.3	35.1	38.7	24.1	4.6
Upper middle income	74	84	93	43	59	74	30	8	29	2.2	9.4	12.6	2.8	6.6
High income	98	99	99	96	96	96	<5	9	...	0.7	2.8	1.4	1.4	7.8

Global

Global	76	82	90	47	56	64	41	11	37	7.8	24.7	24.9	15.1	6.7

[a.] Progress on sanitation and drinking-water: 2014 Update. Joint Monitoring Programme for Water Supply and Sanitation. New York: UNICEF and Geneva: World Health Organization; 2014. In preparation.

[b.] These estimates are modelled according to Bonjour S, Adair-Rohani H, Wolf J, Bruce NG, Mehta S, Prüss-Ustün A et al. Solid Fuel Use for Household Cooking: Country and Regional Estimates for 1980–2010. Environ Health Perspect. 2013;121(7):784–90. doi:10.1289/ehp.1205987 based on the WHO Household Energy database (available at: http://apps.who.int/ghodata/). This database contains compiled information on cooking-fuel use and cooking practices from about 716 nationally representative data sources, including all Demographic and Health Surveys (Macro International), Multiple Indicator Cluster Surveys (UNICEF), World Health Surveys (WHO) and Living Standards Measurement Studies (World Bank) as well as national censuses/surveys and national energy statistics.

[c.] Blencowe H, Cousens S, Oestergaard MZ, Chou D, Moller A-B, Narwal R et al. National, regional, and worldwide estimates of preterm birth rates in the year 2010 with time trends since 1990 for selected countries: a systematic analysis and implications. Lancet. 9 June 2012;379(9832):2162–72. doi:10.1016/S0140-6736(12)60820-4. See the paper for income groupings used.

[d.] WHO Global Data Bank on Infant and Young Child Feeding [online database]. Geneva: World Health Organization; 2014 (http://www.who.int/nutrition/databases/infantfeeding).

[e.] WHO Global Database on Child Growth and Malnutrition [online database]. Geneva: World Health Organization; 2012 (http://www.who.int/nutgrowthdb/database/en, accessed 15 January 2014). 2012 Joint child malnutrition estimates – Levels and trends. New York: UNICEF, Geneva: WHO and Washington, DC: The World Bank (http://www.who.int/nutgrowthdb/estimates2012). For the reference period 1990–1995, figures refer to the first available survey year in the period. For the reference period 2006–2012, figures refer to the latest available survey year in the period. Wasted is calculated as the prevalence of low weight-for-height less than –2 standard deviations; underweight is the prevalence of weight-for-age less than –2 standard deviations; stunting is the prevalence of height-for-age less than –2 standard deviations; and overweight is the prevalence of weight-for-height above +2 standard deviations (using the WHO Child Growth Standards median). Global estimates refer to 2012 for wasted, stunting and overweight, and 1990 and 2012 for underweight. For more information, see the above databases.

[f.] Percentage of population aged 25 years and over with fasting glucose ≥ 126 mg/dl (7.0 mmol/l) or on medication for raised blood glucose. Global status report on noncommunicable diseases 2010. Geneva: World Health Organization; 2011 (http://www.who.int/nmh/publications/ncd_report2010). See Annex 4: Country estimates of NCD mortality and selected risk factors, 2008. Figures reported are age-standardized point estimates, and uncertainty ranges are available at the Global Health Observatory website (http://www.who.int/gho). Income-group aggregates are based on the 2008 World Bank list of economies.

[g.] Percentage of population aged 25 years and over with raised blood pressure (systolic blood pressure ≥ 140 or diastolic blood pressure ≥ 90). Global Health Observatory. Geneva: World Health Organization; 2011. Figures reported are age-standardized point estimates, and uncertainty ranges are available at the Global Health Observatory website (http://www.who.int/gho). Income-group aggregates are based on the 2008 World Bank list of economies.

Prevalence of raised fasting blood glucose[f] (≥ 25 years) (%)		Prevalence of raised blood pressure[g] (≥ 25 years) (%)		Adults aged ≥20 years who are obese[h] (%)		Alcohol consumption among adults aged ≥15 years[i] (litres of pure alcohol per person per year)	Prevalence of smoking any tobacco product among adults aged ≥15 years[j] (%)		Prevalence of current tobacco use among adolescents aged 13–15 years[k] (%)		Prevalence of condom use by adults aged 15–49 years during higher-risk sex[l] (%)		Population aged 15–24 years with comprehensive correct knowledge of HIV/AIDS[m] (%)		
											MDG 6				
Male	Female	Male	Female	Male	Female		Male	Female	Male	Female	Male	Female	Male	Female	
2008		2008		2008		2010	2011		2006–2012		2006–2010		2006–2010		
4.7	4.1	17.0	13.1	0.7	1.3	0.1	8	<1	5	2	7	2	5	3	Minimum
9.9	9.5	34.6	28.3	14.9	22.1	6.5	32	7	22	14	27	29	34	29	Median
25.5	31.9	50.3	42.4	67.5	74.7	17.5	67	50	58	42	74	66	89	90	Maximum
8.3	9.2	38.1	35.5	5.3	11.1	6.0	22	7	...	...	...	...	35	29	African Region
11.5	9.9	26.3	19.7	23.5	29.7	8.4	26	16	18	14	...	...	...	...	Region of the Americas
9.9	9.8	25.4	24.2	1.7	3.7	3.5	34	4	22	8	...	...	36	20	South-East Asia Region
9.6	8.0	33.1	25.6	20.4	23.1	10.9	38	19	...	...	...	...	...	...	European Region
11.0	11.6	30.7	29.1	13.0	24.5	0.7	38	4	21	10	...	...	...	...	Eastern Mediterranean Region
9.2	8.6	28.7	23.7	5.1	6.8	6.8	47	3	...	...	...	...	...	...	Western Pacific Region
8.2	8.4	32.9	29.9	2.6	5.1	3.1	29	4	17	10	...	...	37	30	Low income
9.8	9.8	28.7	26.0	4.7	8.4	4.1	32	4	21	8	...	...	36	21	Lower middle income
10.4	10.3	35.3	28.3	19.5	28.9	6.7	46	6	...	...	...	...	...	...	Upper middle income
10.0	7.1	24.8	17.4	21.8	21.6	10.3	31	19	...	...	...	...	...	...	High income
9.8	9.2	29.2	24.8	10.0	14.0	6.2	36	8	20	10	...	...	...	...	Global

Table 5

h. Percentage of population aged 20 years and over with a body mass index ≥ 30.00 kg/m². Global status report on noncommunicable diseases 2010. Geneva: World Health Organization; 2011 (http://www.who.int/nmh/publications/ncd_report2010). See Annex 4: Country estimates of NCD mortality and selected risk factors, 2008. Figures reported are age-standardized point estimates, and uncertainty ranges are available at the Global Health Observatory website (http://www.who.int/gho). Income-group aggregates are based on the 2008 World Bank list of economies.

i. WHO Global Information System on Alcohol and Health [online database]. Geneva: World Health Organization; 2012 (http://apps.who.int/gho/data/node.main.GISAH?showonly=GISAH). Definition of indicator: total (sum of three year average recorded and unrecorded) amount of alcohol consumed per adult (15+ years) over a calendar year, in litres of pure alcohol. Recorded alcohol consumption refers to official statistics (production, import, export, and sales or taxation data), while the unrecorded alcohol consumption refers to alcohol which is not taxed and is outside the usual system of governmental control.

j. WHO Report on the Global Tobacco Epidemic, 2013. Geneva: World Health Organization; 2013 (http://www.who.int/tobacco/global_report/2013/en/). See Technical Note II: Smoking prevalence in WHO Member States Definition of indicator: smoking at the time of the survey any form of tobacco, including cigarettes, cigars, pipes, bidis, etc. Note: these estimates cannot be used to form a time series with previously published estimates for past years because the quality and quantity of source data increase significantly each year.

k. WHO report on the Global Tobacco Epidemic, 2013. Geneva: World Health Organization; 2013 (http://www.who.int/tobacco/global_report/2013/en/). Global Youth Tobacco Survey data relate to most-recent survey for each country between 2006 and 2012 on tobacco use in any form in the past 30 days.

l. Percentage of women and men aged 15–49 years who had more than one sexual partner in the past 12 months reporting the use of a condom during their last sexual intercourse. AIDSinfo [online database]. Geneva: UNAIDS (http://aidsinfoonline.org/devinfo/libraries/aspx/Home.aspx, accessed 1 February 2014).

m. Percentage of women and men aged 15–24 years who both correctly identify ways of preventing the sexual transmission of HIV and reject major misconceptions about HIV transmission. AIDSinfo [online database]. Geneva: UNAIDS (http://aidsinfoonline.org/devinfo/libraries/aspx/Home.aspx, accessed 1 February 2014).

n. No country data available. Estimate modelled using data from other countries and specific country characteristics.

o. Figure refers to the state as it existed prior to the independence of South Sudan in July 2011.

p. Data refer to children at 6 months. Breastfeeding Report Card 2012, United States: Outcome Indicators [online database]. Atlanta: United States Centers for Disease Control and Prevention (http://www.cdc.gov/breastfeeding/data/reportcard2.htm).

6. Health systems

Table 6 presents data on the resources available to health systems, such as workforce (physicians, nurses and midwives, other health-care workers); infrastructure (hospitals, and hospital and psychiatric beds); medical technologies and devices (radiotherapy, computed tomography units and mammography units); and access to essential medicines.[1] Such data are essential in enabling governments to determine how best to meet the health-related needs of their populations. For example, mental health services depend primarily on trained human resources such as mental health specialists (for example, psychiatrists), psychosocial workers (for example, psychologists) and non-specialist health workers such as primary care staff. The density of psychiatrists is the most widely available and reliable indicator of the human resources available to mental health services, and provides a crude proxy of mental health system capacity.

Estimates of health personnel densities refer to the active health workforce – i.e. those currently participating in the health labour market. Data are derived from multiple sources, including national population censuses, labour-force and employment surveys, health-facility assessments, and routine administrative information systems.[2] Due to the wide diversity of available information sources, there is considerable variability in the coverage and quality of data. Figures may be underestimated or over-estimated where it is not possible to determine whether or not they include health workers in the private sector, or to identify the double counting of health workers holding two or more jobs at different locations. In addition, health service providers may be working outside the health-care sector, working in unpaid and/or unregulated conditions, or not currently engaged in the national health labour market.

The density of hospital beds can be used to indicate the availability of inpatient services. Statistics on hospital-bed density are generally drawn from routine administrative records but in some settings only public-sector beds are included. The density of psychiatric beds provides an estimate of national capacity to treat serious mental disorders that require brief or extended inpatient care. The density of psychiatric beds in any country should be interpreted alongside other resources for mental health care, since beds very often account for a high proportion of all the resources allocated to mental health care.

Medical devices are indispensable in the prevention, diagnosis or treatment of a disease and in rehabilitation and palliative care. As essential basic equipment is still not available everywhere, a United Nations Commission on Life Saving Commodities will be addressing the availability of basic neonatal resuscitation units – along with 13 other commodities. At present, the density of computed tomography scanners, radiotherapy equipment and mammography units acts as an indicator of the availability of expensive high-end equipment for diagnostic imaging and cancer radiotherapy.

---

[1] MDG 8; Target 8.E: In cooperation with pharmaceutical companies, provide access to affordable essential drugs in developing countries.

[2] These include registries on public expenditure, staffing and payroll, as well as records of professional training, registration and licensure.

Data on the availability of medicines are poor in most developing countries. However, data on the availability and consumer prices for selected generic medicines have been derived from surveys conducted using WHO/Health Action International (HAI) standard methods between 2001 and 2012. In individual surveys, availability is reported as the percentage of medicine outlets in which a medicine was found on the day of data collection. As baskets of medicines differ by country, results are not strictly comparable across countries. The consumer price ratio is an expression of how much more – or less – the local medicine price is than the international reference price.

Table 6

Member State	Density of health workforce (per 10 000 population)					Infrastructures and technologies		
	Physicians[a]	Nursing and midwifery personnel[a,b]	Dentistry personnel[a,c]	Pharmaceutical personnel[a,d]	Psychiatrists[e]	Hospitals[f] (per 10 000 population)	Hospital beds[g] (per 10 000 population)	Psychiatric beds[e] (per 10 000 population)
			2006–2013			2006–2010	2013	2006–2012	2006–2010
Afghanistan	2.3	5.0	<0.05 [j]	0.6	...	0.4 [k]	5	...
Albania	11.5	39.9	...	...	0.2	1.4	26	2.1
Algeria	12.1	19.5	3.3	2.4	0.2	...	...	1.4
Andorra	...	...	...	...	0.7	...	25	1.4
Angola	1.7	16.6	...	...	<0.05	...	...	...
Antigua and Barbuda	...	...	...	...	0.1	1.1 [k]	21	12.4
Argentina	...	...	...	...	...	...	47	2.8
Armenia	26.9	49.1	4.2 [j]	0.4 [j]	0.4	4.0	39	4.8
Australia	32.7	106.5	5.4 [j]	10.2 [j]	1.3	...	39	3.9
Austria	48.3	79.1	5.7 [j]	6.9 [j]	2.0	...	76	4.0
Azerbaijan	34.3	66.9	2.6 [j]	1.8 [j]	0.5	8.0 [k]	47	4.3
Bahamas	28.2	41.4	3.4	4.8	...	1.1	29	...
Bahrain	9.1	24.1	2.3	1.5 [j]	0.8	...	21	2.8
Bangladesh	3.6	2.2	0.3 [j]	0.6 [j]	<0.05	0.2	6	0.1
Barbados	...	...	...	...	0.4	1.1	62	21.2
Belarus	37.6	105.3	5.4 [j]	3.1 [j]	0.9	7.4 [k]	113	6.3
Belgium	29.9	157.8	7.2 [j]	11.9 [j]	...	...	65	...
Belize	8.3	19.6	0.4 [j]	3.9 [j]	0.1	2.1	11	0.1
Benin	0.6	7.7	<0.05 [j]	<0.05 [j]	<0.05	0.4 [k]	5	0.2
Bhutan	2.6	9.8	0.3	0.2 [j]	<0.05	1.7 [k]	18	...
Bolivia (Plurinational State of)	4.7	10.1	1.1 [j]	0.7 [j]	0.1	1.1	11	...
Bosnia and Herzegovina	...	...	...	...	0.5	1.0	35	2.4
Botswana	3.4	28.4	...	...	<0.05	1.3 [k]	18	2.2
Brazil	18.9	76.0	11.8 [j]	5.4 [j]	0.3	...	23	1.9
Brunei Darussalam	15.0	77.3	2.3 [j]	1.2 [j]	<0.05	1.4	28	1.0
Bulgaria	38.1	46.8	9.0 [j]	...	0.7	...	64	6.9
Burkina Faso	0.5	5.7	<0.05 [j]	0.2	<0.05	0.3	4	...
Burundi	...	...	...	0.2	<0.05	0.5 [k]	19	...
Cabo Verde	3.0	4.5	0.1 [j]	0.1 [j]	0.1	1.0	21	0.9
Cambodia	2.3	7.9	0.2 [j]	1.0 [j]	<0.05	0.6 [k]	7	<0.05
Cameroon	0.8	4.4	<0.05 [j]	<0.05 [j]	<0.05	0.8	13	0.1
Canada	20.7	92.9	12.6	10.3	1.3	2.3 [k]	27	...
Central African Republic	0.5	2.6	<0.05	<0.05	<0.05	0.5	10	0.1
Chad	0.4	1.9	...	...	<0.05	0.7	...	0.0
Chile	10.2	1.4	<0.05 [j]	<0.05 [j]	0.6	1.0 [k]	21	0.5
China	14.6	15.1	...	2.6 [j]	0.1	...	38	1.4
Colombia	14.7	6.2	9.2 [j]	...	...	...	15	...
Comoros	...	...	...	...	<0.05	0.7 [k]	...	0.0
Congo	1.0	8.2	...	0.2	<0.05	...	...	...
Cook Islands	13.3	64.4	10.6	4.4	...	...	...	...
Costa Rica	11.1	7.7	1.2 [j]	1.8 [j]	0.2	0.8	12	2.3
Côte d'Ivoire	1.4	4.8	0.1 [j]	0.2 [j]	<0.05	1.7	...	...
Croatia	28.4	58.0	7.2 [j]	7.0 [j]	1.0	1.5 [k]	58	9.6
Cuba	67.2	90.5	10.7 [j]	...	1.1	2.0 [k]	53	6.8
Cyprus	22.9	44.6	7.0 [j]	1.7 [j]	0.7	7.5	35	2.2
Czech Republic	36.2	84.3	7.1 [j]	7.6 [j]	1.2	1.3	68	10.5
Democratic People's Republic of Korea	...	...	...	...	...	6.9 [k]	132	...
Democratic Republic of the Congo	...	...	...	<0.05 [j]	<0.05	0.4 [k]	...	...

Infrastructures and technologies			Essential medicines				Member State
			MDG 8				
Computed tomography units[f] (per million population)	Radiotherapy units[f] (per million population)	Mammography units[f] (per million females aged 50 to 69 years)	Median availability of selected generic medicines[h] (%)		Median consumer price ratio of selected generic medicines[i]		
			Public	Private	Public	Private	
2013	2013	2013	2001–2009				
0.2	0.0	0.0	…	…	…	…	Afghanistan
5.4	0.3	54.4	…	…	…	…	Albania
…	0.4[l]	…	…	…	…	…	Algeria
…	…	…	…	…	…	…	Andorra
0.4	<0.05[k]	6.3[k]	…	…	…	…	Angola
22.2	…	272.1	…	…	…	…	Antigua and Barbuda
…	2.8[l]	…	…	…	…	…	Argentina
3.0	1.3	22.5	…	…	…	3.4	Armenia
…	4.0[k]	…	…	…	…	…	Australia
28.5[k]	5.4[k]	…	…	…	…	…	Austria
1.1[k]	1.6[k]	30.7[k]	…	…	…	…	Azerbaijan
13.2	2.6	106.6	…	…	…	…	Bahamas
…	…	…	…	…	…	…	Bahrain
…	0.1[l]	…	…	…	…	…	Bangladesh
7.0[k]	3.5[k]	29.0[k]	…	…	…	…	Barbados
6.2[k]	3.1[k]	17.5[k]	…	…	…	…	Belarus
…	8.3[l]	…	…	…	…	…	Belgium
12.1	0.0	258.0	…	…	…	…	Belize
0.3	0.0	16.1	…	…	…	…	Benin
1.3	0.0	0.0	…	…	…	…	Bhutan
…	0.6[l]	…	31.9	86.7	3.5	4.5	Bolivia (Plurinational State of)
16.5	2.9	182.7	…	…	…	…	Bosnia and Herzegovina
1.0[k]	0.0[k]	19.1[k]	…	…	…	…	Botswana
…	1.7[l]	…	0.0[m]	76.7[m]	…[n]	11.3[m]	Brazil
7.2	…	91.9	…	…	…	…	Brunei Darussalam
…	2.1[l]	…	…	…	…	…	Bulgaria
0.6	0.0	13.6	87.1	72.1	2.2	2.9	Burkina Faso
0.2	0.0	2.7	…	…	…	…	Burundi
2.0	0.0	140.6	…	…	…	…	Cabo Verde
1.2	0.1	…	…	…	…	…	Cambodia
0.6	0.1	17.4	60.0	52.5	2.2	13.6	Cameroon
13.8	8.1[l]	…	…	…	…	…	Canada
0.0	0.0	4.7	…	…	…	…	Central African Republic
0.1[o]	…	4.7	31.3	13.6	3.9	15.1	Chad
12.6	0.9[k]	32.2[k]	…	…	…	…	Chile
…	1.1[l]	…	15.5[p]	13.3[p]	1.6[p]	1.4[p]	China
…	1.4[l]	…	86.7	87.9	…[n]	3.1	Colombia
1.4	0.0	31.3	…	…	…	…	Comoros
…	…	…	21.2	31.3	6.5	11.5	Congo
…	…	…	…	…	…	…	Cook Islands
5.1	2.3	150.3	…	…	…	…	Costa Rica
0.7	0.0	0.0	…	…	…	…	Côte d'Ivoire
14.9	3.0	206.5	…	…	…	…	Croatia
4.8[k]	1.2	15.6[k]	…	…	…	…	Cuba
25.4	2.6	329.6	…	…	…	…	Cyprus
13.0	4.9	97.0	…	…	…	…	Czech Republic
…	0.2[l]	…	…	…	…	…	Democratic People's Republic of Korea
0.1	<0.05	0.7	55.6	65.4	2.0	2.3	Democratic Republic of the Congo

Table 6

Member State	Density of health workforce (per 10 000 population)				Psychiatrists[e]	Infrastructures and technologies		
	Physicians[a]	Nursing and midwifery personnel[a,b]	Dentistry personnel[a,c]	Pharmaceutical personnel[a,d]		Hospitals[f] (per 10 000 population)	Hospital beds[g] (per 10 000 population)	Psychiatric beds[e] (per 10 000 population)
	2006–2013				2006–2010	2013	2006–2012	2006–2010
Denmark	34.2	160.9	8.1[j]	...	1.4	1.0[k]	35	...
Djibouti	2.3	8.0	1.2[j]	3.2[j]	...	...	14	...
Dominica	...	...	...	...	0.3	5.6	38	...
Dominican Republic	14.9	13.3	1.9[j]	...	0.1	...	17	0.3
Ecuador	16.9	19.8	2.4[j]	0.5[j]	0.1	0.3[k]	16	1.2
Egypt	28.3	35.2	4.2[j]	16.7[j]	0.1	0.6[k]	5	1.0
El Salvador	16.0	4.1	6.5[j]	3.2[j]	<0.05	0.5[k]	11	0.1
Equatorial Guinea	...	...	...	...	...	...	21	...
Eritrea	...	...	...	...	<0.05	0.4	7	...
Estonia	32.6	64.6	8.8[j]	6.2[j]	1.4	1.9[k]	53	...
Ethiopia	0.3	2.5	...	0.3	<0.05	0.2	63	<0.05
Fiji	4.3	22.4	2.0[j]	0.9[j]	<0.05	0.0	20	1.6
Finland	29.1	108.3	8.0[j]	11.2[j]	2.8	1.4	55	7.6
France	31.8	93.0	6.6[j]	11.0[j]	2.2	...	64	9.5
Gabon	...	...	...	...	<0.05	3.5	63	0.8
Gambia	1.1	8.7	0.3	0.5	<0.05	0.7[k]	11	0.6
Georgia	42.4	32.2	...	...	0.7	2.2	26	2.9
Germany	38.1	114.9	8.0[j]	6.2[j]	...	...	82	...
Ghana	1.0	9.3	0.1	0.7	<0.05	1.4	9	0.7
Greece	...	...	...	...	1.3	...	48	2.4
Grenada	6.6	38.3	1.8[j]	8.5[j]	0.2	0.9	35	...
Guatemala	9.3	9.0	1.8[j]	...	0.1	0.3[k]	6	0.3
Guinea	...	...	...	...	<0.05	0.4	3	0.1
Guinea-Bissau	0.7	5.9	0.1	0.1	...	56.4	...	...
Guyana	2.1	5.3	0.6	1.2	0.1	3.4	20	3.2
Haiti	...	...	...	...	<0.05	0.2	...	0.2
Honduras	...	...	...	...	0.1	0.4[k]	7	0.5
Hungary	29.6	63.9	5.3[j]	5.7[j]	0.7	1.0[k]	72	7.5
Iceland	34.8	155.9	8.2[j]	10.9[j]	2.0	3.6[k]	32	4.3
India	7.0	17.1	1.0[j]	5.0[j]	<0.05	...	7	0.2
Indonesia	2.0	13.8	1.0	1.0[j]	<0.05	0.4	9	...
Iran (Islamic Republic of)	...	...	...	5.4	0.1	...	1	0.9
Iraq	6.1	...	1.5[j]	1.7[j]	<0.05	1.0	13	0.5
Ireland	27.2	...	...	11.7	0.6	...	29	7.4
Israel	33.5	49.3	7.8[j]	7.7[j]	0.8	0.6	33	4.7
Italy	40.9	...	...	...	0.8	2.1	34	1.1
Jamaica	4.1	10.9	0.9	0.6	0.1	0.8[k]	17	1.8
Japan	23.0	114.9	7.9[j]	21.5[j]	1.0	...	137	27.8
Jordan	25.6	40.5	9.0[j]	21.4[j]	0.1	1.9	18	...
Kazakhstan	35.8	82.5	4.2[j]	8.3[j]	0.6	3.5	72	6.3
Kenya	1.8	7.9	0.2[j]	1.6	<0.05	1.5	14	...
Kiribati	3.8	37.1	1.7[j]	2.1[j]	...	0.0	13	...
Kuwait	17.9	45.5	3.5[j]	3.0[j]	0.3	...	22	3.3
Kyrgyzstan	19.6	61.2	1.8[j]	0.5[j]	0.4	2.6[k]	48	3.5
Lao People's Democratic Republic	1.8	8.8	0.4[j]	1.2[j]	...	2.2[k]	15	...
Latvia	28.8	47.3	6.5[j]	6.1[j]	1.1	1.6[k]	59	12.2
Lebanon	32.0	27.2	14.7[j]	15.7[j]	0.1	3.1	35	4.1
Lesotho	...	...	...	...	<0.05	...	...	0.3
Liberia	0.1	2.7	<0.05[j]	0.8	<0.05	0.4[k]	8	...

Infrastructures and technologies			Essential medicines — MDG 8				Member State
Computed tomography units[f] (per million population)	Radiotherapy units[f] (per million population)	Mammography units[f] (per million females aged 50 to 69 years)	Median availability of selected generic medicines[h] (%)		Median consumer price ratio of selected generic medicines[i]		
			Public	Private	Public	Private	
2013	2013	2013	2001–2009				
23.8	9.6	138.4	...	...	...	...	Denmark
...	...	...	...	...	...	...	Djibouti
13.9	0.0	206.7	...	...	...	...	Dominica
...	1.2[l]	...	...	...	...	...	Dominican Republic
1.6[k]	0.1[k]	...	41.7	71.7	...[n]	5.0	Ecuador
...	0.8[l]	...	...	...	...	...	Egypt
4.7	1.1	70.0	53.8	69.2	...[n]	28.3	El Salvador
...	...	...	...	...	...	...	Equatorial Guinea
0.3	0.0	16.6	...	...	...	...	Eritrea
15.5	2.3	...	...	...	...	...	Estonia
0.4	<0.05	...	...	...	...	...	Ethiopia
3.4	0.0	28.8	...	75.0	...	2.7	Fiji
20.1[k]	7.4[k]	223.2[k]	...	...	...	...	Finland
...	7.5[l]	...	...	...	...	...	France
3.6	0.6	73.1	...	...	...	...	Gabon
1.1	0.0[o]	16.5	...	...	...	...	Gambia
8.8	1.4	40.7	...	...	...	...	Georgia
...	6.4[l]	...	...	...	...	...	Germany
0.2[k]	0.1[k]	...	17.9	44.6	2.4	3.8	Ghana
33.2	4.3	438.4	...	...	...	...	Greece
18.9	0.0	134.6	...	...	...	...	Grenada
...	0.6[l]	...	...	...	...	...	Guatemala
0.0[k]	0.0[k]	0.0[k]	...	...	...	...	Guinea
0.0	0.0	0.0	...	...	...	...	Guinea-Bissau
3.8[o]	1.3[o]	70.0[o]	...	...	...	...	Guyana
0.3[o]	...	19.5	17.6	54.3	4.8	7.3	Haiti
2.1	0.7	50.9	...	...	...	...	Honduras
6.6	1.8	103.6	...	...	...	...	Hungary
39.4	6.1	139.0	...	...	...	...	Iceland
...	0.4[l]	...	22.1	76.8	...[n]	1.9[q]	India
...	0.1[l]	...	65.5	57.8	1.8	2.0	Indonesia
...	0.9[l]	...	96.7	96.7	1.3	1.3	Iran (Islamic Republic of)
2.2[k]	0.2[k]	35.4[k]	...	...	...	...	Iraq
4.5[k]	3.9[k]	23.2[k]	...	...	...	...	Ireland
7.5	3.4	112.3	...	...	...	...	Israel
...	6.4[l]	...	...	...	...	...	Italy
1.4[k]	1.1	51.3	...	...	...	...	Jamaica
101.2	7.2[l]	227.3	...	...	...	...	Japan
5.5	0.8	129.1	27.8	80.0	0.9	10.5	Jordan
1.5[k]	1.3[k]	22.1[k]	0.0	70.0	4.8	3.7	Kazakhstan
0.2	<0.05	6.8[k]	37.7	72.4	2.0	3.3	Kenya
0.0	0.0	0.0	...	...	...	...	Kiribati
...	1.2[l]	...	12.0	0.0	...[n]	15.7	Kuwait
0.9	0.5[l]	16.4[k]	...[r]	70.0	...[r]	3.4	Kyrgyzstan
0.7	0.0	0.0	...	...	...	...	Lao People's Democratic Republic
...	5.4[l]	...	...	...	...	...	Latvia
25.1	1.9	370.2	0.0	83.8	...[n]	6.1	Lebanon
...	...	...	...	...	...	...	Lesotho
...	...	...	...	...	...	...	Liberia

Table 6

133

Member State	Density of health workforce (per 10 000 population)					Infrastructures and technologies		
	Physicians[a]	Nursing and midwifery personnel[a,b]	Dentistry personnel[a,c]	Pharmaceutical personnel[a,d]	Psychiatrists[e]	Hospitals[f] (per 10 000 population)	Hospital beds[g] (per 10 000 population)	Psychiatric beds[e] (per 10 000 population)
			2006–2013		2006–2010	2013	2006–2012	2006–2010
Libya	19.0	68.0	6.0[j]	3.6[j]	...	2.6	37	...
Lithuania	41.2	71.7	7.5[j]	7.4[j]	1.8	2.2	70	...
Luxembourg	28.2	124.7	8.4[j]	7.3[j]	2.1	1.1	54	9.0
Madagascar	1.6	...	<0.05[j]	...	<0.05	0.5	2	0.1
Malawi	0.2	3.4	...	0.2[j]	<0.05	0.4[k]	13	...
Malaysia	12.0	32.8	3.6	4.3	0.1	0.5[k]	19	1.8
Maldives	14.2	50.4	0.9[j]	6.7[j]	0.2	6.7	43	0.0
Mali	0.8	4.3	0.1	0.1[j]	<0.05	0.5[k]	1	0.1
Malta	35.0	70.9	4.5[j]	11.6[j]	0.3	0.9	48	14.5
Marshall Islands	4.4	17.4	1.6[j]	1.5[j]	0.2	3.8	27	0.0
Mauritania	1.3	6.7	0.3	0.4	<0.05	1.0	...	...
Mauritius	...	...	...	...	0.2	1.0[k]	34	5.5
Mexico	21.0	25.3	1.2[j]	...	0.2	3.5[k]	15	0.4
Micronesia (Federated States of)	1.8	33.2	3.5	...	0.1	4.8	32	0.0
Monaco	71.7	172.2	10.4[j]	27.1[j]	3.6	10.6	138	17.3
Mongolia	27.6	35.0	1.9[j]	4.0[j]	0.1	2.5[k]	68	...
Montenegro	19.8	52.5	0.4[j]	1.5[j]	0.7	2.1[k]	40	5.8
Morocco	6.2	8.9	0.8[j]	2.7[j]	0.1	...	9	0.7
Mozambique	0.4	4.1	...	0.6[j]	<0.05	...	7	0.2
Myanmar	6.1	10.0	0.7	...	<0.05	0.6[k]	6	...
Namibia	3.7	27.8	0.4[j]	1.8	<0.05	1.9	...	0.8
Nauru	7.1	70.7	2.1	0.7[j]	<0.05	9.9[k]	50	2.0
Nepal	...	...	...	1.4	<0.05	0.4[k]	50	0.2
Netherlands	...	83.8	...	2.0[j]	1.9	0.8[k]	47	13.1
New Zealand	27.4	108.7	4.6[j]	10.1[j]	1.0	...	23	2.1
Nicaragua	...	...	...	...	0.1	1.0[k]	9	...
Niger	0.2	1.4	<0.05[j]	<0.05	<0.05	0.5	...	0.1
Nigeria	4.1	16.1	0.2[j]	1.1	<0.05	...	...	...
Niue	30.0	160.0	40.0	10.0[j]	<0.05	...	52	0.0
Norway	37.4	134.0	8.6[j]	2.6[j]	3.1	...	33	...
Oman	22.2	50.0	2.6[j]	10.7	0.2	1.3[k]	17	0.3
Pakistan	8.3	5.7	0.6[j]	...	<0.05	0.5	6	0.3
Palau	13.8	57.1	2.5[j]	0.5[j]	0.5	...	48	3.9
Panama	15.5	24.0	3.1[j]	...	...	0.9	22	...
Papua New Guinea	0.5	4.6	...	0.5[j]	<0.05	1.6	...	0.2
Paraguay	...	...	...	...	0.1	2.4[k]	13	0.5
Peru	11.3	15.1	1.5[j]	0.5[j]	0.1	...	15	...
Philippines	...	...	...	8.9	<0.05	1.8	5	...
Poland	22.0	58.4	3.4[j]	6.9[j]	0.5	0.9[k]	65	5.4
Portugal	...	...	...	7.4[j]	...	...	34	...
Qatar	77.4	118.7	5.8[j]	12.6[j]	0.2	...	12	0.4
Republic of Korea	21.4	50.1	4.5[j]	6.7[j]	0.5	3.4	103	19.1
Republic of Moldova	28.6	64.9	4.8[j]	5.3[j]	0.5	2.1	62	5.9
Romania	23.9	55.1	6.2[j]	6.8[j]	0.6	1.7[k]	61	7.5
Russian Federation	43.1	85.2	3.2[j]	0.8[j]	1.2	...	97	11.1
Rwanda	0.6	6.9	0.1	0.1	<0.05	...	...	0.4
Saint Kitts and Nevis	...	...	...	...	0.2	7.4	23	2.3
Saint Lucia	...	...	...	...	0.2	1.6	16	...

Table 6

Infrastructures and technologies			Essential medicines				Member State
			MDG 8				
Computed tomography units[f] (per million population)	Radiotherapy units[f] (per million population)	Mammography units[f] (per million females aged 50 to 69 years)	Median availability of selected generic medicines[h] (%)		Median consumer price ratio of selected generic medicines[i]		
			Public	Private	Public	Private	
2013	2013	2013	2001–2009				
9.7	1.0	…	…	…	…	…	Libya
20.2	3.6	82.5	…	…	…	…	Lithuania
18.9	3.8	168.3	…	…	…	…	Luxembourg
0.1	<0.05	6.2	…	…	…	…	Madagascar
0.3	0.0	0.0[k]	…	…	…	…	Malawi
6.4	1.4	86.7	25.0	43.8	…[n]	6.6	Malaysia
5.8	0.0	57.1	…	…	…	…	Maldives
0.2[k]	0.1	5.4	81.0	70.0	1.8	5.4	Mali
9.3	4.7	99.7	…	…	…	…	Malta
19.0	0.0	142.7	…	…	…	…	Marshall Islands
1.5	0.3[l]	22.4	…	…	…	…	Mauritania
6.4	2.4	49.7	88.8	70.0	…[n]	5.9	Mauritius
3.7	0.5	74.5	46.2[s]	50.0[s]	…[n]	4.7[s]	Mexico
0.0	0.0	0.0	…	…	…	…	Micronesia (Federated States of)
132.2	26.4	599.3	…	…	…	…	Monaco
8.1	0.7[k]	33.3	100.0	80.0	2.6	4.2	Mongolia
16.1	3.2	196.5	…	…	…	…	Montenegro
1.2[k]	0.4[k]	18.5[k]	0.0	57.5	…[n]	9.8	Morocco
…	…	…	…	…	…	…	Mozambique
0.1[k]	0.1[k]	0.7[k]	…	…	…	…	Myanmar
4.8	0.4	42.3	…	…	…	…	Namibia
…	…	…	…	…	…	…	Nauru
…	0.2[l]	…	…	…	…	…	Nepal
12.2	7.2	…	…	…	…	…	Netherlands
…	6.2[l]	…	…	…	…	…	New Zealand
0.5[k]	0.3[k]	…	50.0	87.1	…[n]	5.7	Nicaragua
0.2	0.0	10.9	…	…	…	…	Niger
…	0.1[l]	…	26.2	36.4	3.5	4.3	Nigeria
…	…	…	…	…	…	…	Niue
…	8.1[l]	…	…	…	…	…	Norway
6.9	0.6	149.8	96.7	70.3	…[n]	7.4	Oman
0.3	0.1	1.6	3.3	31.3	…[n]	2.3	Pakistan
…	…	…	…	…	…	…	Palau
9.6	1.6	278.5	…	…	…	…	Panama
0.4	0.1	8.5	…	…	…	…	Papua New Guinea
1.0	0.6	7.3[k]	…	…	…	…	Paraguay
…	1.1[l]	…	61.5	60.9	1.4	5.6	Peru
1.1	0.2	13.1	15.4	26.5	6.4	5.6	Philippines
10.6[k]	2.7[k]	100.7[k]	…	…	…	…	Poland
27.4	4.1	272.0	…	…	…	…	Portugal
8.3	0.9	225.1	…	…	…	…	Qatar
35.4	3.0[o]	402.3	…	…	…	…	Republic of Korea
5.4	0.6	41.0	46.0	56.0	5.2	4.7	Republic of Moldova
5.4	1.2	41.8	…	…	…	…	Romania
…	2.3[l]	…	100.0[t]	100.0[t]	2.7[t]	4.1[t]	Russian Federation
…	…	…	…	…	…	…	Rwanda
18.5	0.0	149.4	…	…	…	…	Saint Kitts and Nevis
11.0	0.0	131.1	…	…	…	…	Saint Lucia

Member State	Density of health workforce (per 10 000 population)					Infrastructures and technologies		
	Physicians[a]	Nursing and midwifery personnel[a,b]	Dentistry personnel[a,c]	Pharmaceutical personnel[a,d]	Psychiatrists[e]	Hospitals[f] (per 10000 population)	Hospital beds[g] (per 10000 population)	Psychiatric beds[e] (per 10000 population)
			2006–2013			2006–2010	2013	2006–2012	2006–2010
Saint Vincent and the Grenadines	...	...	...	...	0.2	0.0	52	...
Samoa	4.5	18.5	3.4	3.1	0.1	4.2	...	0.0
San Marino	51.3	88.9	...	7.2[j]	1.6	3.2[k]	38	...
Sao Tome and Principe	...	...	...	...	0.1	...	29	3.6
Saudi Arabia	7.7	23.4	0.9[j]	0.6[j]	0.3	1.0[k]	21	1.2
Senegal	0.6	4.2	0.1[j]	0.1	<0.05	0.2[k]	...	0.3
Serbia	21.1	...	2.3[j]	2.1[j]	1.0	1.1[k]	...	...
Seychelles	...	...	...	...	0.2	1.1[k]	36	...
Sierra Leone	0.2	1.7	<0.05[j]	0.2	<0.05	...	...	0.3
Singapore	19.2	63.9	3.3[j]	3.9[j]	0.3	0.5	20	4.2
Slovakia	30.0	...	5.0[j]	4.7[j]	1.1	1.5[k]	60	6.9
Slovenia	25.2	84.6	6.3[j]	5.6[j]	0.7	1.3	46	7.7
Solomon Islands	2.2	20.5	...	...	...	...	13	...
Somalia	0.4	1.1	...	0.1[j]	<0.05	...	...	0.6
South Africa	7.8	49.0	2.0	4.1	<0.05	0.7[k]	...	2.2
South Sudan	...	...	...	...	...	...	...	...
Spain	37.0	50.8	...	10.3[j]	0.9	1.6	31	4.3
Sri Lanka	6.8	16.4	0.8	0.4[j]	<0.05	...	36	0.9
Sudan	2.8	8.4	0.2[j]	0.1[j]	<0.05[v]	1.3	8	0.1[v]
Suriname	...	...	...	...	0.1	0.4	31	5.7
Swaziland	1.7	16.0	0.4	0.5	<0.05	0.8	21	1.3
Sweden	32.7	110.5	8.3[j]	...	0.4	...	27	3.5
Switzerland	39.4	173.6	5.4[j]	5.5[j]	4.1	...	50	...
Syrian Arab Republic	15.0	18.6	7.9[j]	8.1[j]	<0.05	...	15	0.6
Tajikistan	19.0	44.8	1.8[j]	...	0.1	4.7[k]	55	2.1
Thailand	3.9	20.8	2.6	1.3[j]	<0.05	1.8	21	1.3
The former Yugoslav Republic of Macedonia	26.2	...	7.0[j]	15.9	1.0	...	45	6.4
Timor-Leste	0.7	11.1	0.4	1.1	<0.05	...	59	...
Togo	0.5	2.7	<0.05	<0.05[j]	<0.05	0.6[k]	7	0.2
Tonga	5.6	38.8	3.6	0.9[j]	0.2	3.8[k]	26	2.1
Trinidad and Tobago	11.8	35.6	2.2[j]	4.9[j]	0.2	...	27	7.7
Tunisia	12.2	32.8	2.9[j]	3.0[j]	0.2	2.3	21	0.9
Turkey	17.1	24.0	2.9[j]	3.5[j]	0.2	1.5	25	1.0
Turkmenistan	...	...	1.2[j]	1.7[j]	...	...	40	...
Tuvalu	10.9	58.2	3.6	1.8	...	...	...	...
Uganda	...	...	...	0.3	<0.05	0.4	5	0.3
Ukraine	35.3	76.0	6.8[j]	0.4[j]	1.0	...	90	9.4
United Arab Emirates	19.3	40.9	4.3[j]	5.9[j]	<0.05	...	11	0.2
United Kingdom	27.9	88.3	5.4[j]	6.7[j]	1.5	...	29	5.0
United Republic of Tanzania	0.1	2.4	0.1	<0.05	<0.05	...	7	0.3
United States of America	24.5	...	...	8.8[j]	0.8	...	29	3.4
Uruguay	37.4	55.5	7.0[j]	5.3	1.7	3.9[k]	25	4.6
Uzbekistan	23.8	119.7	1.8[j]	0.4[j]	0.3	...	44	1.8
Vanuatu	1.2	17.0	0.1[j]	0.1[j]	<0.05	2.4	18	0.2
Venezuela (Bolivarian Republic of)	...	...	...	...	...	...	9	...
Viet Nam	11.6	11.4	...	3.1	0.1	...	20	1.8
Yemen	2.0	6.8	0.4	0.9	...	3.0	7	...
Zambia	0.7	7.8	0.2[j]	1.3	<0.05	0.5	20	0.3
Zimbabwe	0.6	12.5	0.1[j]	1.9	<0.05	0.5	17	1.0

Infrastructures and technologies			Essential medicines MDG 8				Member State
Computed tomography units[f] (per million population)	Radiotherapy units[f] (per million population)	Mammography units[f] (per million females aged 50 to 69 years)	Median availability of selected generic medicines[h] (%)		Median consumer price ratio of selected generic medicines[i]		
			Public	Private	Public	Private	
2013	2013	2013	2001–2009				
0.0	0.0	229.9	...	...	...	...	Saint Vincent and the Grenadines
5.3	0.0	91.2	...	...	...	...	Samoa
31.8	0.0	229.1	...	...	...	...	San Marino
...	...	...	56.3	22.2	2.4	13.8	Sao Tome and Principe
3.8[k]	0.1[k]	40.6[k]	...	...	...	...	Saudi Arabia
0.4[k]	0.1[k]	5.2[k]	...	...	...	...	Senegal
13.7	1.5	84.6	...	...	...	...	Serbia
10.8[k]	...	127.7[k]	...	...	...	...	Seychelles
0.3	...	...	...	...	...	...	Sierra Leone
8.9	3.5	127.6	...	...	...	...	Singapore
...	4.8[l]	...	...	...	...	...	Slovakia
13.5[k]	5.8[k]	136.2[k]	...	...	...	...	Slovenia
...	...	...	...	...	...	...	Solomon Islands
...	...	...	...	...	...	...	Somalia
1.0[k]	0.6[k]	7.8[k]	...	71.7[u]	...	6.5[u]	South Africa
...	...	...	...	...	...	...	South Sudan
13.9	4.2	...	...	...	...	...	Spain
1.2	0.1	...	...	...	...	1.1	Sri Lanka
1.1	0.2	12.2	51.7[w]	77.1[w]	4.4[w]	4.7[w]	Sudan
7.4	3.7	93.6	...	...	...	...	Suriname
2.4	0.0	33.6	...	...	...	...	Swaziland
...	6.9[l]	...	...	...	...	...	Sweden
...	...	...	...	...	...	...	Switzerland
...	0.3[l]	...	...[r]	98.2	...[r]	2.5	Syrian Arab Republic
1.1[k]	0.1[k]	12.6[k]	75.0	85.0	2.4	2.3	Tajikistan
6.0	1.0	27.9	75.0	28.6	2.6	3.3	Thailand
...	...	...	...	...	...	...	The former Yugoslav Republic of Macedonia
...	...	...	...	...	...	...	Timor-Leste
0.7	...	10.4	...	...	...	...	Togo
0.0	0.0	0.0	...	...	...	...	Tonga
3.0[k]	3.0	35.2[k]	...	...	...	...	Trinidad and Tobago
8.9	1.6	22.6[k]	64.3	95.1	...[n]	6.8	Tunisia
14.5	2.0	230.4	...	...	...	...	Turkey
...	...	...	...	...	...	...	Turkmenistan
...	...	...	...	...	...	...	Tuvalu
0.5	0.1	4.4	20.0	80.0	...[n]	2.6	Uganda
...	2.4[l]	...	88.6	91.4	3.7	3.0	Ukraine
...	0.6[l]	...	61.1	73.9	...[n]	13.8	United Arab Emirates
...	5.0[l]	...	...	...	...	...	United Kingdom
0.1	0.1[k]	6.1	23.4	47.9	1.3	2.7	United Republic of Tanzania
...	12.4[l]	...	...	...	...	...	United States of America
12.9	3.8	172.4	...	...	...	...	Uruguay
...	0.6[l]	...	...	82.5	...	2.0	Uzbekistan
0.0	0.0	0.0	...	...	...	...	Vanuatu
...	2.5[l]	...	...	...	...	...	Venezuela (Bolivarian Republic of)
...	0.4[l]	...	...	...	...	...	Viet Nam
3.6	0.1	17.6	5.0	90.0	1.1	3.5	Yemen
0.2	0.1	4.6	...	...	...	...	Zambia
0.4	0.4	6.9	...	...	...	...	Zimbabwe

Table 6

137

6. Health systems

	Density of health workforce (per 10 000 population)				Psychiatrists[e]	Infrastructures and technologies		
	Physicians[a]	Nursing and midwifery personnel[a,b]	Dentistry personnel[a,c]	Pharmaceutical personnel[a,d]		Hospitals[f] (per 10 000 population)	Hospital beds[g] (per 10 000 population)	Psychiatric beds[e] (per 10 000 population)
	2006–2013				2006–2010	2013	2006–2012	2006–2010
Ranges of country values								
Minimum	0.1	1.1	<0.05	<0.05	<0.05	0.0	1	0.0
Median	12.8	28.4	2.9	2.4	2.0	1.1	26	1.7
Maximum	77.4	173.6	40.0	27.1	4.1	56.4	138	27.8
WHO region								
African Region	2.6	12.0	0.5	0.9	<0.05	0.8	...	0.6
Region of the Americas	20.8	45.8	6.9	6.7	0.5	...	23	2.3
South-East Asia Region	5.9	15.3	1.0	3.8	<0.05	...	10	0.3
European Region	33.1	80.5	5.0	5.1	1.1	...	53	6.3
Eastern Mediterranean Region	11.4	16.1	1.9	6.1	0.1	0.9	8	0.6
Western Pacific Region	15.3	25.1	...	4.5	0.2	...	43	3.9
Income group								
Low income	2.4	5.4	0.3	0.5	<0.05	0.8	21	0.2
Lower middle income	7.8	17.8	1.2	4.2	0.1	...	10	0.6
Upper middle income	15.5	25.3	...	3.1	0.2	...	32	2.2
High income	29.4	86.9	5.8	8.4	1.0	...	54	8.3
Global	14.1	29.2	2.7	4.3	0.3	...	27	2.5

a. WHO Global Health Workforce Statistics (http://who.int/hrh/statistics/hwfstats/en/). See this source for the latest updates, disaggregated health workforce statistics and metadata descriptors. Due to variability of data sources and national occupation titles, the figures provided may not always be comparable with regards to coverage and quality. In general, the denominator data for health workforce density (i.e. national population estimates) were obtained from the World Population Prospects database of the United Nations Population Division. In some cases the official report provided only workforce density indicators, from which estimates of the stock were calculated.

b. Figures include nursing personnel and midwifery personnel, whenever available. In many countries, nurses trained with midwifery skills are counted and reported as nurses. This makes the distinction between nursing personnel and midwifery personnel difficult to draw.

c. Figures include dentists, dental technicians/assistants and related occupations. Due to variability of data sources, the professional-level and associate-level occupations may not always be distinguishable.

d. Figures include pharmacists, pharmaceutical technicians/assistants and related occupations. Due to variability of data sources, the professional-level and associate-level occupations may not always be distinguishable.

e. Mental health atlas 2011. Geneva: World Health Organization; 2011 (http://www.who.int/mental_health/publications/mental_health_atlas_2011/). Income-group aggregates are based on the 2011 World Bank list of economies.

f. Data are derived from the WHO Baseline country survey on medical devices 2013 conducted in 2013. Geneva: World Health Organization; 2013. Densities were computed by adding both public-sector and private-sector data unless otherwise noted. Hospitals include district, rural, provincial, specialized, teaching and research hospitals. Radiotherapy units include Linear Accelerators and Cobalt-60 units.

g. PAHO/WHO Country Representative and National Authorities. Data provided by Member States on basic indicators via an online data-entry tool. Washington, DC; 2014. As of January 2014; European health for all database (HFA-DB). Copenhagen: WHO Regional Office for Europe; 2014 (http://data.euro.who.int/hfadb/); Western Pacific Country Health Information Profiles 2014 Revision. Manila: WHO Regional Office for the Western Pacific; 2014 (http://hiip.wpro.who.int/portal/default.aspx); Regional Health Observatory. Cairo: WHO Regional Office for the Eastern Mediterranean; 2014 (http://rho.emro.who.int/rhodata/); additional data compiled by the WHO Regional Office for Africa (as of January 2011) and the WHO Regional Office for South-East Asia (as of January 2014). Depending on the source and means of monitoring, data may not be exactly comparable across countries. See above sources for country-specific details.

h. Surveys of medicine prices and availability using WHO/HAI standard methodology conducted between 2001 and 2012 (available at: http://www.haiweb.org/medicineprices/). In individual surveys, availability is reported as the percentage of medicine outlets in which a medicine was found on the day of data collection. As baskets of medicines differ by individual country, results are not exactly comparable across countries. Median availability is determined for the specific list of medicines in each survey, and does not account for alternate dosage forms or strengths of these products or for therapeutic alternatives. Public-sector data may be limited by the fact that the list of survey medicines may not correspond to national essential

Infrastructures and technologies			Essential medicines				
			MDG 8				
Computed tomography units[f] (per million population)	Radiotherapy units[f] (per million population)	Mammography units[f] (per million females aged 50 to 69 years)	Median availability of selected generic medicines[h] (%)		Median consumer price ratio of selected generic medicines[i]		
			Public	Private	Public	Private	
2013	2013	2013	2001–2009				
0.0	0.0	0.0	0.0	0.0	0.9	1.1	Minimum
3.8	0.6	35.4	46.0	70.2	2.4	4.4	Median
132.2	26.4	599.3	100.0	100.0	6.5	28.3	Maximum
0.4	0.1	7.4	…	…	…	…	African Region
…	5.3	…	…	…	…	…	Region of the Americas
…	0.3	…	…	…	…	…	South-East Asia Region
…	4.0	…	…	…	…	…	European Region
1.9	0.4	20.9	…	…	…	…	Eastern Mediterranean Region
…	1.5	…	…	…	…	…	Western Pacific Region
0.3	0.1	5.0	…	…	…	…	Low income
…	0.4	…	…	…	…	…	Lower middle income
…	1.2	…	…	…	…	…	Upper middle income
…	6.8	…	…	…	…	…	High income
…	1.8	…	…	…	…	…	Global

Table 6

medicines lists (EMLs) where these exist, and some public-sector facilities may not be expected to stock all of the survey medicines. This has been addressed in the revised edition of the survey tool, which allows public-sector data to be analysed by EML status and level of care.

i. Surveys of medicine prices and availability using WHO/HAI standard methodology conducted between 2001 and 2012 (available at: http://www.haiweb.org/medicineprices/). Consumer price ratio = ratio of median local unit price to the Management Sciences for Health (MSH) international reference price of selected generic medicines. Data are unadjusted for differences in the MSH reference price year used, exchange-rate fluctuations, national inflation rates, variations in purchasing power parities, levels of development or other factors. In each survey, median consumer price ratios are obtained for the basket of medicines surveyed and found in at least four medicine outlets. As baskets of medicines differ by individual country, results are not exactly comparable across countries. However, data on specific medicines are publicly available at the above HAI website, and matched basket comparisons on a subset of medicines can be made.

j. Separate figures were not reported for associate-level professionals and hence may not be comparable with previous publications.

k. Refers to public sector only.

l. Data derived from the Directory of Radiotherapy Centres (DIRAC) from the International Atomic Energy Agency (IAEA) – http://www-naweb.iaea.org/nahu/dirac/query3.asp. This source does not specify if data are derived from the public or private sector, and was only taken into account if a country participating in the WHO Baseline country survey on medical devices did not provide such data.

m. Based on a survey of medicine prices and availability in Rio Grande do Sul State, Brazil.

n. Medicines are provided free to patients in the public sector.

o. Refers to the private sector only.

p. Simple average of three surveys of medicine prices and availability in China (Shaanxi, Shandong and Shanghai provinces).

q. Simple average across seven state surveys.

r. No public-sector medicine outlets available.

s. Based on a survey in Mexico City, Mexico.

t. Based on a survey in Tatarstan province, Russian Federation.

u. Based on a survey of medicine prices and availability in Gauteng province, South Africa.

v. Figure refers to the state as it existed prior to the independence of South Sudan in July 2011.

w. Simple average of four surveys in Sudan (Gadarif, Khartoum, North Kordofan and Northern states).

7. Health expenditure

Table 7 presents data on government expenditure on health and on private expenditure on health, including externally funded expenditure on health. Sub-components of government expenditure on health ("social security expenditure") and private expenditure on health ("out-of-pocket expenditure"; and "private prepaid plans") are also included. These data are generated from information that has been collected by WHO since 1999. The most comprehensive and consistent data on health financing are generated from national health accounts (NHAs) that collect expenditure information within an internationally recognized framework. NHAs trace financing as it flows from funding sources to decision-makers (who decide upon the use of the funds) and then to the providers and beneficiaries of health services. Not all countries maintain or update NHAs – in such cases, data are obtained through technical contacts in the country or from publicly available documents and reports. Missing values are estimated using various accounting techniques depending upon the data available for each country.[1] WHO sends all such estimates to the respective ministries of health every year for validation.

Table 7

---

[1] To obtain the latest updates, a full series or more-disaggregated health expenditures including metadata and sources, see: http://www.who.int/nha/.

Member State	Health expenditure ratios[a]											
	Total expenditure on health as % of gross domestic product		General government expenditure on health as % of total expenditure on health[b]		Private expenditure on health as % of total expenditure on health[b]		General government expenditure on health as % of total government expenditure		External resources for health as % of total expenditure on health		Social security expenditure on health as % of general government expenditure on health	
	2000	2011	2000	2011	2000	2011	2000	2011	2000	2011	2000	2011
Afghanistan[f,g]	…	8.4	…	19.0	…	81.0	…	3.5	…	19.4	…	0
Albania	6.4	6.0	36.1	47.9	63.9	52.1	7.1	9.8	6.0	1.0	20.4	74.1
Algeria[f]	3.5	4.4	73.3	82.0	26.7	18.0	8.8	9.0	0.1	0	35.5	31.6
Andorra	6.2	7.2	64.8	73.6	35.2	26.4	19.1	…	0	…	88.1	57.4
Angola[f]	3.4	3.4	49.5	62.6	50.5	37.4	2.9	5.6	2.5	2.3	0	0
Antigua and Barbuda[f]	4.0	5.5	69.0	73.7	31.0	26.3	11.4	15.8	…	3.6	0	11.1
Argentina[f]	9.2	7.9	53.9	66.5	46.1	33.5	14.7	21.7	0	0.8	59.6	64.1
Armenia	6.3	3.7	18.2	52.2	81.8	47.8	5.3	7.4	8.7	8.0	0	0
Australia[h]	8.1	9.0	66.8	67.6	33.2	32.4	15.1	17.2	0	…	0	0
Austria	10.0	11.3	75.6	75.3	24.4	24.7	14.6	16.9	0	…	59.0	53.6
Azerbaijan[i]	4.7	5.0	18.6	21.6	81.4	78.4	5.4	3.7	4.0	0.7	0	0
Bahamas	5.2	7.5	48.1	45.6	51.9	54.4	14.8	15.7	0	…	1.8	2.2
Bahrain[f]	3.5	3.8	67.3	69.9	32.7	30.1	10.7	8.7	0	0	0.4	1.6
Bangladesh	2.8	3.8	39.0	38.2	61.0	61.8	7.6	9.8	6.9	6.8	0	0
Barbados	6.3	7.2	65.8	66.0	34.2	34.0	11.7	10.3	4.0	1.7	0	0.2
Belarus	6.1	4.9	75.5	70.5	24.5	29.5	10.1	13.0	0.1	0.3	0	0
Belgium	8.1	10.5	74.6	75.9	25.4	24.1	12.3	15.0	0	…	85.4	86.2
Belize[f]	4.0	5.8	52.6	66.5	47.4	33.5	6.5	13.4	2.1	4.2	0	13.5
Benin[f]	4.3	4.5	44.2	52.1	55.8	47.9	10.0	10.8	17.0	35.3	0.5	0.4
Bhutan[f,j]	6.7	3.7	79.3	83.9	20.7	16.1	12.2	8.0	21.3	17.2	0	0
Bolivia (Plurinational State of)[f]	6.1	5.0	60.1	70.8	39.9	29.2	9.8	7.9	6.0	4.9	62.0	42.9
Bosnia and Herzegovina	7.1	9.9	56.7	71.3	43.3	28.7	11.4	16.6	9.0	2.4	97.7	90.1
Botswana[f]	4.7	5.2	62.2	61.6	37.8	38.4	7.3	8.0	0.5	10.0	…	…
Brazil	7.2	8.9	40.3	45.7	59.7	54.3	4.1	8.7	0.5	0.3	0	0
Brunei Darussalam[k]	3.0	2.2	86.5	92.0	13.5	8.0	6.3	6.2	…	…	…	…
Bulgaria	6.2	7.3	60.9	55.3	39.1	44.7	9.1	11.3	1.9	…	12.0	68.4
Burkina Faso	5.1	6.4	39.6	49.5	60.4	50.5	8.8	12.4	13.9	25.7	0.8	0.2
Burundi[f,j]	6.3	9.0	30.6	63.3	69.4	36.7	7.3	13.6	18.7	46.4	29.5	12.4
Cabo Verde[m]	4.8	4.0	73.3	75.5	26.7	24.5	9.9	8.8	13.0	18.0	34.9	25.2
Cambodia	6.3	5.6	20.5	22.6	79.5	77.4	8.7	6.2	8.6	15.0	…	…
Cameroon[f]	4.4	5.4	21.0	34.7	79.0	65.3	6.1	8.5	4.2	4.4	3.9	2.6
Canada	8.8	10.9	70.4	70.4	29.6	29.6	15.1	17.4	…	…	2.0	2.0
Central African Republic[f]	4.3	3.9	50.2	51.4	49.8	48.6	12.9	12.5	19.1	35.8	…	…
Chad[f,j]	6.3	2.8	42.5	29.6	57.5	70.4	13.1	3.3	24.9	20.5	…	…
Chile	7.7	7.1	43.3	48.4	56.7	51.6	14.1	14.8	0	0	15.0	11.4
China	4.6	5.1	38.3	55.9	61.7	44.1	10.9	12.5	0.1	0.1	57.2	67.0
Colombia[f]	5.9	6.5	79.3	75.2	20.7	24.8	19.3	20.2	0.3	0.2	66.8	83.4
Comoros[f,j]	3.5	3.6	43.7	40.2	56.3	59.8	9.3	6.5	21.3	29.9	0	0
Congo	2.1	2.5	57.5	67.5	42.5	32.5	4.8	6.5	4.6	11.5	0	0
Cook Islands[f]	3.4	3.6	90.1	91.0	9.9	9.0	9.9	11.7	2.2	5.4	0	0
Costa Rica[f]	7.1	10.2	78.6	74.7	21.4	25.3	24.1	28.0	0.9	0.9	80.7	81.0
Côte d'Ivoire[f]	6.5	6.8	28.5	24.5	71.5	75.5	10.0	8.5	4.2	11.1	2.0	6.3
Croatia	7.8	6.8	86.1	82.5	13.9	17.5	14.5	15.1	0.4	0	97.6	94.3
Cuba	6.1	10.0	90.8	94.7	9.2	5.3	10.8	14.0	0.2	0.2	0	…
Cyprus	5.8	7.4	41.7	43.3	58.3	56.7	6.5	6.9	0	…	0	1.6
Czech Republic	6.3	7.5	90.3	84.2	9.7	15.8	13.7	14.6	0	…	89.5	92.3
Democratic People's Republic of Korea	…	…	…	…	…	…	…	…	…	…	…	…
Democratic Republic of the Congo[f]	4.8	6.1	4.2	50.8	95.8	49.2	1.8	11.5	2.8	39.9	…	…
Denmark	8.7	10.9	83.9	85.3	16.1	14.7	13.6	16.1	0	…	0	0

Health expenditure ratios[a]				Per capita health expenditures[a]								Member State
Out-of-pocket expenditure as % of private expenditure on health		Private prepaid plans as % of private expenditure on health		Per capita total expenditure on health at average exchange rate[d] (US$)		Per capita total expenditure on health[e] (PPP int. $)		Per capita government expenditure on health at average exchange rate[d] (US$)		Per capita government expenditure on health[e] (PPP int. $)		
2000	2011	2000	2011	2000	2011	2000	2011	2000	2011	2000	2011	
...	94.0	...	0	...	48	...	43	...	9	...	8	Afghanistan[f,g]
99.9	99.7	0	...	70	243	248	534	25	116	89	256	Albania
96.7	94.7	3.1	5.1	60	233	181	366	44	191	133	300	Algeria[f]
75.5	73.9	22.3	24.0	1330	3053	1978	3050	862	2247	1282	2245	Andorra
71.4	70.1	0	0	22	178	74	198	11	111	37	124	Angola[f]
86.8	85.0	13.2	15.0	408	703	592	1061	281	518	409	782	Antigua and Barbuda[f]
63.0	62.8	30.7	27.8	710	866	841	1393	383	576	453	927	Argentina[f]
94.5	98.4	...	1.6	39	127	127	225	7	66	23	118	Armenia
59.7	59.9	21.8	24.4	1713	5991	2246	3890	1144	4052	1500	2631	Australia[h]
62.1	62.2	19.4	16.4	2403	5643	2898	4795	1818	4251	2192	3613	Austria
77.7	89.0	0.3	0.7	30	359	102	503	6	77	19	109	Azerbaijan[i]
40.2	54.0	58.6	45.1	1107	1622	1424	2325	532	740	684	1060	Bahamas
68.0	59.9	25.2	22.0	476	766	802	820	320	535	540	574	Bahrain[f]
95.1	96.6	0.1	0.3	10	27	24	67	4	10	9	26	Bangladesh
77.3	100	22.7	...	602	935	792	1450	396	617	521	956	Barbados
57.1	90.4	0.1	0.8	64	311	317	740	48	219	239	522	Belarus
80.9	81.7	15.4	17.5	1845	4914	2248	4079	1377	3730	1677	3096	Belgium
82.3	69.8	2.7	16.8	139	264	208	434	73	175	109	288	Belize[f]
99.9	91.2	0.1	7.2	15	34	47	68	7	18	21	36	Benin[f]
100	94.7	0	1.2	52	94	166	227	41	79	131	190	Bhutan[f,j]
81.6	88.3	8.1	8.8	60	115	188	248	36	82	113	175	Bolivia (Plurinational State of)[f]
100	96.9	...	0.8	103	471	314	887	59	336	178	632	Bosnia and Herzegovina
36.7	12.7	4.1	79.9	152	404	401	814	95	249	249	502	Botswana[f]
63.6	57.8	34.3	40.4	265	1119	502	1035	107	512	203	474	Brazil
98.8	97.8	0.6	1.1	543	917	1274	1179	470	844	1102	1085	Brunei Darussalam[k]
100	96.8	...	1.0	98	522	385	1080	60	288	235	597	Bulgaria
94.3	76.1	1.0	2.2	12	39	41	82	5	19	16	41	Burkina Faso
73.0	69.7	0.2	1.0	7	21	22	47	2	13	7	30	Burundi[f,l]
95.2	93.7	2.6	3.1	59	153	92	165	43	116	68	125	Cabo Verde[m]
89.6	80.3	0.2	0.4	19	49	59	129	4	11	12	29	Cambodia
94.4	94.3	...	...	26	64	72	120	5	22	15	42	Cameroon[f]
53.7	48.5	38.8	43.3	2090	5656	2520	4541	1470	3982	1773	3197	Canada
92.9	90.5	1.2	1.8	11	19	29	32	5	10	15	16	Central African Republic[f]
96.2	96.7	0.4	0.2	10	25	41	41	4	7	18	12	Chad[f,j]
63.8	64.0	36.2	36.0	390	1022	738	1478	169	495	320	716	Chile
95.6	78.8	1.0	6.4	43	274	107	423	16	153	41	236	China
59.0	64.0	41.0	36.0	148	466	346	657	117	350	274	494	Colombia[f]
100	100	0	0	13	31	35	43	6	13	15	17	Comoros[f,j]
98.9	96.0	0.8	3.6	22	85	59	107	13	58	34	72	Congo
100	100	0	0	175	511	243	412	158	464	219	374	Cook Islands[f]
88.2	91.0	2.3	5.0	287	883	510	1243	226	659	401	928	Costa Rica[f]
79.1	77.0	3.9	3.5	42	84	107	126	12	21	30	31	Côte d'Ivoire[f]
100	78.6	...	5.2	377	992	847	1362	325	818	730	1123	Croatia
100	100	0	0	166	605	147	429	151	573	134	406	Cuba
95.7	87.0	4.3	10.8	744	2123	1107	2233	310	919	461	966	Cyprus
100	93.2	0	0.8	361	1545	981	1968	326	1301	886	1657	Czech Republic
...	...	...	...	...	...	...	...	...	...	...	...	Democratic People's Republic of Korea
76.8	70.0	0	2.4	14	15	12	24	<1	8	<1	12	Democratic Republic of the Congo[f]
90.9	87.2	8.7	12.2	2613	6521	2511	4456	2191	5563	2106	3801	Denmark

Table 7

7. Health expenditure

Member State	Health expenditure ratios[a]											
	Total expenditure on health as % of gross domestic product		General government expenditure on health as % of total expenditure on health[b]		Private expenditure on health as % of total expenditure on health[b]		General government expenditure on health as % of total government expenditure		External resources for health as % of total expenditure on health		Social security expenditure on health as % of general government expenditure on health	
	2000	2011	2000	2011	2000	2011	2000	2011	2000	2011	2000	2011
Djibouti	5.8	8.7	67.8	57.4	32.2	42.6	12.0	14.1	32.6	12.6	11.3	9.5
Dominica	5.0	6.0	69.0	71.0	31.0	29.0	6.6	12.3	3.7	5.2	0	0.8
Dominican Republic[f]	6.3	5.4	34.5	49.3	65.5	50.7	15.9	14.2	2.0	5.1	17.0	25.8
Ecuador[f]	3.6	6.9	31.2	36.1	68.8	63.9	6.4	6.4	4.1	0.3	28.0	34.5
Egypt	5.4	4.9	40.5	40.7	59.5	59.3	7.3	6.3	1.0	0.5	24.3	19.4
El Salvador[f]	8.1	6.8	46.1	63.6	53.9	36.4	14.8	14.7	0.9	5.5	47.7	42.5
Equatorial Guinea[l,n]	2.4	4.5	77.4	54.2	22.6	45.8	8.7	7.0	7.2	2.1	0	0
Eritrea[l,o]	4.5	2.7	39.1	50.5	60.9	49.5	2.6	3.6	29.8	71.6	0	0
Estonia	5.3	5.8	77.4	80.5	22.6	19.5	11.3	12.3	0.3	…	86.3	86.4
Ethiopia[f]	4.3	4.1	53.6	50.0	46.4	50.0	8.9	11.1	16.5	51.8	0	0
Fiji[f]	3.9	3.8	83.6	65.3	16.4	34.7	11.3	9.2	7.4	7.8	0	0
Finland	7.2	9.0	71.3	75.4	28.7	24.6	10.6	12.3	0	…	19.5	19.0
France	10.1	11.6	79.4	76.8	20.6	23.2	15.5	15.9	0	…	94.3	92.3
Gabon[f]	2.9	3.4	40.3	52.9	59.7	47.1	5.3	7.2	2.3	1.0	14.2	27.1
Gambia[f]	4.5	4.7	27.6	62.3	72.4	37.7	10.0	11.2	15.4	61.6	0	0
Georgia[p]	6.9	9.4	17.0	18.1	83.0	81.9	6.9	5.3	1.2	2.8	46.0	68.8
Germany	10.4	11.3	79.5	76.5	20.5	23.5	18.3	19.1	0	…	87.2	88.6
Ghana[f]	4.8	5.3	49.4	55.9	50.6	44.1	8.0	12.5	14.3	13.2	0	21.6
Greece	7.9	9.0	60.0	66.1	40.0	33.9	10.1	11.4	…	…	45.9	64.0
Grenada	6.6	6.5	52.0	48.3	48.0	51.7	13.2	11.0	…	2.9	0	0.4
Guatemala[f]	5.6	6.7	40.2	35.4	59.8	64.6	17.0	15.7	3.4	2.1	51.2	41.8
Guinea[f]	5.6	6.0	19.4	24.3	80.6	75.7	6.4	6.8	14.0	12.2	1.1	4.5
Guinea-Bissau[f,l,q]	4.9	6.3	10.5	26.8	89.5	73.2	2.3	7.8	30.0	47.3	5.4	1.5
Guyana	5.8	6.8	84.7	67.3	15.3	32.7	10.8	15.6	3.9	16.3	7.1	2.7
Haiti[f]	6.1	8.5	27.7	21.5	72.3	78.5	16.0	5.5	9.4	86.2	0	0
Honduras	6.6	8.4	54.2	49.4	45.8	50.6	18.1	17.0	2.5	3.4	13.7	26.2
Hungary	7.2	7.9	70.7	65.0	29.3	35.0	10.6	10.3	0	…	83.9	83.7
Iceland	9.5	9.2	81.1	80.7	18.9	19.3	18.4	15.6	0	…	33.4	36.1
India[f]	4.3	3.9	26.0	30.5	74.0	69.5	7.4	8.2	0.5	1.1	18.3	15.8
Indonesia[f]	2.0	2.9	36.1	37.9	63.9	62.1	4.5	6.2	…	1.2	6.3	18.2
Iran (Islamic Republic of)[r]	4.6	4.6	41.6	49.5	58.4	50.5	10.6	10.5	0	0	57.8	50.2
Iraq[l,s]	0.8	2.7	4.8	75.1	95.2	24.9	0.1	4.9	54.9	1.4	0	0
Ireland	6.1	8.8	75.1	67.0	24.9	33.0	14.7	12.4	…	…	1.2	0.5
Israel	7.4	7.6	64.0	61.2	36.0	38.8	9.2	10.4	…	…	67.0	71.5
Italy	7.9	9.2	74.2	77.8	25.8	22.2	12.7	14.4	0	…	0.1	0.2
Jamaica[f]	5.5	5.2	52.6	53.6	47.4	46.4	6.6	8.6	1.8	1.7	0	0.3
Japan	7.6	10.0	80.8	82.1	19.2	17.6	15.9	19.4	0	…	84.9	87.6
Jordan[f,t]	9.7	8.8	48.0	65.5	52.0	34.5	13.7	17.8	4.5	2.8	9.7	28.2
Kazakhstan	4.2	3.9	50.9	57.9	49.1	42.1	9.2	10.5	7.4	0.7	…	…
Kenya[f]	4.7	4.4	46.3	39.4	53.7	60.6	10.6	5.9	8.0	40.0	10.9	13.1
Kiribati[f]	7.9	10.8	94.9	82.0	5.1	18.0	8.8	10.3	28.5	3.0	0	0
Kuwait	2.5	2.6	76.3	82.4	23.7	17.6	5.2	5.6	0	0	0	0
Kyrgyzstan	4.7	6.2	44.3	59.9	55.7	40.1	12.0	11.6	6.0	10.8	10.0	64.1
Lao People's Democratic Republic[f,u]	3.3	2.8	35.1	49.4	64.9	50.6	5.8	6.1	29.2	23.4	1.2	4.9
Latvia	6.0	6.0	54.4	57.1	45.6	42.9	8.7	8.9	0.5	…	…	…
Lebanon	10.9	7.4	29.5	38.0	70.5	62.0	7.6	9.5	2.1	0.9	46.3	49.7
Lesotho	6.9	11.7	50.2	77.5	49.8	22.5	6.3	14.5	3.0	26.5	0	0
Liberia[f,l]	5.9	15.6	24.5	29.7	75.5	70.3	6.7	19.1	9.2	54.0	0	0
Libya[l]	3.4	3.9	49.1	77.3	50.9	22.7	6.0	4.5	0	0.1	…	…

144

Health expenditure ratios[a]				Per capita health expenditures[a]								Member State
Out-of-pocket expenditure as % of private expenditure on health		Private prepaid plans as % of private expenditure on health		Per capita total expenditure on health at average exchange rate[d] (US$)		Per capita total expenditure on health[e] (PPP int. $)		Per capita government expenditure on health at average exchange rate[d] (US$)		Per capita government expenditure on health[e] (PPP int. $)		
2000	2011	2000	2011	2000	2011	2000	2011	2000	2011	2000	2011	
98.5	99.2	1.5	0.8	44	119	90	218	30	68	61	125	Djibouti
88.9	84.5	11.1	15.5	231	402	369	758	159	285	255	538	Dominica
71.9	78.9	18.7	17.9	173	293	323	521	60	145	112	257	Dominican Republic[f]
85.3	86.5	4.8	10.9	53	362	198	665	16	131	62	240	Ecuador[f]
97.4	97.7	0.4	1.7	79	137	199	308	32	56	81	125	Egypt
94.6	88.0	5.4	12.0	179	252	371	467	82	160	171	297	El Salvador[f]
82.2	94.9	0	0	57	1051	181	1327	44	570	140	719	Equatorial Guinea[l,n]
100	100	0	0	7	12	22	15	3	6	8	8	Eritrea[l,o]
88.5	91.3	0	1.3	213	928	509	1294	165	747	394	1041	Estonia
79.2	79.9	0.5	1.5	5	14	20	43	3	7	11	21	Ethiopia[f]
63.5	64.7	26.2	24.7	80	167	133	181	67	109	112	118	Fiji[f]
77.7	75.7	8.8	8.5	1700	4411	1855	3382	1212	3327	1322	2551	Finland
34.4	32.1	61.6	59.7	2209	4968	2553	4128	1754	3813	2027	3169	France
84.9	84.9	11.7	11.7	118	401	339	516	48	212	136	273	Gabon[f]
54.1	48.1	2.3	3.1	29	24	66	87	8	15	18	54	Gambia[f]
99.4	79.3	0.6	11.8	45	310	143	526	8	56	24	95	Georgia[p]
51.0	50.8	40.2	39.9	2387	4996	2679	4474	1898	3819	2131	3420	Germany
64.4	67.5	10.6	6.3	13	83	46	99	6	46	23	55	Ghana[f]
85.9	91.3	5.5	8.4	918	2304	1453	2322	551	1522	872	1534	Greece
100	97.8	…	…	339	481	476	694	176	232	248	335	Grenada
89.4	82.6	4.2	5.7	96	215	197	329	39	76	79	117	Guatemala[f]
99.5	92.7	0	0.7	19	27	43	62	4	7	8	15	Guinea[f]
54.7	56.5	0	0	16	35	86	72	2	9	9	19	Guinea-Bissau[f,l,q]
86.1	92.3	0.3	0.2	56	221	127	217	47	149	108	146	Guyana
69.7	3.5	…	…	26	62	62	101	7	13	17	22	Haiti[f]
95.0	92.0	5.0	8.0	76	187	169	335	41	92	92	165	Honduras
89.8	74.5	0.6	7.4	326	1096	852	1690	230	713	603	1099	Hungary
100	92.9	0	…	2961	4051	2761	3361	2400	3268	2238	2711	Iceland
91.8	86.3	1.1	4.6	20	62	66	146	5	19	17	44	India[f]
72.9	76.3	6.4	3.6	15	99	47	132	6	38	17	50	Indonesia[f]
96.2	95.8	3.6	3.9	231	326	379	874	96	161	158	432	Iran (Islamic Republic of)[r]
100	100	…	…	7	160	16	110	<1	120	<1	83	Iraq[l,s]
60.8	42.2	30.9	38.0	1572	4306	1774	3703	1180	2883	1332	2480	Ireland
68.5	65.3	8.7	26.5	1454	2373	1722	2186	930	1453	1102	1338	Israel
96.7	92.7	3.5	4.9	1527	3339	2029	3017	1134	2599	1506	2348	Italy
65.0	71.0	30.0	25.6	189	273	327	395	100	146	172	212	Jamaica[f]
80.1	80.6	12.7	13.5	2834	4656	1969	3415	2290	3824	1591	2804	Japan
74.9	76.8	5.3	18.1	171	386	309	494	82	253	149	324	Jordan[f,t]
98.9	98.7	0.2	0.2	52	458	204	534	27	265	104	309	Kazakhstan
80.4	76.7	6.6	9.3	19	35	53	73	9	14	25	29	Kenya[f]
2.5	0.5	0	0	65	181	167	257	62	149	158	211	Kiribati[f]
93.0	90.4	7.0	9.6	494	1349	925	1190	377	1112	706	981	Kuwait
89.3	86.0	…	…	13	71	62	152	6	42	27	91	Kyrgyzstan
91.8	78.2	0	…	11	35	39	75	4	18	14	37	Lao People's Democratic Republic[f,u]
96.8	86.4	3.2	5.7	197	826	479	1141	107	472	261	651	Latvia
80.7	72.2	16.8	25.8	579	646	961	1003	171	246	284	382	Lebanon
71.1	69.0	…	…	29	146	72	219	14	113	36	169	Lesotho
50.3	30.0	…	0.7	11	59	18	92	3	18	4	27	Liberia[f,l]
100	100	0	0	252	211	436	181	124	163	214	140	Libya[l]

145

Table 7

7. Health expenditure

Member State	Health expenditure ratios[a]											
	Total expenditure on health as % of gross domestic product		General government expenditure on health as % of total expenditure on health[b]		Private expenditure on health as % of total expenditure on health[b]		General government expenditure on health as % of total government expenditure		External resources for health as % of total expenditure on health		Social security expenditure on health as % of general government expenditure on health	
	2000	2011	2000	2011	2000	2011	2000	2011	2000	2011	2000	2011
Lithuania	6.5	6.7	69.7	71.4	30.3	28.6	11.6	12.7	1.7	3.3	88.3	84.9
Luxembourg	7.5	6.7	85.1	84.1	14.9	15.9	16.9	13.5	...	...	71.0	80.5
Madagascar[f]	5.0	4.1	49.3	55.9	50.7	44.1	15.5	13.5	14.9	35.5	...	...
Malawi[f]	6.1	8.3	45.8	72.4	54.2	27.6	7.6	17.8	26.8	56.5	0	0
Malaysia[f]	3.0	3.8	55.8	55.2	44.2	44.8	5.2	6.2	0.7	0	0.7	0.9
Maldives[f]	7.1	8.1	57.6	44.4	42.4	55.6	11.1	9.3	2.7	0.8	0	22.2
Mali[f]	6.3	6.8	32.9	43.8	67.1	56.2	8.9	12.3	7.8	25.4	1.5	0.7
Malta	6.6	8.7	72.5	63.9	27.5	36.1	12.1	13.3	...	...	...	...
Marshall Islands[f]	22.5	16.0	87.9	83.0	12.1	17.0	21.1	22.9	33.1	36.4	35.0	15.2
Mauritania	6.0	5.9	66.5	65.2	33.5	34.8	12.9	10.1	11.2	9.7	8.7	11.1
Mauritius	3.7	4.9	52.0	48.2	48.0	51.8	8.7	9.7	1.4	4.5	...	...
Mexico[f]	5.1	6.0	46.6	50.3	53.4	49.7	16.6	15.1	1.0	0.8	67.6	55.7
Micronesia (Federated States of)	7.8	13.7	93.9	91.0	6.1	9.0	10.9	19.1	71.5	68.8	21.4	17.1
Monaco[i]	3.3	4.4	87.1	88.6	12.9	11.4	14.2	18.8	0	...	98.1	98.7
Mongolia[f]	4.7	6.0	82.1	63.3	17.9	36.7	10.9	8.4	28.0	4.2	24.1	21.5
Montenegro[v]	7.5	7.2	69.0	58.2	31.0	41.8	16.9	9.1	...	0.9	99.0	89.3
Morocco	4.2	6.3	29.4	33.1	70.6	66.9	4.8	6.0	0.5	0.3	0	24.5
Mozambique[f]	6.2	6.4	70.0	44.0	30.0	56.0	17.0	7.7	25.3	72.6	0.3	33.1
Myanmar[w]	2.1	1.8	14.2	15.9	85.8	84.1	8.6	1.5	1.1	7.1	2.9	3.0
Namibia[f]	6.1	8.6	68.9	61.3	31.1	38.7	13.9	13.9	3.8	12.0	1.8	2.5
Nauru[f]	13.3	8.1	94.4	88.0	5.6	12.0	11.2	9.9	12.7	39.6	0	0
Nepal[f,x]	5.0	6.1	24.6	45.3	75.4	54.7	7.6	13.6	15.3	13.2	0	0
Netherlands	8.0	11.9	63.1	79.5	36.9	13.4	11.4	19.1	0	...	93.9	90.5
New Zealand	7.6	10.3	78.0	82.7	22.0	17.3	15.6	20.3	0	...	0	9.4
Nicaragua	5.4	7.6	53.5	54.3	46.5	45.7	13.1	19.1	7.8	10.8	27.0	35.2
Niger[f]	6.4	6.8	23.6	33.2	76.4	66.8	8.4	10.3	21.4	21.8	3.3	1.7
Nigeria[f]	4.6	5.7	33.5	34.0	66.5	66.0	4.2	6.7	16.2	5.1	0	...
Niue[k]	7.9	10.6	98.5	98.9	1.5	1.1	6.6	8.4	4.5	76.7	0	0
Norway	9.1	9.9	83.6	85.1	16.4	14.9	18.0	19.3	...	...	15.5	12.2
Oman	3.1	2.4	81.8	81.7	18.2	18.3	7.0	5.3	0	0	0	...
Pakistan[f,y]	3.0	3.0	21.7	31.0	78.3	69.0	3.5	4.7	0.8	7.0	5.8	3.1
Palau[f]	12.0	9.0	58.5	74.7	41.5	25.3	12.0	16.4	25.6	34.4	0	0
Panama	7.8	7.9	68.1	68.2	31.9	31.8	21.3	12.8	1.0	0.4	50.0	35.6
Papua New Guinea[f]	4.0	4.2	81.7	77.7	18.3	22.3	9.9	10.2	23.8	20.5	0	0
Paraguay	8.1	8.9	39.9	38.6	60.1	61.4	17.7	11.2	2.8	2.6	52.4	34.8
Peru	4.7	4.7	58.7	56.9	41.3	43.1	14.9	15.0	1.1	1.2	49.5	52.2
Philippines[z]	3.2	4.4	47.6	36.9	52.4	63.1	8.4	10.2	3.5	1.0	14.7	24.6
Poland	5.5	6.9	70.0	70.3	30.0	29.2	9.4	11.1	0	0.1	82.6	85.4
Portugal	9.3	10.2	66.6	65.0	33.4	35.0	14.9	13.5	0	...	1.7	1.9
Qatar[f]	2.2	1.9	72.3	78.6	27.7	21.4	5.0	4.9	0	...	0	0
Republic of Korea	4.3	7.4	50.4	55.3	49.6	44.7	9.7	13.5	0	...	77.3	78.9
Republic of Moldova[aa]	6.7	11.4	48.5	45.5	51.5	54.5	8.9	13.3	14.7	9.6	...	84.9
Romania	4.3	5.6	81.2	79.2	18.8	20.8	9.1	11.3	...	...	81.9	82.1
Russian Federation	5.4	6.1	59.9	59.8	40.1	40.2	12.7	10.1	0.2	...	40.3	47.1
Rwanda	4.2	11.0	39.2	59.3	60.8	40.7	8.5	24.0	52.0	46.2	6.4	10.5
Saint Kitts and Nevis[f]	4.3	5.8	60.4	37.9	39.6	62.1	9.6	6.5	5.4	1.7	0.5	0.3
Saint Lucia	5.6	7.6	52.6	46.6	47.4	53.4	11.7	11.1	0.3	1.6	4.9	4.3
Saint Vincent and the Grenadines	3.7	4.9	82.3	81.7	17.7	18.3	10.8	11.7	0.3	3.3	0	0
Samoa[f]	6.0	7.0	76.8	88.5	23.2	11.5	13.7	13.5	16.2	22.6	0.3	0.5

Health expenditure ratios[a]				Per capita health expenditures[a]								Member State
Out-of-pocket expenditure as % of private expenditure on health		Private prepaid plans as % of private expenditure on health		Per capita total expenditure on health at average exchange rate[d] (US$)		Per capita total expenditure on health[e] (PPP int. $)		Per capita government expenditure on health at average exchange rate[d] (US$)		Per capita government expenditure on health[e] (PPP int. $)		
2000	2011	2000	2011	2000	2011	2000	2011	2000	2011	2000	2011	
86.2	97.7	0.3	2.2	212	887	560	1352	148	634	390	966	Lithuania
79.0	72.3	13.1	20.1	3495	7751	4037	6020	2973	6516	3434	5061	Luxembourg
76.9	82.0	5.3	8.9	12	19	39	39	6	10	19	22	Madagascar[f]
40.5	53.9	8.1	16.0	9	30	36	74	4	22	16	53	Malawi[f]
77.6	79.0	11.3	18.0	120	384	282	619	67	212	157	341	Malaysia[f]
54.5	88.3	3.6	6.5	162	525	274	707	93	233	158	314	Maldives[f]
99.1	99.6	0.1	0.4	16	51	51	85	5	22	17	37	Mali[f]
96.9	93.8	3.1	6.3	643	1900	1248	2444	466	1215	904	1563	Malta
75.2	75.2	24.8	24.8	466	567	333	414	409	470	292	343	Marshall Islands[f]
94.5	94.5	0.6	0.6	24	51	76	107	16	33	51	70	Mauritania
74.6	91.5	8.3	1.7	146	450	308	767	76	217	160	370	Mauritius
95.3	91.6	4.7	8.4	328	609	509	1004	153	306	237	505	Mexico[f]
100	97.5	0	0	170	412	209	506	159	375	197	460	Micronesia (Federated States of)
54.3	61.2	45.7	38.8	2685	7180	3091	5937	2339	6359	2693	5258	Monaco[i]
66.9	93.1	0	0	22	190	92	288	18	120	75	182	Mongolia[f]
91.1	91.0	...	...	121	522	491	985	83	304	339	573	Montenegro[v]
76.6	88.3	23.4	11.7	54	195	110	321	16	65	32	106	Morocco
40.6	9.0	...	...	15	33	27	61	10	14	19	27	Mozambique[f]
100	93.7	0	0	3	19	12	23	<1	3	2	4	Myanmar[w]
18.2	17.9	77.3	61.2	126	486	243	612	87	298	168	375	Namibia[f]
58.4	58.4	0	0	386	365	431	243	365	321	407	214	Nauru[f]
91.2	83.6	0.1	...	12	41	46	85	3	19	11	39	Nepal[f,x]
24.3	41.4	43.0	38.7	1932	5997	2349	5118	1218	4769	1482	4070	Netherlands
69.9	63.2	28.5	27.6	1052	3715	1606	3175	821	3072	1253	2625	New Zealand
91.6	92.4	0.6	2.7	54	124	132	292	29	67	71	159	Nicaragua
89.1	88.4	3.4	2.3	10	25	31	42	2	8	7	14	Niger[f]
92.7	95.6	5.1	3.1	17	85	60	143	6	29	20	49	Nigeria[f]
100	100	0	0	318	1820	814	2618	313	1799	802	2588	Niue[k]
93.8	90.1	...	...	3432	9908	3309	6106	2867	8436	2765	5198	Norway
64.4	59.3	21.3	22.4	264	610	657	688	216	498	537	562	Oman
81.0	90.2	0.4	0.6	15	36	49	83	3	11	11	26	Pakistan[f,y]
73.4	46.1	26.6	38.9	908	923	1566	1588	532	689	917	1187	Palau[f]
81.3	85.4	18.7	14.6	295	664	542	1181	201	453	369	806	Panama
56.0	55.9	5.5	5.5	26	74	69	113	21	58	56	87	Papua New Guinea[f]
86.6	91.4	13.4	8.6	124	352	329	550	49	136	131	212	Paraguay
81.3	87.1	15.0	9.6	96	283	230	483	57	161	135	275	Peru
77.2	83.5	11.1	11.7	33	105	76	182	16	39	36	67	Philippines[z]
100	76.2	0.8	2.4	247	920	583	1452	173	646	409	1021	Poland
72.8	78.1	9.8	13.3	1070	2302	1659	2615	712	1497	1105	1700	Portugal
100	63.8	...	24.3	652	1738	1437	1595	471	1366	1039	1254	Qatar[f]
79.5	78.8	10.1	12.4	491	1652	744	2198	247	914	375	1217	Republic of Korea
83.3	82.8	...	0.1	24	224	98	436	11	102	47	199	Republic of Moldova[aa]
100	97.8	...	0.6	72	480	248	864	59	380	201	684	Romania
74.7	87.9	8.1	7.0	96	803	369	1354	57	480	221	809	Russian Federation
40.7	49.4	0.9	...	9	62	24	138	3	37	9	82	Rwanda
94.2	88.8	5.8	9.1	392	820	533	1046	237	311	322	396	Saint Kitts and Nevis[f]
98.1	98.9	1.9	1.1	272	513	452	860	143	239	238	400	Saint Lucia
100	100	...	...	137	310	237	519	113	253	195	424	Saint Vincent and the Grenadines
81.6	62.6	0	0	80	245	165	309	61	217	127	273	Samoa[f]

Table 7

Member State	Health expenditure ratios[a]											
	Total expenditure on health as % of gross domestic product		General government expenditure on health as % of total expenditure on health[b]		Private expenditure on health as % of total expenditure on health[b]		General government expenditure on health as % of total government expenditure		External resources for health as % of total expenditure on health		Social security expenditure on health as % of general government expenditure on health	
	2000	2011	2000	2011	2000	2011	2000	2011	2000	2011	2000	2011
San Marino	5.3	5.5	85.8	85.8	14.2	14.2	20.4	13.6	0	...	100	85.0
Sao Tome and Principe	8.9	7.6	43.2	34.2	56.8	65.8	9.0	5.6	34.8	25.0	0	0
Saudi Arabia [f]	4.2	3.5	72.1	67.3	27.9	32.7	8.6	5.7	0	0	...	...
Senegal [f]	4.6	5.0	40.9	55.8	59.1	44.2	10.1	9.6	16.2	16.8	7.4	4.0
Serbia [v,ab]	7.4	10.3	70.0	62.1	30.0	37.9	13.5	14.1	1.1	0.7	92.5	93.2
Seychelles	4.8	3.6	82.7	94.8	17.3	5.2	7.3	9.5	4.3	8.7	5.0	5.2
Sierra Leone [f]	18.4	16.3	21.5	16.2	78.5	83.8	14.2	12.3	5.2	18.2	0	0
Singapore	2.7	4.2	45.0	33.3	55.0	66.7	6.2	8.9	0	0	4.8	15.5
Slovakia	5.5	7.9	89.4	70.9	10.6	29.1	9.4	14.7	0.9	...	98.2	89.6
Slovenia	8.3	8.9	74.0	73.7	26.0	26.3	13.1	12.8	0.2	...	93.7	93.4
Solomon Islands [f]	4.6	7.7	94.3	96.7	5.7	3.3	20.7	21.6	13.1	48.7	0	0
Somalia [i]	2.4	...	44.8	...	55.2	...	4.2	...	40.1	...	0	...
South Africa [f]	8.3	8.7	41.3	47.7	58.7	52.3	13.2	12.9	0.3	2.1	3.3	2.8
South Sudan	...	1.7	...	41.3	...	58.7	...	4.0	...	19.5	...	...
Spain	7.2	9.3	71.6	73.0	28.4	27.0	13.2	15.0	0	...	9.6	6.3
Sri Lanka	3.7	3.3	48.4	42.1	51.6	57.9	6.8	6.5	0.3	2.9	0.3	0.1
Sudan [f,j]	3.4	6.7	27.1	30.2	72.9	69.8	8.3	10.9	4.4	4.2	8.3	11.1
Suriname	8.7	6.0	53.4	49.8	46.6	50.2	11.7	11.9	9.9	4.1	33.8	41.7
Swaziland	5.3	8.3	56.3	69.4	43.7	30.6	10.5	18.1	5.8	20.0	0	0
Sweden	8.2	9.5	84.9	81.6	15.1	18.4	12.6	15.1	0	...	0	...
Switzerland	9.9	11.0	55.4	64.9	44.6	35.1	15.4	21.1	0	...	72.8	70.8
Syrian Arab Republic [ac]	4.9	3.4	40.4	46.3	59.6	53.7	6.5	5.3	0.1	1.2	...	...
Tajikistan	4.6	5.8	20.4	29.6	79.6	70.4	6.5	6.2	2.3	14.3	...	...
Thailand f	3.4	4.1	56.1	77.7	43.9	22.3	11.0	15.3	0	0.5	9.4	9.3
The former Yugoslav Republic of Macedonia	8.7	6.9	57.7	63.6	42.3	36.4	15.0	13.7	2.8	1.1	97.4	91.9
Timor-Leste [ad]	5.1	4.6	67.9	75.3	32.1	24.7	18.9	2.9	27.8	54.1	...	0
Togo [f]	5.3	8.0	28.5	52.2	71.5	47.8	8.5	15.4	5.9	17.4	11.7	6.5
Tonga [f,j]	4.8	5.0	70.5	83.5	29.5	16.5	15.4	12.6	22.2	26.2	0	0
Trinidad and Tobago [f]	4.0	5.3	45.4	49.2	54.6	50.8	6.4	7.2	7.2	1.0	0	0
Tunisia [f]	5.4	7.0	54.9	59.4	45.1	40.6	8.1	13.3	0.9	0.8	28.9	56.3
Turkey	4.9	6.1	62.9	72.7	37.1	27.3	9.8	12.8	0.1	0.5	55.5	57.0
Turkmenistan [i,ae]	3.9	2.1	81.8	63.8	18.2	36.2	13.7	8.7	1.4	1.1	6.5	6.5
Tuvalu [f]	11.0	17.6	100	99.9	0	0.1	5.9	17.2	44.0	17.4	0	0
Uganda [f]	6.6	9.3	26.8	25.0	73.2	75.0	7.3	10.1	28.3	27.6	0	0
Ukraine	5.6	7.3	51.8	55.7	48.2	44.3	10.2	11.8	0.5	0.4	0	0.6
United Arab Emirates	2.2	3.1	76.7	69.5	23.3	30.5	7.7	9.3	0	0	0	0
United Kingdom	7.0	9.4	79.1	82.8	20.9	17.2	15.1	16.0	0	...	...	...
United Republic of Tanzania [f]	3.4	7.4	43.4	37.4	56.6	62.6	9.4	10.2	27.8	40.2	0	...
United States of America	13.6	17.7	43.0	47.8	57.0	52.2	17.4	20.3	...	...	79.2	86.0
Uruguay [f]	11.2	8.6	54.6	69.5	45.4	30.5	20.5	21.8	...	0.2	27.4	45.2
Uzbekistan	5.3	5.6	47.5	50.9	52.5	49.1	8.7	9.0	6.7	2.0	...	...
Vanuatu [f]	3.6	3.8	76.6	87.3	23.4	12.7	10.5	14.0	2.5	24.8	0	0
Venezuela (Bolivarian Republic of)	5.7	4.5	41.5	36.6	58.5	63.4	8.0	6.3	0.7	0	34.6	32.2
Viet Nam [f]	5.3	6.8	30.9	45.2	69.1	54.8	6.6	10.1	2.6	2.6	19.7	39.6
Yemen [f]	4.1	5.0	54.0	26.8	46.0	73.2	8.0	4.3	7.9	4.1	0	0
Zambia [f]	5.6	6.2	51.3	63.6	48.7	36.4	12.2	16.4	17.8	27.8	0	0
Zimbabwe	...	...	...	...	...	...	...	...	...	...	...	...

Out-of-pocket expenditure as % of private expenditure on health 2000	2011	Private prepaid plans as % of private expenditure on health 2000	2011	Per capita total expenditure on health at average exchange rate (US$) 2000	2011	Per capita total expenditure on health (PPP int. $) 2000	2011	Per capita government expenditure on health at average exchange rate (US$) 2000	2011	Per capita government expenditure on health (PPP int. $) 2000	2011	Member State
94.9	95.9	5.1	4.1	2161	3553	2469	3235	1855	3050	2120	2777	San Marino
76.1	85.2	0	0	46	108	311	143	20	37	134	49	Sao Tome and Principe
66.1	58.8	10.6	18.6	398	721	754	898	287	486	543	605	Saudi Arabia[f]
91.6	77.4	7.1	21.1	22	54	60	94	9	30	25	53	Senegal[f]
84.2	95.5	...	0.8	51	622	313	1172	35	387	219	728	Serbia[v,ab]
99.1	88.2	...	5.4	371	413	813	877	307	392	672	832	Seychelles
95.2	91.4	0.6	0.2	28	82	121	192	6	13	26	31	Sierra Leone[f]
95.7	94.1	0	3.6	662	2144	954	2556	298	714	430	851	Singapore
89.2	77.4	...	0	208	1415	604	1917	186	1004	540	1360	Slovakia
44.1	44.8	51.0	50.1	831	2171	1452	2423	615	1600	1074	1786	Slovenia
56.7	56.7	0	0	48	124	91	230	45	119	86	223	Solomon Islands[f]
100	...	0	...	7	...	17	...	3	...	8	...	Somalia[f]
22.2	13.8	72.4	81.1	246	670	551	930	102	319	228	443	South Africa[f]
...	94.8	...	3.7	...	32	...	35	...	13	...	14	South Sudan
83.1	76.6	13.7	20.6	1045	2978	1546	2984	749	2175	1107	2180	Spain
80.8	83.0	2.8	4.1	32	93	101	183	16	39	49	77	Sri Lanka
90.9	95.7	2.4	1.0	15	119	49	164	4	36	13	50	Sudan[f,i]
44.0	27.1	0.8	15.5	167	490	385	504	89	244	206	251	Suriname
42.4	42.9	18.9	19.2	75	270	197	436	42	188	111	303	Swaziland
91.1	88.1	...	1.5	2282	5419	2289	3938	1937	4423	1943	3214	Sweden
74.0	73.4	23.8	24.4	3541	9248	3230	5673	1963	6001	1790	3681	Switzerland
100	100	...	...	59	102	161	...	24	47	65	...	Syrian Arab Republic[ac]
99.0	85.4	...	0.1	6	48	40	120	1	14	8	36	Tajikistan
76.9	55.8	12.8	30.8	67	214	168	372	38	166	94	289	Thailand f
100	100	...	...	153	344	508	784	88	219	293	499	The former Yugoslav Republic of Macedonia
11.7	15.4	0	0	19	46	52	79	13	35	35	59	Timor-Leste[ad]
88.2	84.6	4.7	4.2	14	43	42	75	4	22	12	39	Togo[f]
77.5	67.8	10.6	17.9	92	219	162	247	65	183	114	206	Tonga[f,j]
86.3	81.3	7.1	14.4	260	935	509	1370	118	460	231	674	Trinidad and Tobago[f]
80.1	86.7	17.8	10.7	123	304	293	652	67	180	161	387	Tunisia[f]
74.6	64.4	11.8	7.3	196	644	436	1047	124	469	274	762	Turkey
100	100	...	...	44	114	137	195	36	73	112	125	Turkmenistan[l,ae]
100	100	0	0	161	639	225	477	161	639	225	476	Tuvalu[f]
56.7	64.8	0.1	0.2	16	41	45	123	4	10	12	31	Uganda[f]
91.4	93.6	1.1	2.1	36	262	184	528	18	146	95	294	Ukraine
69.4	63.2	20.2	27.3	752	1375	865	1430	577	955	664	993	United Arab Emirates
53.3	56.8	17.6	6.0	1761	3659	1830	3364	1394	3031	1448	2787	United Kingdom
83.5	52.6	4.5	1.5	10	38	25	108	4	14	11	40	United Republic of Tanzania[f]
25.0	22.0	59.1	62.5	4790	8467	4790	8467	2062	4047	2062	4047	United States of America
31.2	45.4	14.9	68.7	773	1174	953	1294	422	816	520	899	Uruguay[f]
99.7	94.0	0	5.6	29	91	76	193	14	46	36	98	Uzbekistan
71.6	56.7	10.7	20.6	52	125	122	172	40	109	93	151	Vanuatu[f]
90.9	96.3	3.2	3.7	273	487	481	575	113	178	199	210	Venezuela (Bolivarian Republic of)
95.6	83.2	...	...	20	93	72	227	6	42	22	103	Viet Nam[f]
94.6	98.6	2.2	1.3	25	63	88	108	14	17	47	29	Yemen[f]
80.4	66.4	0.9	3.6	18	87	52	99	9	55	27	63	Zambia[f]
...	...	...	...	...	...	...	...	...	...	...	...	Zimbabwe

Table 7

7. Health expenditure

	Total expenditure on health as % of gross domestic product		General government expenditure on health as % of total expenditure on health[b]		Health expenditure ratios[a] Private expenditure on health as % of total expenditure on health[b]		General government expenditure on health as % of total government expenditure		External resources for health as % of total expenditure on health		Social security expenditure on health as % of general government expenditure on health	
	2000	2011	2000	2011	2000	2011	2000	2011	2000	2011	2000	2011
Ranges of country values												
Minimum	0.8	1.7	4.2	15.9	1.5	0.1	0.1	1.5	0	0	0	0
Median	5.6	6.5	55.2	61.6	45.1	38.4	10.1	11.3	2.7	4.5	5.0	10.0
Maximum	22.5	17.7	100	99.9	95.8	84.1	24.1	28.0	71.5	86.2	100	98.7
WHO region												
African Region	5.6	6.2	43.5	48.3	56.5	51.7	8.7	9.7	6.5	11.8	8.2	8.0
Region of the Americas	11.5	14.1	45.0	49.5	55.0	50.5	14.7	18.1	0.1	0.1	67.2	71.9
South-East Asia Region	3.6	3.7	32.0	36.7	68.8	63.3	7.3	8.7	0.8	1.5	13.2	13.6
European Region	7.9	9.0	74.2	73.9	25.8	25.8	14.0	14.9	0.1	0.1	52.5	51.3
Eastern Mediterranean Region	4.1	4.2	48.1	51.0	51.9	49.0	7.4	7.4	1.0	1.1	18.3	23.7
Western Pacific Region	5.9	6.6	63.9	65.0	36.1	34.9	13.6	14.8	0.2	0.1	68.1	69.1
Income group												
Low income	4.0	5.2	40.5	38.9	64.0	61.1	8.4	9.2	14.0	28.9	1.9	4.3
Lower middle income	4.1	4.4	33.7	36.6	66.3	63.4	7.1	8.1	2.4	2.3	15.0	16.4
Upper middle income	5.4	5.8	47.2	56.2	52.8	43.8	8.8	11.8	0.6	0.4	43.1	50.3
High income	9.8	11.9	59.3	61.3	40.7	38.6	15.3	17.0	0	0	62.7	65.4
Global	8.2	9.1	56.3	58.8	43.7	41.1	13.6	15.2	0.3	0.4	58.8	60.6

a. Health expenditure series. Geneva: World Health Organization (latest updates and more information on countries are available at: http://apps.who.int/nha/database/DataExplorerRegime.aspx). All the indicators refer to expenditures by financing agent except external resources which is a financing source. WHO regional, income-group and global aggregates are calculated using absolute amounts in national currency units converted to Purchasing Power Parity (PPP) equivalents unless otherwise noted. For health expenditure ratios, values smaller than 0.05% may appear as zero. For per capita indicators, when the value is less than 0.5 it is represented as < 1. In countries where the fiscal year begins in July, expenditure data have been allocated to the later calendar year (for example, 2011 data will cover the fiscal year 2010–11), unless otherwise stated for the country. Absolute values of expenditures are expressed in nominal terms (current prices).

b. In some cases, the sum of general government and private expenditures on health may not add up to 100% because of rounding.

c. Care needs to be taken in interpreting external resource figures. Most are taken from the OECD DAC/CRS database except where a reliable full NHA study has been done. These are disbursements to recipient countries as reported by donors, lagged one year to account for the delay between disbursement and expenditure. Disbursement data are not available prior to 2002 and commitments are used instead.

d. National currency unit per US$ are calculated using the average exchange rates for the year. WHO regional, income-group and global aggregates are calculated using constant US$.

e. PPP series resulting from the 2005 International comparison project (ICP) estimated by the World Bank has been used. In countries where this is not available, PPPs are estimated by WHO.

f. A new basis for these estimates was provided by new NHA reports, surveys, National Accounts series, accessed information and/or country consultations.

g. Non-profit institutions (such as NGOs) serving households are accounted for in "external assistance" and recorded under government expenditure. Gross domestic product (GDP) includes both licit and illicit GDPs (for example, opium). Government expenditures include external assistance (external budget).

h. About 30% of the expenditure in residential facilities for care of the aged has a health purpose, but this is difficult to estimate routinely and so is not included under health at present. Such health-purpose expenditure was about US$ 2.1 billion in 2005–06 or 0.2% of GDP.

i. Adjustments for currency change (from old to new manat) were made for the entire Azerbaijan series starting from World Health Statistics 2008.

j. Fiscal year starts in July and expenditure data have been allocated to the later calendar year (i.e. 2007 data cover the fiscal year 2006–07).

k. Fiscal year starts in April and expenditure data have been allocated to the earlier calendar year (i.e. 2006 data cover the fiscal year 2006–07).

l. Estimates should be viewed with caution as these are derived from scarce data.

m. The national accounts data have been revised from 2002 onward. The new data are obtained through a new computation methodology that uses an updated input–output table (International Monetary Fund, World Economic Outlook).

n. Increases in government expenditure on health are due to investment in capital expenditures.

o. The change in the trend of out-of-pocket expenditure in 2008 was driven by a large decrease in total private consumption in 2008 and a large increase in 2009.

p. As a result of recent health-care reforms in Georgia, public compulsory insurance

Health expenditure ratios[a]				Per capita health expenditures[a]								
Out-of-pocket expenditure as % of private expenditure on health		Private prepaid plans as % of private expenditure on health		Per capita total expenditure on health at average exchange rate[d] (US$)		Per capita total expenditure on health[e] (PPP int. $)		Per capita government expenditure on health at average exchange rate[d] (US$)		Per capita government expenditure on health[e] (PPP int. $)		
2000	2011	2000	2011	2000	2011	2000	2011	2000	2011	2000	2011	
2.5	0.5	0	0	3	12	12	15	<1	3	<1	4	Minimum
84.5	84.6	4.2	5.6	111	344	248	511	65	191	158	298	Median
100	100	77.3	81.1	4790	9908	4790	8467	2973	8436	3434	5258	Maximum
56.2	56.6	34.6	31.7	35	99	89	158	15	49	39	76	African Region
32.3	30.1	53.7	56.5	1879	3482	2013	3542	838	1726	905	1754	Region of the Americas
88.9	84.3	2.4	5.2	20	69	61	142	6	26	20	52	South-East Asia Region
67.0	68.8	22.6	20.9	931	2370	1207	2311	703	1782	895	1709	European Region
88.2	88.9	5.6	7.0	93	195	173	327	46	107	83	166	Eastern Mediterranean Region
86.1	78.4	7.2	9.6	286	679	293	710	208	472	187	461	Western Pacific Region
84.1	76.2	1.3	1.5	10	30	28	64	4	11	11	25	Low income
89.6	87.1	2.6	4.4	25	82	76	163	8	31	26	60	Lower middle income
80.2	74.2	15.7	17.2	112	408	224	586	53	226	106	330	Upper middle income
38.5	37.6	47.5	49.0	2253	4586	2370	4319	1334	2875	1405	2648	High income
49.5	49.7	38.6	38.2	485	1007	568	1053	280	613	320	619	Global

Table 7

has since 2008 been implemented by private insurance companies. The voucher cost of this insurance is treated as general government health expenditure.

q. Government expenditures show fluctuations due to variations in capital investment.

r. Exchange rate changed in 2002 from multiple to a managed floating exchange rate. Inter-bank market rate used prior to 2002.

s. The estimates do not include expenditures for Northern Iraq. The break in the series was due to changed sources.

t. The public expenditure on health includes contributions from the United Nations Relief and Works Agency for Palestine Refugees in the Near East (UNRWA) made to Palestinian refugees residing in Jordanian territories.

u. Fiscal year starts in October and expenditure data have been allocated to the later calendar year (i.e. 2007 data cover the fiscal year 2006–07).

v. After the declaration of independence on 3 June 2006, Serbia and Montenegro became separate states. Health expenditures for previous years have been estimated separately for each of the two countries.

w. The market exchange rate is used to estimate the per capita figures. A new basis for these estimates was provided by new NHA reports, surveys, National Accounts series, accessed information and/or country consultations.

x. Changes in population data between the United Nations Population Division's World Population Prospects: the 2010 Revision and World Population Prospects: the 2012 Revision led to changes in per capita levels.

y. Total level of government expenditure on health increased due to the inclusion of local government expenditure, as well as a more-comprehensive estimation of regional expenditure on health.

z. The 2005–2011 NHA were computed based on revised estimation methodologies

developed by the National Statistical Coordination Board (NSCB) Technical Staff following an extensive review in 2012 of the input data by NHA component and the computational procedures (see http://www.nscb.gov.ph/stats/pnha/technotes.asp). This major revision involved the expansion of the coverage of the NHA in 2005–2011 compared with previous years.

aa. The health expenditure data as well as the population data after 2000 do not include Transdniestria. Data on GDP and private final consumption expenditure exclude Transdniestria from 1995.

ab. The estimates do not include the expenditures of the provinces of Kosovo and Metohia, which are under the administration of the United Nations.

ac. The exchange rate used for the Syrian Arab Republic is the rate for non-commercial transactions from the Central Bank of Syria.

ad. GDP does not include the income from petroleum. The country became independent in 2002. However, NHA estimates have been produced for previous years based on the available macro data. Until 2007, the fiscal year ended in June. There was then a transition period in the second quarter of 2007 to make the fiscal year equal to the calendar year. Expenditure data have been allocated exceptionally to the previous calendar year (i.e. 2005 data covers the fiscal year 2005–06). Drop in health expenditures from previous years is mainly due to revision of out-of-pocket expenditure estimates.

ae. On 1 January 2009 Turkmenistan introduced the new manat ISO code TMT. The exchange rate between the old and the new currency is 1 TMT = 5000 TMM. The entire health expenditure series has been adjusted.

8. Health inequities

In general, the global reporting of health indicators focuses on national averages. However, data on the distribution of health and health services within countries and between population subgroups are equally important. Such data help to identify health inequities – unfair and avoidable differences in health and health service provision.

Health inequity is not only detrimental to the most vulnerable, but can be seen across the social gradient. Measuring and tracking disaggregated health data are key components of incorporating gender, equity and human-rights aspects into health systems, and advancing a health-in-all-policies agenda. It also provides evidence and feedback for strengthening equity-oriented initiatives such as the movement towards universal health coverage. Table 8 covers data from 83 countries collected during Demographic and Health Surveys (DHS) and Multiple Indicator Cluster Surveys (MICS) conducted between 2005 and 2011.

Six health indicators are presented – modern contraceptive prevalence; antenatal care coverage; births attended by skilled health personnel; DTP3 immunization coverage among 1-year-olds; children < 5 years of age who are stunted; and under-five mortality rate – with data disaggregated according to urban or rural residence, household wealth, maternal educational level and, where applicable, by the sex of the child.

For household wealth and maternal educational level, point estimates are shown for subgroups with the highest and lowest levels of these measures. A complete set of disaggregated data on these and other health indicators is available at the Health Equity Monitor of the WHO Global Health Observatory.[1]

Table 8

---

[1] Health Equity Monitor, Global Health Observatory [online database]. Geneva: World Health Organization (http://www.who.int/gho/health_equity/en/index.html).

| Member State | Source | Contraceptive prevalence: modern methods[a] (%) | | | | | | Antenatal care coverage: at least 4 visits[a,b] (%) | | | | | | Births attended by skilled health personnel[a,c] (%) | | | | | |
| | | Place of residence | | Wealth quintile | | Educational level of woman | | Place of residence | | Wealth quintile | | Educational level of woman | | Place of residence | | Wealth quintile | | Educational level of woman | |
		Rural	Urban	Lowest	Highest	None	Secondary or higher	Rural	Urban	Lowest	Highest	None	Secondary or higher	Rural	Urban	Lowest	Highest	None	Secondary or higher
Afghanistan		...	...	...	...	...	...	...	...	...	...	...	...	...	...	...	...	...	...
Albania	DHS 2008–2009	10	12	11	14	...e	13	57	82	49	91	...e	80	99	100	98	100	...e	100
Algeria		...	...	...	...	...	...	...	...	...	...	...	...	...	...	...	...	...	...
Andorra		...	...	...	...	...	...	...	...	...	...	...	...	...	...	...	...	...	...
Angola		...	...	...	...	...	...	...	...	...	...	...	...	...	...	...	...	...	...
Antigua and Barbuda		...	...	...	...	...	...	...	...	...	...	...	...	...	...	...	...	...	...
Argentina		...	...	...	...	...	...	...	...	...	...	...	...	...	...	...	...	...	...
Armenia	DHS 2010	19	33	21	38	...e	27	89	96	88	96	...e	93	99	100	99	100	...e	100
Australia		...	...	...	...	...	...	...	...	...	...	...	...	...	...	...	...	...	...
Austria		...	...	...	...	...	...	...	...	...	...	...	...	...	...	...	...	...	...
Azerbaijan	DHS 2006	10	18	11	21	6	15	30	60	20	74	...e	46	81	97	78	100	83 g	89
Bahamas		...	...	...	...	...	...	...	...	...	...	...	...	...	...	...	...	...	...
Bahrain		...	...	...	...	...	...	...	...	...	...	...	...	...	...	...	...	...	...
Bangladesh	DHS 2007	46	52	47	49	46	48	16	38	8	47	7	35	13	37	5	51	5	33
Barbados		...	...	...	...	...	...	...	...	...	...	...	...	...	...	...	...	...	...
Belarus		...	...	...	...	...	...	...	...	...	...	...	...	...	...	...	...	...	...
Belgium		...	...	...	...	...	...	...	...	...	...	...	...	...	...	...	...	...	...
Belize	MICS 2006	...	...	...	...	...	...	...	...	...	...	...	...	93	99	84	98 g	...e	99
Benin	DHS 2006	5	9	2	13	4	16	55	71	40	88	54	85	74	86	56	97	72	98
Bhutan	MICS 2010	66	64	69	62	67	57	73	87	64	92	74	88	54	89	34	95	54	94
Bolivia (Plurinational State of)	DHS 2008	26	40	23	47	22	43	60	81	50	91	49	85	51	88	38	99	40	91
Bosnia and Herzegovina	MICS 2006	9	16	4	20	3 g	14	...	...	...	...	...	...	100	100	99	100	...e	100
Botswana		...	...	...	...	...	...	...	...	...	...	...	...	...	...	...	...	...	...
Brazil		...	...	...	...	...	...	...	...	...	...	...	...	...	...	...	...	...	...
Brunei Darussalam		...	...	...	...	...	...	...	...	...	...	...	...	...	...	...	...	...	...
Bulgaria		...	...	...	...	...	...	...	...	...	...	...	...	...	...	...	...	...	...
Burkina Faso	DHS 2010	11	31	7	34	11	44	31	45	24	47	31	57	62	94	47	93	63	97
Burundi	DHS 2010	17	29	15	26	14	34	33	39	34	37	32	46	58	88	51	81	52	91
Cabo Verde		...	...	...	...	...	...	...	...	...	...	...	...	...	...	...	...	...	...
Cambodia	DHS 2010	36	31	35	31	34	34	55	80	43	83	40	78	67	95	49	97	47	91
Cameroon	DHS 2011	9	21	2	26	3	25	50	77	33	86	35	82	47	87	19	97	23	93
Canada		...	...	...	...	...	...	...	...	...	...	...	...	...	...	...	...	...	...
Central African Republic	MICS 2006	3	18	1	23	2	29	...	...	...	...	...	...	35	83	27	89	34	88
Chad		...	...	...	...	...	...	...	...	...	...	...	...	...	...	...	...	...	...
Chile		...	...	...	...	...	...	...	...	...	...	...	...	...	...	...	...	...	...
China		...	...	...	...	...	...	...	...	...	...	...	...	...	...	...	...	...	...
Colombia	DHS 2010	72	73	68	75	63	73	81	91	79	96	61	92	86	98	84	99	71	98
Comoros		...	...	...	...	...	...	...	...	...	...	...	...	...	...	...	...	...	...
Congo		...	...	...	...	...	...	...	...	...	...	...	...	...	...	...	...	...	...
Cook Islands		...	...	...	...	...	...	...	...	...	...	...	...	...	...	...	...	...	...
Costa Rica		...	...	...	...	...	...	...	...	...	...	...	...	...	...	...	...	...	...
Côte d'Ivoire	MICS 2006	6	15	4	19	6	22	...	...	...	...	...	...	40	84	29	95	47	87
Croatia		...	...	...	...	...	...	...	...	...	...	...	...	...	...	...	...	...	...
Cuba	MICS 2010–2011	78	72	...	...	...e	73	...	...	...	...	...	...	...	...	...	...	...	...
Cyprus		...	...	...	...	...	...	...	...	...	...	...	...	...	...	...	...	...	...
Czech Republic		...	...	...	...	...	...	...	...	...	...	...	...	...	...	...	...	...	...
Democratic People's Republic of Korea		...	...	...	...	...	...	...	...	...	...	...	...	...	...	...	...	...	...
Democratic Republic of the Congo	MICS 2010	4	10	1	14	2	10	39	57	38	62	33	56	67	94	60	96	60	88
Denmark		...	...	...	...	...	...	...	...	...	...	...	...	...	...	...	...	...	...

DTP3 immunization coverage among 1-year-olds[a] (%)								Children aged <5 years who are stunted[a] (%)								Under-five mortality rate[a,d] (probability of dying by age 5 per 1000 live births) MDG 4								Member State
Sex		Place of residence		Wealth quintile		Educational level of mother		Sex		Place of residence		Wealth quintile		Educational level of mother		Sex		Place of residence		Wealth quintile		Educational level of mother		
Male	Female	Rural	Urban	Lowest	Highest	None	Secondary or higher	Male	Female	Rural	Urban	Lowest	Highest	None	Secondary or higher	Male	Female	Rural	Urban	Lowest	Highest	None	Secondary or higher	
...	...	...	...	...	...	...	...	...	...	...	...	...	...	...	...	...	...	...	...	...	...	...	...	Afghanistan
97	98	97	99	100	97 [g]	... [e]	97	18	21	19	20	27	13	... [e]	17	27	16	28	13	34	13	... [f]	19	Albania
...	...	...	...	...	...	...	...	...	...	...	...	...	...	...	...	...	...	...	...	...	...	...	...	Algeria
...	...	...	...	...	...	...	...	...	...	...	...	...	...	...	...	...	...	...	...	...	...	...	...	Andorra
...	...	...	...	...	...	...	...	...	...	...	...	...	...	...	...	...	...	...	...	...	...	...	...	Angola
...	...	...	...	...	...	...	...	...	...	...	...	...	...	...	...	...	...	...	...	...	...	...	...	Antigua and Barbuda
...	...	...	...	...	...	...	...	...	...	...	...	...	...	...	...	...	...	...	...	...	...	...	...	Argentina
95	95	94	96	88	97 [g]	... [e]	95	20	18	22	17	26	19	... [e]	19	21	22	26	19	26	22	... [f]	22	Armenia
...	...	...	...	...	...	...	...	...	...	...	...	...	...	...	...	...	...	...	...	...	...	...	...	Australia
...	...	...	...	...	...	...	...	...	...	...	...	...	...	...	...	...	...	...	...	...	...	...	...	Austria
31	29	22	39	21	64	... [e]	31	27	24	30	20	33	15	... [e]	25	64	49	63	51	63	38	... [f]	57	Azerbaijan
...	...	...	...	...	...	...	...	...	...	...	...	...	...	...	...	...	...	...	...	...	...	...	...	Bahamas
...	...	...	...	...	...	...	...	...	...	...	...	...	...	...	...	...	...	...	...	...	...	...	...	Bahrain
91	91	91	92	92	95	85	95	44	42	45	36	54	26	51	33	75	71	76	62	85	43	91	52	Bangladesh
...	...	...	...	...	...	...	...	...	...	...	...	...	...	...	...	...	...	...	...	...	...	...	...	Barbados
...	...	...	...	...	...	...	...	...	...	...	...	...	...	...	...	...	...	...	...	...	...	...	...	Belarus
...	...	...	...	...	...	...	...	...	...	...	...	...	...	...	...	...	...	...	...	...	...	...	...	Belgium
77	65	70	72	73 [g]	... [e]	73	... [e]	24	21	28	15	38	8	26	... [e]	...	...	...	...	...	...	...	...	Belize
66	69	62	77	50	87	62	91	46	40	47	36	50	29	47	27	139	132	145	115	151	83	143	79	Benin
...	...	...	...	...	...	...	...	33	34	36	28	41	21	37	23	...	...	...	...	...	...	...	...	Bhutan
87	85	87	85	86	86	85	90	28	26	39	17	46	6	50	15	79	71	98	54	116	31	134	43	Bolivia (Plurinational State of)
90	88	90	86	80	90	... [e]	91	13	11	12	11	18	8	... [e]	11	...	...	...	...	...	...	...	...	Bosnia and Herzegovina
...	...	...	...	...	...	...	...	...	...	...	...	...	...	...	...	...	...	...	...	...	...	...	...	Botswana
...	...	...	...	...	...	...	...	...	...	...	...	...	...	...	...	...	...	...	...	...	...	...	...	Brazil
...	...	...	...	...	...	...	...	...	...	...	...	...	...	...	...	...	...	...	...	...	...	...	...	Brunei Darussalam
...	...	...	...	...	...	...	...	...	...	...	...	...	...	...	...	...	...	...	...	...	...	...	...	Bulgaria
90	89	89	92	83	93	89	92	37	32	37	21	42	18	37	11	153	141	155	104	174	95	155	61	Burkina Faso
96	96	96	91	94	94	96	93	63	53	60	38	70	42	62	31	134	116	129	79	148	80	138	44	Burundi
...	...	...	...	...	...	...	...	...	...	...	...	...	...	...	...	...	...	...	...	...	...	...	...	Cabo Verde
85	85	84	90	74	93	67	92	41	37	41	27	49	22	46	31	76	59	75	29	91	30	86	35	Cambodia
69	69	61	80	45	88	46	84	35	29	40	21	49	12	46	19	135	121	153	93	184	72	175	76	Cameroon
...	...	...	...	...	...	...	...	...	...	...	...	...	...	...	...	...	...	...	...	...	...	...	...	Canada
39	39	29	55	22	63	24	63	46	40	47	38	49	31	47	36	...	...	...	...	...	...	...	...	Central African Republic
...	...	...	...	...	...	...	...	...	...	...	...	...	...	...	...	...	...	...	...	...	...	...	...	Chad
...	...	...	...	...	...	...	...	...	...	...	...	...	...	...	...	...	...	...	...	...	...	...	...	Chile
...	...	...	...	...	...	...	...	...	...	...	...	...	...	...	...	...	...	...	...	...	...	...	...	China
91	90	88	91	85	93	79	91	14	12	17	12	20	7	31	11	24	19	24	21	29	13	53	18	Colombia
...	...	...	...	...	...	...	...	...	...	...	...	...	...	...	...	...	...	...	...	...	...	...	...	Comoros
...	...	...	...	...	...	...	...	...	...	...	...	...	...	...	...	...	...	...	...	...	...	...	...	Congo
...	...	...	...	...	...	...	...	...	...	...	...	...	...	...	...	...	...	...	...	...	...	...	...	Cook Islands
...	...	...	...	...	...	...	...	...	...	...	...	...	...	...	...	...	...	...	...	...	...	...	...	Costa Rica
78	77	71	89	60	96	73	87	44	37	46	32	47	27	43	31	...	...	...	...	...	...	...	...	Côte d'Ivoire
...	...	...	...	...	...	...	...	...	...	...	...	...	...	...	...	...	...	...	...	...	...	...	...	Croatia
99	96	93	99	...	...	... [e]	97	...	...	...	...	...	...	...	...	...	...	...	...	...	...	...	...	Cuba
...	...	...	...	...	...	...	...	...	...	...	...	...	...	...	...	...	...	...	...	...	...	...	...	Cyprus
...	...	...	...	...	...	...	...	...	...	...	...	...	...	...	...	...	...	...	...	...	...	...	...	Czech Republic
...	...	...	...	...	...	...	...	...	...	...	...	...	...	...	...	...	...	...	...	...	...	...	...	Democratic People's Republic of Korea
63	61	57	77	48	80	54	73	47	40	47	34	47	26	50	35	...	...	...	...	...	...	...	...	Democratic Republic of the Congo
...	...	...	...	...	...	...	...	...	...	...	...	...	...	...	...	...	...	...	...	...	...	...	...	Denmark

Table 8

Member State	Source	Contraceptive prevalence: modern methods[a] (%)						Antenatal care coverage: at least 4 visits[a,b] (%)						Births attended by skilled health personnel[a,c] (%)					
		Place of residence		Wealth quintile		Educational level of woman		Place of residence		Wealth quintile		Educational level of woman		Place of residence		Wealth quintile		Educational level of woman	
		Rural	Urban	Lowest	Highest	None	Secondary or higher	Rural	Urban	Lowest	Highest	None	Secondary or higher	Rural	Urban	Lowest	Highest	None	Secondary or higher
Djibouti	MICS 2006	4	18	...	...	12	33	...	...	...	...	...	...	40	95	...	...	92	96
Dominica		...	...	...	...	...	...	...	...	...	...	...	...	...	...	...	...	...	...
Dominican Republic	DHS 2007	73	69	67	69	68	67	94	95	90	97	88	97	97	98	95	99	90	99
Ecuador		...	...	...	...	...	...	...	...	...	...	...	...	...	...	...	...	...	...
Egypt	DHS 2008	55	62	52	62	56	58	58	81	42	89	46	76	72	90	55	97	60	87
El Salvador		...	...	...	...	...	...	...	...	...	...	...	...	...	...	...	...	...	...
Equatorial Guinea		...	...	...	...	...	...	...	...	...	...	...	...	...	...	...	...	...	...
Eritrea		...	...	...	...	...	...	...	...	...	...	...	...	...	...	...	...	...	...
Estonia		...	...	...	...	...	...	...	...	...	...	...	...	...	...	...	...	...	...
Ethiopia	DHS 2011	23	50	13	48	22	55	14	46	8	46	12	65	5	52	2	46	5	74
Fiji		...	...	...	...	...	...	...	...	...	...	...	...	...	...	...	...	...	...
Finland		...	...	...	...	...	...	...	...	...	...	...	...	...	...	...	...	...	...
France		...	...	...	...	...	...	...	...	...	...	...	...	...	...	...	...	...	...
Gabon		...	...	...	...	...	...	...	...	...	...	...	...	...	...	...	...	...	...
Gambia	MICS 2005–2006	...	...	...	...	...	...	...	...	...	...	...	...	43	83	28	89	51	85
Georgia		...	...	...	...	...	...	...	...	...	...	...	...	...	...	...	...	...	...
Germany		...	...	...	...	...	...	...	...	...	...	...	...	...	...	...	...	...	...
Ghana	DHS 2008	15	19	12	21	11	19	72	88	63	94	68	88	43	84	24	95	36	78
Greece		...	...	...	...	...	...	...	...	...	...	...	...	...	...	...	...	...	...
Grenada		...	...	...	...	...	...	...	...	...	...	...	...	...	...	...	...	...	...
Guatemala		...	...	...	...	...	...	...	...	...	...	...	...	...	...	...	...	...	...
Guinea		...	...	...	...	...	...	...	...	...	...	...	...	...	...	...	...	...	...
Guinea-Bissau	MICS 2006	2	15	1	19	3	26	...	...	...	...	...	...	27	69	19	79	28	80
Guyana	DHS 2009	40	40	31	45	21	41	77	82	72	83	59 [g]	82	90	98	81	96	71	94
Haiti	DHS 2005–2006	22	28	15	29	19	31	46	67	33	82	36	79	15	47	6	68	9	60
Honduras	DHS 2005–2006	51	62	41	65	46	62	76	87	69	96	62	93	50	90	33	99	37	96
Hungary		...	...	...	...	...	...	...	...	...	...	...	...	...	...	...	...	...	...
Iceland		...	...	...	...	...	...	...	...	...	...	...	...	...	...	...	...	...	...
India	DHS 2005–2006	45	56	35	58	46	50	28	62	12	77	16	63	38	74	19	89	26	75
Indonesia	DHS 2007	58	57	50	58	40	59	76	90	61	96	44	90	63	88	44	95	31	87
Iran (Islamic Republic of)		...	...	...	...	...	...	...	...	...	...	...	...	...	...	...	...	...	...
Iraq	MICS 2006	27	36	...	...	29	39	...	...	...	...	...	...	78	95	...	...	79	96
Ireland		...	...	...	...	...	...	...	...	...	...	...	...	...	...	...	...	...	...
Israel		...	...	...	...	...	...	...	...	...	...	...	...	...	...	...	...	...	...
Italy		...	...	...	...	...	...	...	...	...	...	...	...	...	...	...	...	...	...
Jamaica		...	...	...	...	...	...	...	...	...	...	...	...	...	...	...	...	...	...
Japan		...	...	...	...	...	...	...	...	...	...	...	...	...	...	...	...	...	...
Jordan	DHS 2007	36	43	35	47	36	42	91	95	90	98	76	95	99	99	98	100	94	99
Kazakhstan	MICS 2006	44	52	40	57	... [e]	49	...	...	...	...	...	...	100	100	100	100	... [e]	100
Kenya	DHS 2008–2009	37	47	17	48	12	52	44	60	36	63	35	64	37	75	20	81	19	73
Kiribati		...	...	...	...	...	...	...	...	...	...	...	...	...	...	...	...	...	...
Kuwait		...	...	...	...	...	...	...	...	...	...	...	...	...	...	...	...	...	...
Kyrgyzstan	MICS 2005–2006	45	47	47	49	... [e]	46	...	...	...	...	...	...	96	100	93	100	... [e]	97
Lao People's Democratic Republic	MICS 2006	...	...	...	...	...	...	...	...	...	...	...	...	11	68	3	81	3	63
Latvia		...	...	...	...	...	...	...	...	...	...	...	...	...	...	...	...	...	...
Lebanon		...	...	...	...	...	...	...	...	...	...	...	...	...	...	...	...	...	...
Lesotho	DHS 2009	41	57	29	61	28	55	66	83	58	85	68	79	54	88	35	90	40	80
Liberia	DHS 2007	7	16	3	17	7	18	61	76	55	78	62	77	32	79	26	81	36	76
Libya		...	...	...	...	...	...	...	...	...	...	...	...	...	...	...	...	...	...

MDG 4																								
DTP3 immunization coverage among 1-year-olds[a] (%)								Children aged <5 years who are stunted[a] (%)								Under-five mortality rate[a,d] (probability of dying by age 5 per 1000 live births)								Member State
Sex		Place of residence		Wealth quintile		Educational level of mother		Sex		Place of residence		Wealth quintile		Educational level of mother		Sex		Place of residence		Wealth quintile		Educational level of mother		
Male	Female	Rural	Urban	Lowest	Highest	None	Secondary or higher	Male	Female	Rural	Urban	Lowest	Highest	None	Secondary or higher	Male	Female	Rural	Urban	Lowest	Highest	None	Secondary or higher	
61	59	44 [g]	61	...	...	58	67	35	31	40	33	...	...	33	37	...	...	...	...	...	...	...	...	Djibouti
...	...	...	...	...	...	...	...	...	...	...	...	...	...	...	...	...	...	...	...	...	...	...	...	Dominica
76	73	74	75	67	85	54	78	11	8	13	8	16	4	14	8	40	34	38	37	53	27	56	29	Dominican Republic
...	...	...	...	...	...	...	...	...	...	...	...	...	...	...	...	...	...	...	...	...	...	...	...	Ecuador
97	98	97	99	97	99	97	99	31	27	30	27	30	27	30	28	38	28	36	29	48	19	44	26	Egypt
...	...	...	...	...	...	...	...	...	...	...	...	...	...	...	...	...	...	...	...	...	...	...	...	El Salvador
...	...	...	...	...	...	...	...	...	...	...	...	...	...	...	...	...	...	...	...	...	...	...	...	Equatorial Guinea
...	...	...	...	...	...	...	...	...	...	...	...	...	...	...	...	...	...	...	...	...	...	...	...	Eritrea
...	...	...	...	...	...	...	...	...	...	...	...	...	...	...	...	...	...	...	...	...	...	...	...	Estonia
35	39	33	62	26	64	32	73	46	43	46	31	49	29	47	20	121	97	114	82	136	84	120	36	Ethiopia
...	...	...	...	...	...	...	...	...	...	...	...	...	...	...	...	...	...	...	...	...	...	...	...	Fiji
...	...	...	...	...	...	...	...	...	...	...	...	...	...	...	...	...	...	...	...	...	...	...	...	Finland
...	...	...	...	...	...	...	...	...	...	...	...	...	...	...	...	...	...	...	...	...	...	...	...	France
...	...	...	...	...	...	...	...	...	...	...	...	...	...	...	...	...	...	...	...	...	...	...	...	Gabon
84	88	86	86	89	89	86	87	29	27	32	19	37	15	29	19	...	...	...	...	...	...	...	...	Gambia
...	...	...	...	...	...	...	...	...	...	...	...	...	...	...	...	...	...	...	...	...	...	...	...	Georgia
...	...	...	...	...	...	...	...	...	...	...	...	...	...	...	...	...	...	...	...	...	...	...	...	Germany
89	89	91	87	89	93	85	91	29	26	32	20	33	14	30	24	93	75	90	75	102	60	102	67	Ghana
...	...	...	...	...	...	...	...	...	...	...	...	...	...	...	...	...	...	...	...	...	...	...	...	Greece
...	...	...	...	...	...	...	...	...	...	...	...	...	...	...	...	...	...	...	...	...	...	...	...	Grenada
...	...	...	...	...	...	...	...	...	...	...	...	...	...	...	...	...	...	...	...	...	...	...	...	Guatemala
...	...	...	...	...	...	...	...	...	...	...	...	...	...	...	...	...	...	...	...	...	...	...	...	Guinea
65	64	62	71	57	78	61	77	48	48	51	41	49	37	51	36	...	...	...	...	...	...	...	...	Guinea-Bissau
82	87	84	88	77	86	...[e]	86	20	17	21	11	31	10	23	15	41	39	38	46	33	44	...[f]	36	Guyana
53	55	50	61	46	72	48	69	31	26	34	19	40	7	39	12	105	99	114	77	124	55	122	65	Haiti
93	93	94	92	94	88	89	93	31	28	38	17	50	7	54	9	39	34	43	29	50	20	53	19	Honduras
...	...	...	...	...	...	...	...	...	...	...	...	...	...	...	...	...	...	...	...	...	...	...	...	Hungary
...	...	...	...	...	...	...	...	...	...	...	...	...	...	...	...	...	...	...	...	...	...	...	...	Iceland
58	53	51	69	34	82	37	78	48	48	51	40	60	26	57	36	82	88	93	60	117	39	106	49	India
66	68	61	75	46	82	29	76	...	...	...	...	...	...	...	...	55	46	60	38	77	31	93	37	Indonesia
...	...	...	...	...	...	...	...	...	...	...	...	...	...	...	...	...	...	...	...	...	...	...	...	Iran (Islamic Republic of)
63	58	50	68	...	...	46	75	29	26	31	25	...	...	30	23	...	...	...	...	...	...	...	...	Iraq
...	...	...	...	...	...	...	...	...	...	...	...	...	...	...	...	...	...	...	...	...	...	...	...	Ireland
...	...	...	...	...	...	...	...	...	...	...	...	...	...	...	...	...	...	...	...	...	...	...	...	Israel
...	...	...	...	...	...	...	...	...	...	...	...	...	...	...	...	...	...	...	...	...	...	...	...	Italy
...	...	...	...	...	...	...	...	...	...	...	...	...	...	...	...	...	...	...	...	...	...	...	...	Jamaica
...	...	...	...	...	...	...	...	...	...	...	...	...	...	...	...	...	...	...	...	...	...	...	...	Japan
97	98	97	98	97	98	89	98	16	13	17	14	18	9	26	14	22	23	27	21	30	27	27	21	Jordan
98	97	96	99	98	98	...[e]	97	18	17	20	15	21	12	...[e]	17	...	...	...	...	...	...	...	...	Kazakhstan
83	90	86	88	78	90	82	92	37	33	37	27	44	25	39	25	90	77	85	75	97	69	86	58	Kenya
...	...	...	...	...	...	...	...	...	...	...	...	...	...	...	...	...	...	...	...	...	...	...	...	Kiribati
...	...	...	...	...	...	...	...	...	...	...	...	...	...	...	...	...	...	...	...	...	...	...	...	Kuwait
46	49	37	64	25	72	...[e]	48	19	18	21	15	20	14	...[e]	18	...	...	...	...	...	...	...	...	Kyrgyzstan
40	42	38	56	29	59	29	57	48	47	51	32	58	23	55	31	...	...	...	...	...	...	...	...	Lao People's Democratic Republic
...	...	...	...	...	...	...	...	...	...	...	...	...	...	...	...	...	...	...	...	...	...	...	...	Latvia
...	...	...	...	...	...	...	...	...	...	...	...	...	...	...	...	...	...	...	...	...	...	...	...	Lebanon
84	84	82	91	73	88	...[e]	88	41	35	40	29	45	28	41 [g]	31	123	87	111	89	107	81	...[f]	89	Lesotho
49	52	41	70	30	72	47	70	41	35	42	29	43	25	40	28	147	131	144	129	137	115	149	116	Liberia
...	...	...	...	...	...	...	...	...	...	...	...	...	...	...	...	...	...	...	...	...	...	...	...	Libya

Table 8

Member State	Source	Contraceptive prevalence: modern methods[a] (%)						Antenatal care coverage: at least 4 visits[a,b] (%)						Births attended by skilled health personnel[a,c] (%)					
		Place of residence		Wealth quintile		Educational level of woman		Place of residence		Wealth quintile		Educational level of woman		Place of residence		Wealth quintile		Educational level of woman	
		Rural	Urban	Lowest	Highest	None	Secondary or higher	Rural	Urban	Lowest	Highest	None	Secondary or higher	Rural	Urban	Lowest	Highest	None	Secondary or higher
Lithuania		...	...	...	...	...	...	...	...	...	...	...	...	...	...	...	...	...	...
Luxembourg		...	...	...	...	...	...	...	...	...	...	...	...	...	...	...	...	...	...
Madagascar	DHS 2008–2009	28	36	18	36	18	34	46	71	35	75	37	67	39	82	22	90	23	76
Malawi	DHS 2010	41	50	35	48	37	49	45	49	41	51	44	52	69	84	63	89	62	88
Malaysia		...	...	...	...	...	...	...	...	...	...	...	...	...	...	...	...	...	...
Maldives	DHS 2009	28	26	29	26	36	20	87	80	88	80	83	86	93	99	89	99	85	99
Mali	DHS 2006	4	13	3	16	5	23	28	55	23	64	31	70	12	67	9	75	22	78
Malta		...	...	...	...	...	...	...	...	...	...	...	...	...	...	...	...	...	...
Marshall Islands		...	...	...	...	...	...	...	...	...	...	...	...	...	...	...	...	...	...
Mauritania	MICS 2007	3	14	1	16	4	19	...	...	...	...	...	...	39	90	21	95	45	92
Mauritius		...	...	...	...	...	...	...	...	...	...	...	...	...	...	...	...	...	...
Mexico		...	...	...	...	...	...	...	...	...	...	...	...	...	...	...	...	...	...
Micronesia (Federated States of)		...	...	...	...	...	...	...	...	...	...	...	...	...	...	...	...	...	...
Monaco		...	...	...	...	...	...	...	...	...	...	...	...	...	...	...	...	...	...
Mongolia		...	...	...	...	...	...	...	...	...	...	...	...	...	...	...	...	...	...
Montenegro	MICS 2005–2006	15	18	8	23	...[e]	19	...	...	...	...	...	...	98	100	98	100	...[e]	99
Morocco		...	...	...	...	...	...	...	...	...	...	...	...	...	...	...	...	...	...
Mozambique	MICS 2008	8	22	5	30	6	33	...	...	...	...	...	...	46	78	37	89	41	90
Myanmar		...	...	...	...	...	...	...	...	...	...	...	...	...	...	...	...	...	...
Namibia	DHS 2006–2007	43	64	30	68	32	63	68	73	64	77	51	75	73	94	60	98	50	92
Nauru		...	...	...	...	...	...	...	...	...	...	...	...	...	...	...	...	...	...
Nepal	DHS 2011	42	50	36	49	49	37	48	72	28	84	29	75	32	73	11	82	19	63
Netherlands		...	...	...	...	...	...	...	...	...	...	...	...	...	...	...	...	...	...
New Zealand		...	...	...	...	...	...	...	...	...	...	...	...	...	...	...	...	...	...
Nicaragua		...	...	...	...	...	...	...	...	...	...	...	...	...	...	...	...	...	...
Niger	DHS 2006	3	18	2	16	3	29	11	35	9	35	12	54	8	71	5	59	13	81
Nigeria	DHS 2008	7	17	3	22	3	19	34	69	16	81	22	71	28	65	8	86	12	77
Niue		...	...	...	...	...	...	...	...	...	...	...	...	...	...	...	...	...	...
Norway		...	...	...	...	...	...	...	...	...	...	...	...	...	...	...	...	...	...
Oman		...	...	...	...	...	...	...	...	...	...	...	...	...	...	...	...	...	...
Pakistan	DHS 2006–2007	18	30	12	32	19	28	20	48	10	64	17	61	30	60	16	77	27	74
Palau		...	...	...	...	...	...	...	...	...	...	...	...	...	...	...	...	...	...
Panama		...	...	...	...	...	...	...	...	...	...	...	...	...	...	...	...	...	...
Papua New Guinea		...	...	...	...	...	...	...	...	...	...	...	...	...	...	...	...	...	...
Paraguay		...	...	...	...	...	...	...	...	...	...	...	...	...	...	...	...	...	...
Peru	DHS 2004–2008	40	53	34	54	34	53	84	94	78	97	80	94	54	94	38	99	46	92
Philippines	DHS 2008	33	35	26	33	9	36	73	83	61	93	32	84	48	78	26	94	11	73
Poland		...	...	...	...	...	...	...	...	...	...	...	...	...	...	...	...	...	...
Portugal		...	...	...	...	...	...	...	...	...	...	...	...	...	...	...	...	...	...
Qatar		...	...	...	...	...	...	...	...	...	...	...	...	...	...	...	...	...	...
Republic of Korea		...	...	...	...	...	...	...	...	...	...	...	...	...	...	...	...	...	...
Republic of Moldova		...	...	...	...	...	...	...	...	...	...	...	...	...	...	...	...	...	...
Romania		...	...	...	...	...	...	...	...	...	...	...	...	...	...	...	...	...	...
Russian Federation		...	...	...	...	...	...	...	...	...	...	...	...	...	...	...	...	...	...
Rwanda	DHS 2010	45	47	39	50	37	52	35	40	34	43	33	43	67	82	61	86	57	88
Saint Kitts and Nevis		...	...	...	...	...	...	...	...	...	...	...	...	...	...	...	...	...	...
Saint Lucia		...	...	...	...	...	...	...	...	...	...	...	...	...	...	...	...	...	...
Saint Vincent and the Grenadines		...	...	...	...	...	...	...	...	...	...	...	...	...	...	...	...	...	...
Samoa		...	...	...	...	...	...	...	...	...	...	...	...	...	...	...	...	...	...

DTP3 immunization coverage among 1-year-olds[a] (%)								Children aged <5 years who are stunted[a] (%)								Under-five mortality rate[a,d] (probability of dying by age 5 per 1000 live births) — MDG 4								Member State
Sex		Place of residence		Wealth quintile		Educational level of mother		Sex		Place of residence		Wealth quintile		Educational level of mother		Sex		Place of residence		Wealth quintile		Educational level of mother		
Male	Female	Rural	Urban	Lowest	Highest	None	Secondary or higher	Male	Female	Rural	Urban	Lowest	Highest	None	Secondary or higher	Male	Female	Rural	Urban	Lowest	Highest	None	Secondary or higher	
...	...	...	...	...	...	...	...	...	...	...	...	...	...	...	...	...	...	...	...	...	...	...	...	Lithuania
...	...	...	...	...	...	...	...	...	...	...	...	...	...	...	...	...	...	...	...	...	...	...	...	Luxembourg
73	73	71	89	54	93	50	89	53	48	51	43	48	43	49	46	85	78	84	63	106	48	97	54	Madagascar
93	94	93	94	91	94	89	97	51	43	48	40	56	35	53	38	137	116	128	113	131	105	136	94	Malawi
...	...	...	...	...	...	...	...	...	...	...	...	...	...	...	...	...	...	...	...	...	...	...	...	Malaysia
98	98	98	98	98	97	98	98	20	16	20	15	21	14	23	15	29	25	28	23	28	21	47	12	Maldives
71	65	65	77	65	78	66	86	40	35	42	27	44	22	40	19	222	206	234	156	233	123	223	102	Mali
...	...	...	...	...	...	...	...	...	...	...	...	...	...	...	...	...	...	...	...	...	...	...	...	Malta
...	...	...	...	...	...	...	...	...	...	...	...	...	...	...	...	...	...	...	...	...	...	...	...	Marshall Islands
56	56	58	52	52	60	50	63	30	27	32	24	34	20	31	18	...	...	...	...	...	...	...	...	Mauritania
...	...	...	...	...	...	...	...	...	...	...	...	...	...	...	...	...	...	...	...	...	...	...	...	Mauritius
...	...	...	...	...	...	...	...	...	...	...	...	...	...	...	...	...	...	...	...	...	...	...	...	Mexico
...	...	...	...	...	...	...	...	...	...	...	...	...	...	...	...	...	...	...	...	...	...	...	...	Micronesia (Federated States of)
...	...	...	...	...	...	...	...	...	...	...	...	...	...	...	...	...	...	...	...	...	...	...	...	Monaco
...	...	...	...	...	...	...	...	...	...	...	...	...	...	...	...	...	...	...	...	...	...	...	...	Mongolia
82	78	84	78	68 [g]	83 [g]	... [e]	83	8	8	9	7	14	5	... [e]	6	...	...	...	...	...	...	...	...	Montenegro
...	...	...	...	...	...	...	...	...	...	...	...	...	...	...	...	...	...	...	...	...	...	...	...	Morocco
73	73	69	85	59	88	66	91	47	41	47	35	51	26	49	25	...	...	...	...	...	...	...	...	Mozambique
...	...	...	...	...	...	...	...	...	...	...	...	...	...	...	...	...	...	...	...	...	...	...	...	Myanmar
84	83	82	86	75	94	62	89	31	26	31	24	38	12	38	23	80	58	75	60	90	30	78	55	Namibia
...	...	...	...	...	...	...	...	...	...	...	...	...	...	...	...	...	...	...	...	...	...	...	...	Nauru
92	91	92	95	88	98	86	97	41	39	42	27	56	25	48	29	62	62	64	45	74	35	73	40	Nepal
...	...	...	...	...	...	...	...	...	...	...	...	...	...	...	...	...	...	...	...	...	...	...	...	Netherlands
...	...	...	...	...	...	...	...	...	...	...	...	...	...	...	...	...	...	...	...	...	...	...	...	New Zealand
...	...	...	...	...	...	...	...	...	...	...	...	...	...	...	...	...	...	...	...	...	...	...	...	Nicaragua
39	41	35	63	31	63	36	66	58	52	58	35	57	40	56	24	220	213	229	139	204	154	221	91	Niger
36	36	27	55	9	77	11	69	43	38	45	31	52	24	51	27	175	166	190	122	217	88	209	107	Nigeria
...	...	...	...	...	...	...	...	...	...	...	...	...	...	...	...	...	...	...	...	...	...	...	...	Niue
...	...	...	...	...	...	...	...	...	...	...	...	...	...	...	...	...	...	...	...	...	...	...	...	Norway
...	...	...	...	...	...	...	...	...	...	...	...	...	...	...	...	...	...	...	...	...	...	...	...	Oman
62	55	54	68	35	78	48	85	...	...	...	...	...	...	...	...	93	94	100	78	120	59	102	62	Pakistan
...	...	...	...	...	...	...	...	...	...	...	...	...	...	...	...	...	...	...	...	...	...	...	...	Palau
...	...	...	...	...	...	...	...	...	...	...	...	...	...	...	...	...	...	...	...	...	...	...	...	Panama
...	...	...	...	...	...	...	...	...	...	...	...	...	...	...	...	...	...	...	...	...	...	...	...	Papua New Guinea
...	...	...	...	...	...	...	...	...	...	...	...	...	...	...	...	...	...	...	...	...	...	...	...	Paraguay
83	79	79	82	77	87	81	82	30	26	45	15	55	7	62	16	37	32	49	24	59	12	51	23	Peru
87	84	83	88	72	94	36 [g]	90	...	...	...	...	...	...	...	...	41	34	46	28	59	17	135 [h]	30	Philippines
...	...	...	...	...	...	...	...	...	...	...	...	...	...	...	...	...	...	...	...	...	...	...	...	Poland
...	...	...	...	...	...	...	...	...	...	...	...	...	...	...	...	...	...	...	...	...	...	...	...	Portugal
...	...	...	...	...	...	...	...	...	...	...	...	...	...	...	...	...	...	...	...	...	...	...	...	Qatar
...	...	...	...	...	...	...	...	...	...	...	...	...	...	...	...	...	...	...	...	...	...	...	...	Republic of Korea
...	...	...	...	...	...	...	...	...	...	...	...	...	...	...	...	...	...	...	...	...	...	...	...	Republic of Moldova
...	...	...	...	...	...	...	...	...	...	...	...	...	...	...	...	...	...	...	...	...	...	...	...	Romania
...	...	...	...	...	...	...	...	...	...	...	...	...	...	...	...	...	...	...	...	...	...	...	...	Russian Federation
97	97	97	96	96	99	96	98	48	40	46	28	54	26	52	23	104	96	103	80	115	75	123	63	Rwanda
...	...	...	...	...	...	...	...	...	...	...	...	...	...	...	...	...	...	...	...	...	...	...	...	Saint Kitts and Nevis
...	...	...	...	...	...	...	...	...	...	...	...	...	...	...	...	...	...	...	...	...	...	...	...	Saint Lucia
...	...	...	...	...	...	...	...	...	...	...	...	...	...	...	...	...	...	...	...	...	...	...	...	Saint Vincent and the Grenadines
...	...	...	...	...	...	...	...	...	...	...	...	...	...	...	...	...	...	...	...	...	...	...	...	Samoa

Table 8

Member State	Source	MDG 5																	
		Contraceptive prevalence: modern methods[a] (%)						Antenatal care coverage: at least 4 visits[a,b] (%)						Births attended by skilled health personnel[a,c] (%)					
		Place of residence		Wealth quintile		Educational level of woman		Place of residence		Wealth quintile		Educational level of woman		Place of residence		Wealth quintile		Educational level of woman	
		Rural	Urban	Lowest	Highest	None	Secondary or higher	Rural	Urban	Lowest	Highest	None	Secondary or higher	Rural	Urban	Lowest	Highest	None	Secondary or higher
San Marino		...	...	...	...	...	...	...	...	...	...	...	...	...	...	...	...	...	...
Sao Tome and Principe	DHS 2008–2009	40	28	31	37	15	32	69	76	58	91	53	82	75	89	74	93	73	88
Saudi Arabia		...	...	...	...	...	...	...	...	...	...	...	...	...	...	...	...	...	...
Senegal	DHS 2010–2011	7	20	4	23	8	26	42	62	32	69	45	67	49	90	30	95	58	88
Serbia	MICS 2010	19	24	11	31	...e	21	94	94	86	96	...e	94	100	100	99	100	...e	100
Seychelles		...	...	...	...	...	...	...	...	...	...	...	...	...	...	...	...	...	...
Sierra Leone	MICS 2010	8	16	5	21	7	23	74	78	68	84	72	82	59	72	44	85	57	79
Singapore		...	...	...	...	...	...	...	...	...	...	...	...	...	...	...	...	...	...
Slovakia		...	...	...	...	...	...	...	...	...	...	...	...	...	...	...	...	...	...
Slovenia		...	...	...	...	...	...	...	...	...	...	...	...	...	...	...	...	...	...
Solomon Islands		...	...	...	...	...	...	...	...	...	...	...	...	...	...	...	...	...	...
Somalia	MICS 2006	0	3	0	4	1	7	...	...	...	...	...	...	15	65	11	77	25	73
South Africa		...	...	...	...	...	...	...	...	...	...	...	...	...	...	...	...	...	...
South Sudan		...	...	...	...	...	...	...	...	...	...	...	...	...	...	...	...	...	...
Spain		...	...	...	...	...	...	...	...	...	...	...	...	...	...	...	...	...	...
Sri Lanka		...	...	...	...	...	...	...	...	...	...	...	...	...	...	...	...	...	...
Sudan		...	...	...	...	...	...	...	...	...	...	...	...	...	...	...	...	...	...
Suriname	MICS 2006	41	47	29	51	14	51	...	...	...	...	...	...	82	95	81	96	75	95
Swaziland	MICS 2010	61	69	55	68	49	68	76	80	72	85	81	80	80	89	65	94	61	88
Sweden		...	...	...	...	...	...	...	...	...	...	...	...	...	...	...	...	...	...
Switzerland		...	...	...	...	...	...	...	...	...	...	...	...	...	...	...	...	...	...
Syrian Arab Republic	MICS 2006	35	48	29	53	34	46	...	...	...	...	...	...	88	98	78	99	77	98
Tajikistan		...	...	...	...	...	...	...	...	...	...	...	...	...	...	...	...	...	...
Thailand	MICS 2005–2006	76	72	79	70	63	71	...	...	...	...	...	...	97	99	93	100	81	99
The former Yugoslav Republic of Macedonia		...	...	...	...	...	...	...	...	...	...	...	...	...	...	...	...	...	...
Timor-Leste	DHS 2009–2010	19	28	15	32	15	25	53	63	41	68	44	65	21	59	11	69	14	50
Togo	MICS 2006	9	14	7	16	7	21	...	...	...	...	...	...	65	94	56	96	65	92
Tonga		...	...	...	...	...	...	...	...	...	...	...	...	...	...	...	...	...	...
Trinidad and Tobago	MICS 2006	...	...	37	45	...e	39	...	...	...	...	...	...	...	...	98	100	...e	98
Tunisia		...	...	...	...	...	...	...	...	...	...	...	...	...	...	...	...	...	...
Turkey		...	...	...	...	...	...	...	...	...	...	...	...	...	...	...	...	...	...
Turkmenistan		...	...	...	...	...	...	...	...	...	...	...	...	...	...	...	...	...	...
Tuvalu		...	...	...	...	...	...	...	...	...	...	...	...	...	...	...	...	...	...
Uganda	DHS 2011	23	39	13	39	16	38	46	57	43	59	45	56	53	89	44	88	38	81
Ukraine	DHS 2007	42	50	36	53	...e	48	83	75	84	76	...e	77	98	99	97	99	...e	99
United Arab Emirates		...	...	...	...	...	...	...	...	...	...	...	...	...	...	...	...	...	...
United Kingdom		...	...	...	...	...	...	...	...	...	...	...	...	...	...	...	...	...	...
United Republic of Tanzania	DHS 2010	25	34	19	38	18	35	39	55	37	59	35	65	42	83	33	90	34	86
United States of America		...	...	...	...	...	...	...	...	...	...	...	...	...	...	...	...	...	...
Uruguay		...	...	...	...	...	...	...	...	...	...	...	...	...	...	...	...	...	...
Uzbekistan	MICS 2006	60	57	61	57	...e	59	...	...	...	...	...	...	100	100	100	100	...e	100
Vanuatu	MICS 2007	36	41	28	44	20	41	...	...	...	...	...	...	72	87	55	90	51	86
Venezuela (Bolivarian Republic of)		...	...	...	...	...	...	...	...	...	...	...	...	...	...	...	...	...	...
Viet Nam	MICS 2010–2011	61	58	65	58	66	59	51	82	27	89	6	66	91	99	72	99	45	97
Yemen	MICS 2006	13	34	5	35	16	30	...	...	...	...	...	...	26	62	17	74	27	61
Zambia	DHS 2007	28	42	31	48	27	44	61	59	59	62	56	63	31	83	27	91	23	73
Zimbabwe	DHS 2010–2011	56	60	52	64	42	60	64	66	60	73	68	68	58	86	48	91	39	75

DTP3 immunization coverage among 1-year-olds[a] (%)								Children aged <5 years who are stunted[a] (%)								Under-five mortality rate[a,d] (probability of dying by age 5 per 1000 live births) — MDG 4								Member State
Male	Female	Rural	Urban	Lowest	Highest	None	Secondary or higher	Male	Female	Rural	Urban	Lowest	Highest	None	Secondary or higher	Male	Female	Rural	Urban	Lowest	Highest	None	Secondary or higher	
...	...	...	...	...	...	...	...	...	...	...	...	...	...	...	...	...	...	...	...	...	...	...	...	San Marino
88	87	86	89	87	91	...[e]	88	29	30	28	30	37	19	27	25	86	55	67	74	86	28	...[f]	46	Sao Tome and Principe
...	...	...	...	...	...	...	...	...	...	...	...	...	...	...	...	...	...	...	...	...	...	...	...	Saudi Arabia
84	81	82	84	75	88	81	95	28	25	31	20	35	15	30	12	90	82	101	61	118	54	96	37	Senegal
...	...	...	...	...	...	...	...	6	7	8	6	9	3	...[e]	8	...	...	...	...	...	...	...	...	Serbia
...	...	...	...	...	...	...	...	...	...	...	...	...	...	...	...	...	...	...	...	...	...	...	...	Seychelles
77	75	75	78	77	80	74	84	47	42	46	41	47	33	47	37	...	...	...	...	...	...	...	...	Sierra Leone
...	...	...	...	...	...	...	...	...	...	...	...	...	...	...	...	...	...	...	...	...	...	...	...	Singapore
...	...	...	...	...	...	...	...	...	...	...	...	...	...	...	...	...	...	...	...	...	...	...	...	Slovakia
...	...	...	...	...	...	...	...	...	...	...	...	...	...	...	...	...	...	...	...	...	...	...	...	Slovenia
...	...	...	...	...	...	...	...	...	...	...	...	...	...	...	...	...	...	...	...	...	...	...	...	Solomon Islands
16	12	7	26	5	29	11	24[g]	43	41	48	32	51	25	45	26	...	...	...	...	...	...	...	...	Somalia
...	...	...	...	...	...	...	...	...	...	...	...	...	...	...	...	...	...	...	...	...	...	...	...	South Africa
...	...	...	...	...	...	...	...	...	...	...	...	...	...	...	...	...	...	...	...	...	...	...	...	South Sudan
...	...	...	...	...	...	...	...	...	...	...	...	...	...	...	...	...	...	...	...	...	...	...	...	Spain
...	...	...	...	...	...	...	...	...	...	...	...	...	...	...	...	...	...	...	...	...	...	...	...	Sri Lanka
...	...	...	...	...	...	...	...	...	...	...	...	...	...	...	...	...	...	...	...	...	...	...	...	Sudan
85	85	87	85	83	86	79	87	12	10	14	8	17	4	23	7	...	...	...	...	...	...	...	...	Suriname
91	90	91	89	90	84	90	90	34	28	33	23	42	14	40	25	...	...	...	...	...	...	...	...	Swaziland
...	...	...	...	...	...	...	...	...	...	...	...	...	...	...	...	...	...	...	...	...	...	...	...	Sweden
...	...	...	...	...	...	...	...	...	...	...	...	...	...	...	...	...	...	...	...	...	...	...	...	Switzerland
73	75	72	75	60	79	53	80	30	27	29	28	36	26	36	24	...	...	...	...	...	...	...	...	Syrian Arab Republic
...	...	...	...	...	...	...	...	...	...	...	...	...	...	...	...	...	...	...	...	...	...	...	...	Tajikistan
93	94	94	92	94	91	93	94	16	15	17	12	21	9	20	14	...	...	...	...	...	...	...	...	Thailand
...	...	...	...	...	...	...	...	...	...	...	...	...	...	...	...	...	...	...	...	...	...	...	...	The former Yugoslav Republic of Macedonia
69	64	65	71	55	73	57	75	60	56	60	49	63	47	63	52	83	76	86	59	87	52	89	66	Timor-Leste
64	62	59	70	58	75	50	79	32	27	35	22	37	19	34	22	...	...	...	...	...	...	...	...	Togo
...	...	...	...	...	...	...	...	...	...	...	...	...	...	...	...	...	...	...	...	...	...	...	...	Tonga
64	71	...	...	66[g]	61[g]	...[e]	69	...	...	...	...	...	...	...	...	...	...	...	...	...	...	...	...	Trinidad and Tobago
...	...	...	...	...	...	...	...	...	...	...	...	...	...	...	...	...	...	...	...	...	...	...	...	Tunisia
...	...	...	...	...	...	...	...	...	...	...	...	...	...	...	...	...	...	...	...	...	...	...	...	Turkey
...	...	...	...	...	...	...	...	...	...	...	...	...	...	...	...	...	...	...	...	...	...	...	...	Turkmenistan
...	...	...	...	...	...	...	...	...	...	...	...	...	...	...	...	...	...	...	...	...	...	...	...	Tuvalu
73	72	72	76	75	75	71	79	37	29	36	18	36	22	40	25	114	97	110	76	124	71	133	79	Uganda
...	...	...	...	...	...	...	...	...	...	...	...	...	...	...	...	23	13	19	18	23h	9	...[i]	19	Ukraine
...	...	...	...	...	...	...	...	...	...	...	...	...	...	...	...	...	...	...	...	...	...	...	...	United Arab Emirates
...	...	...	...	...	...	...	...	...	...	...	...	...	...	...	...	...	...	...	...	...	...	...	...	United Kingdom
88	88	86	97	84	97	79	96	45	38	44	31	48	27	45	22	97	88	92	95	104	84	97	74	United Republic of Tanzania
...	...	...	...	...	...	...	...	...	...	...	...	...	...	...	...	...	...	...	...	...	...	...	...	United States of America
...	...	...	...	...	...	...	...	...	...	...	...	...	...	...	...	...	...	...	...	...	...	...	...	Uruguay
94	93	95	89	94	93	...[e]	93	20	20	20	19	21	16	...[e]	20	...	...	...	...	...	...	...	...	Uzbekistan
64	63	62	69	46	67	37[g]	71	31	20	26	26	28	24	28	25	...	...	...	...	...	...	...	...	Vanuatu
...	...	...	...	...	...	...	...	...	...	...	...	...	...	...	...	...	...	...	...	...	...	...	...	Venezuela (Bolivarian Republic of)
72	76	70	82	59	86	35[g]	77	24	22	27	12	41	6	41	20	...	...	...	...	...	...	...	...	Viet Nam
51	49	44	64	32	78	42	73	...	...	...	...	...	...	...	...	...	...	...	...	...	...	...	...	Yemen
82	80	77	90	78	95	70	90	48	42	48	39	48	34	45	37	151	122	138	131	124	108	146	104	Zambia
72	75	73	76	67	81	...[e]	78	35	27	32	28	35	24	38	30	88	68	78	77	86	57	...[f]	71	Zimbabwe

Table 8

161

8. Health inequities

	MDG 5																	
	Contraceptive prevalence: modern methods[a] (%)						Antenatal care coverage: at least 4 visits[a,b] (%)						Births attended by skilled health personnel[a,c] (%)					
	Place of residence		Wealth quintile		Educational level of woman		Place of residence		Wealth quintile		Educational level of woman		Place of residence		Wealth quintile		Educational level of woman	
	Rural	Urban	Lowest	Highest	None	Secondary or higher	Rural	Urban	Lowest	Highest	None	Secondary or higher	Rural	Urban	Lowest	Highest	None	Secondary or higher
Ranges of country values																		
Minimum	0	3	0	4	1	7	11	35	8	35	6	35	5	37	2	46	3	33
Median	27	35	21	38	19	37	56	74	43	82	44	77	58	88	44	95	43	88
Maximum	78	73	79	75	68	73	94	96	90	98	88	97	100	100	100	100	94	100

[a.] Data are derived from the re-analysis of publicly available Demographic and Health Surveys (DHS) and Multiple Indicator Cluster Surveys (MICS) micro-data, using the standard indicator definitions as published in DHS or UNICEF documentation. The analysis was carried out by the International Center for Analysis and Monitoring of Equity in Health and Nutrition based in the Federal University of Pelotas, Brazil, and updated in December 2013. In some cases there may be slight differences between these results and those reported in DHS or MICS country reports due to differences in the calculation of indicator numerators and/or denominators.

[b.] Data derived from DHS relate to the most recent live births occurring in the five years preceding the survey.

[c.] Data derived from DHS relate to births occurring in the five years preceding the survey. Data derived from MICS relate to births occurring in the two years preceding the survey.

[d.] The under-five mortality rate relates to the decade preceding the survey.

[e.] The figure is not reported as it is based on fewer than 25 cases.

[f.] The figure is not reported as it is based on fewer than 250 unweighted person-years of exposure to the risk of death.

[g.] The figure is based on a small number of cases (25–49 unweighted cases).

[h.] The figure is based on 250–499 unweighted person-years of exposure to the risk of death.

[i.] The figure cannot be calculated.

DTP3 immunization coverage among 1-year-olds[a] (%)								Children aged <5 years who are stunted[a] (%)								Under-five mortality rate[a,d] (probability of dying by age 5 per 1000 live births) MDG 4								
Sex		Place of residence		Wealth quintile		Educational level of mother		Sex		Place of residence		Wealth quintile		Educational level of mother		Sex		Place of residence		Wealth quintile		Educational level of mother	
Male	Female	Rural	Urban	Lowest	Highest	None	Secondary or higher	Male	Female	Rural	Urban	Lowest	Highest	None	Secondary or higher	Male	Female	Rural	Urban	Lowest	Highest	None	Secondary or higher	
6	12	7	26	5	29	11	31	6	7	8	6	9	3	14	6	21	13	19	13	26	9	27	12	Minimum
8	77	76	84	74	87	66	87	34	29	37	27	42	22	41	24	86	76	86	63	102	50	102	53	Median
9	98	98	99	100	99	98	99	63	56	60	49	70	47	63	52	222	213	234	156	233	154	223	116	Maximum

Table 8

163

9. Demographic and socioeconomic statistics

Table 9 presents data on demographic and socioeconomic factors that are major determinants of health. The table includes four MDG-related indicators – adolescent fertility; primary school enrolment; population living in poverty; and cellular phone subscriber rates. The table also includes data on demographics (such as population size, growth and degree of urbanization); crude birth and death rates; coverage of civil registration of births and underlying cause of death; adult literacy; and per capita gross national income. In addition to their intrinsic value, such data are also important in making other statistics comparable across countries. For example, data on disease incidence, prevalence and mortality rates – and on the availability of health-system resources – all require reliable population-based denominators.

These demographic and socioeconomic statistics have been derived from data produced by a range of national and international organizations. The latter include the United Nations Population Division, United Nations International Telecommunication Union (ITU), the United Nations Department of Economic and Social Affairs (UNDESA), the United Nations Educational, Scientific and Cultural Organization (UNESCO), the United Nations Children's Fund (UNICEF) and the World Bank. Estimates are based on a combination of administrative records, population-based surveys, censuses and civil registration data, and on statistical modelling to adjust for missing values. For more information on the sources and methods used for a particular indicator, please refer to the relevant footnotes below and to the website of the relevant organization.

Table 9

Member State	Population[a]						Civil registration coverage (%)		Crude birth rate[a] (per 1000 population)
	Total (000s)	Median age (years)	Aged under 15 (%)	Aged over 60 (%)	Annual growth rate (%)	Living in urban areas (%)	Births[b]	Causes of death[c]	
	2012	2012	2012	2012	2002–2012	2012	2006–2012		2012
Afghanistan	29 825	16	47	4	3.0	24	37	…	35.3
Albania	3 162	33	21	15	−0.3	55	99	…	12.8
Algeria	38 482	27	27	7	1.7	74	99	…	24.6
Andorra	78	…	15	23	0.9	…	>90[i]	>80	9.0[j]
Angola	20 821	16	48	4	3.4	60	…	…	44.8
Antigua and Barbuda	89	30	26	12	1.1	30	…	80	16.6
Argentina	41 087	31	24	15	0.9	93	99[i]	99	16.9
Armenia	2 969	32	20	14	−0.3	64	100	76	13.9
Australia	23 050	37	19	19	1.6	89	>90[i]	100	13.3
Austria	8 464	42	15	24	0.4	68	>90[i]	100	9.5
Azerbaijan	9 309	29	22	8	1.2	54	94	93	18.1
Bahamas	372	32	22	11	1.9	84	…	89	15.4
Bahrain	1 318	30	20	3	5.9	89	…	89	15.6
Bangladesh	154 695	25	31	7	1.2	29	31	…	20.3
Barbados	283	37	19	16	0.5	45	…	100	12.7
Belarus	9 405	39	15	19	−0.5	75	100[i]	100	11.0
Belgium	11 060	41	17	24	0.7	98	>90[i]	100	11.7
Belize	324	23	34	6	2.5	45	95	100	23.8
Benin	10 051	18	43	5	3.0	46	80	…	36.9
Bhutan	742	25	29	7	2.1	36	100	…	19.9
Bolivia (Plurinational State of)	10 496	22	35	7	1.7	67	76[i]	…	25.9
Bosnia and Herzegovina	3 834	39	16	21	−0.2	49	100	89	8.8
Botswana	2 004	22	34	6	1.0	62	72	…	23.8
Brazil	198 656	30	25	11	1.0	85	93[i]	93	15.1
Brunei Darussalam	412	30	26	7	1.7	76	…	93	15.9
Bulgaria	7 278	43	14	26	−0.8	74	>90[i]	100	9.6
Burkina Faso	16 460	17	46	4	2.9	27	77	…	41.4
Burundi	9 850	18	44	4	3.4	11	75	…	45.0
Cabo Verde	494	24	30	7	0.7	63	91	…	20.4
Cambodia	14 865	24	31	8	1.6	20	62	…	25.9
Cameroon	21 700	18	43	5	2.6	53	61	…	37.7
Canada	34 838	40	16	21	1.1	81	>90[i]	100	11.2
Central African Republic	4 525	20	40	6	1.8	39	61	…	34.5
Chad	12 448	16	49	4	3.3	22	16	…	46.4
Chile	17 465	33	21	14	1.0	89	100[i]	98	14.1
China	1 384 770	35	18	13	0.6	52	…	4	13.4
Colombia	47 704	27	28	9	1.5	76	97	98	19.1
Comoros	718	19	42	5	2.5	28	…	…	35.9
Congo	4 337	19	42	5	2.8	64	91	…	38.0
Cook Islands	21	…	31	9	1.1	…	…	82	15.0[j]
Costa Rica	4 805	29	24	10	1.6	65	…	90	15.3
Côte d'Ivoire	19 840	19	41	5	1.7	52	65	…	36.7
Croatia	4 307	42	15	25	−0.3	58	…	100	9.5
Cuba	11 271	40	17	18	0.1	75	100[i]	100	9.6
Cyprus	1 129	35	17	17	1.4	71	>90[i]	85	11.5
Czech Republic	10 660	40	15	23	0.4	73	>90[i]	100	11.1
Democratic People's Republic of Korea	24 763	33	22	13	0.6	60	100	…	14.4
Democratic Republic of the Congo	65 705	17	45	5	2.8	35	28	…	43.2

Crude death rate[c] (per 1000 population)	Total fertility rate[a] (per woman)	MDG 5 Adolescent fertility rate[d] (per 1000 girls aged 15–19 years)	Literacy rate among adults aged ≥15 years[e] (%)	MDG 2 Net primary school enrolment rate[e] (%) Male	Female	Gross national income per capita[f] (PPP int. $)	MDG 1 Population living on <$1 (PPP int. $) a day[g] (%)	MDG 8 Cellular phone subscribers[h] (per 100 population)	Member State
2012	2012	2006–2011	2006–2012	2006–2012		2012	2006–2012	2012	
8.4	5.1	90	…	…	…	1 560	…	60	Afghanistan
9.3	1.8	11	97	…	…	9 280	<2.0	111	Albania
5.7	2.8	4	73	98	96	8 360	…	98	Algeria
8.3	1.4[j]	…	…	…	…	…	…	81	Andorra
14.4	6.0	…	70	97	74	5 400	43.4	47	Angola
6.8	2.1	…	99[k]	87	84	18 920	…	143	Antigua and Barbuda
7.6	2.2	68	98	…	…	…	<2.0	152	Argentina
12.4	1.7	28	100	89	98	8 820	2.5	112	Armenia
6.4	1.9	16	…	96	97	43 300	…	106	Australia
9.3	1.5	9	…	…	…	43 390	…	161	Austria
6.2	1.9	41	100	90[m]	88[m]	9 310	<2.0	109	Azerbaijan
6.0	1.9	41	…	94	99	29 020	…	81	Bahamas
2.2	2.1	14	95	…	…	…	…	161	Bahrain
5.7	2.2	128	58	94[m]	98[m]	2 030	43.3	63	Bangladesh
6.5	1.8	50	…	97[m]	97[m]	25 670	…	123	Barbados
13.0	1.5	21	100	94[n]	94[n]	14 960	<2.0	114	Belarus
9.8	1.9	11	…	99	99	39 860	…	111	Belgium
4.1	2.7	…	…	98	100	7 630	…	53	Belize
9.7	4.9	94	29[o]	100	88	1 550	…	84	Benin
6.5	2.3	59	…	90	93	6 200	<2.0	76	Bhutan
6.9	3.3	89	91	87	87	4 880	15.6	90	Bolivia (Plurinational State of)
9.2	1.3	17	98	…	…	9 650	<2.0	88	Bosnia and Herzegovina
8.1	2.7	51	85	83[n]	85[n]	16 060	…	154	Botswana
6.6	1.8	71	90	…	…	11 530	6.1	125	Brazil
3.5	2.0	18	95	96	95	…	…	114	Brunei Darussalam
14.6	1.5	41	98	98	98	15 450	<2.0	148	Bulgaria
9.8	5.7	130	29	68	65	1 490	44.6	61	Burkina Faso
11.5	6.1	65	87	94	94	550	81.3	23	Burundi
5.2	2.3	…	85	99	96	4 930	…	86	Cabo Verde
5.7	2.9	48	74	100	97	2 330	18.6	129	Cambodia
11.0	4.9	127	71	97	86	2 270	9.6	60	Cameroon
7.1	1.7	14	…	…	…	42 530	…	80	Canada
14.4	4.5	229	57	81	64	1 080	62.8	25	Central African Republic
14.0	6.4	203	35	72	56	1 620	…	35	Chad
5.4	1.8	54	99	93	93	21 310	<2.0	138	Chile
7.1	1.7	6	95	…	…	9 040	11.8	80	China
3.9	2.3	85	94	87	86	9 990	8.2	103	Colombia
8.3	4.8	…	76	86	80	1 210	…	40	Comoros
10.4	5.0	147	…	88	96	3 450	54.1	99	Congo
5.0	2.4[j]	…	…	…	…	…	…	…	Cook Islands
4.4	1.8	67	96	92	93	12 500	3.1	112	Costa Rica
12.7	4.9	128	57	67	56	1 920	23.8	91	Côte d'Ivoire
11.6	1.5	13	99	97	99	20 200	<2.0	115	Croatia
7.9	1.5	51	100	96	97	…	…	15	Cuba
5.5	1.5	4	99	99[m]	99[m]	29 840	…	98	Cyprus
10.0	1.5	10	…	…	…	24 720	…	127	Czech Republic
9.2	2.0	1	100	…	…	…	…	7	Democratic People's Republic of Korea
14.0	6.0	135	61	…	…	390	87.7	31	Democratic Republic of the Congo

167

Table 9

9. Demographic and socioeconomic statistics

Member State	Population[a]						Civil registration coverage (%)		Crude birth rate[a] (per 1000 population)
	Total (000s)	Median age (years)	Aged under 15 (%)	Aged over 60 (%)	Annual growth rate (%)	Living in urban areas (%)	Births[b]	Causes of death[c]	
	2012	2012	2012	2012	2002–2012	2012	2006–2012		2012
Denmark	5 598	41	18	24	0.4	87	>90[i]	98	11.4
Djibouti	860	23	34	6	1.4	77	92	…	27.8
Dominica	72	…	26	12	0.3	…	…	100	16.0[j]
Dominican Republic	10 277	26	31	9	1.4	70	82	57	21.2
Ecuador	15 492	26	30	9	1.7	68	90	85	21.1
Egypt	80 722	25	31	9	1.7	44	…	95	23.5
El Salvador	6 297	24	31	10	0.5	65	99	77	20.2
Equatorial Guinea	736	20	39	5	2.9	40	…	…	35.8
Eritrea	6 131	18	43	4	3.6	22	…	…	37.4
Estonia	1 291	41	16	24	−0.4	70	>90[i]	100	11.0
Ethiopia	91 729	18	43	5	2.7	17	…	…	33.5
Fiji	875	27	29	8	0.7	53	…	100	20.8
Finland	5 408	42	16	26	0.4	84	>90[i]	100	11.2
France	63 937	40	18	24	0.6	86	>90[i]	100	12.4
Gabon	1 633	21	38	7	2.4	87	90	…	32.2
Gambia	1 791	17	46	4	3.2	58	53	…	43.0
Georgia	4 358	37	18	19	−0.6	53	99	87	13.5
Germany	82 800	45	13	27	−0.1	74	>90[i]	100	8.4
Ghana	25 366	20	39	5	2.5	53	63	…	31.3
Greece	11 125	42	15	25	0.1	62	>90[i]	100	9.9
Grenada	105	26	27	10	0.3	39	…	100	19.4
Guatemala	15 083	19	41	7	2.5	50	97	91	31.4
Guinea	11 451	19	42	5	2.4	36	…	…	37.3
Guinea-Bissau	1 664	19	42	5	2.2	45	24	…	37.9
Guyana	795	22	37	5	0.6	28	88	73	20.7
Haiti	10 174	22	35	7	1.4	55	80	…	26.0
Honduras	7 936	22	36	6	2.0	53	94	…	26.1
Hungary	9 976	40	15	23	−0.2	70	>90[i]	100	9.8
Iceland	326	35	21	18	1.3	94	>90[i]	100	14.6
India	1 236 687	26	29	8	1.4	32	41	8	20.7
Indonesia	246 864	27	29	8	1.4	51	67	…	19.2
Iran (Islamic Republic of)	76 424	28	24	8	1.2	69	99[i]	68	19.0
Iraq	32 778	20	41	5	2.6	66	99	65	31.5
Ireland	4 576	35	22	17	1.5	62	>90[i]	100	15.6
Israel	7 644	30	28	15	2.0	92	>90[i]	100	20.6
Italy	60 885	44	14	27	0.6	69	>90[i]	100	9.3
Jamaica	2 769	28	28	11	0.5	52	98	71	18.1
Japan	127 250	46	13	32	0.1	92	>90[i]	100	8.4
Jordan	7 009	23	34	5	3.6	83	99	64	27.7
Kazakhstan	16 271	29	25	10	1.1	53	100	92	20.9
Kenya	43 178	19	42	4	2.7	24	60	…	35.5
Kiribati	101	23	30	9	1.6	44	94	…	23.3
Kuwait	3 250	29	25	4	4.6	98	…	96	20.9
Kyrgyzstan	5 474	24	30	6	0.9	35	96	98	27.0
Lao People's Democratic Republic	6 646	21	36	6	1.8	35	75	…	27.3
Latvia	2 060	41	15	24	−1.2	68	>90[i]	100	10.9
Lebanon	4 647	29	22	12	2.8	87	100	…	13.2
Lesotho	2 052	21	37	6	0.8	28	45	…	27.6

Crude death rate[c] (per 1000 population)	Total fertility rate[a] (per woman)	MDG 5 Adolescent fertility rate[d] (per 1000 girls aged 15–19 years)	Literacy rate among adults aged ≥15 years[e] (%)	MDG 2 Net primary school enrolment rate[e] (%) Male	Female	Gross national income per capita[f] (PPP int. $)	MDG 1 Population living on <$1 (PPP int. $) a day[g] (%)	MDG 8 Cellular phone subscribers[h] (per 100 population)	Member State
2012	2012	2006–2011	2006–2012	2006–2012		2012	2006–2012	2012	
9.6	1.9	5	…	95	97	43 430	…	118	Denmark
9.0	3.5	…	…	62	56	…	…	25	Djibouti
7.2	2.1[j]	48	…	95	97	11 980	…	152	Dominica
4.8	2.5	…	90	90	88	9 660	2.2	87	Dominican Republic
5.3	2.6	…	92	96	98	9 490	4.6	106	Ecuador
6.5	2.8	50	74	…	…	6 450	<2.0	120	Egypt
6.6	2.2	65	84	95	95	6 720	9.0	137	El Salvador
11.9	4.9	…	94	62	62	18 570	…	68	Equatorial Guinea
6.5	4.8	…	69	36	32	550	…	5	Eritrea
11.5	1.6	16	100	97	97	22 500	…	160	Estonia
7.5	4.6	79	39	…	…	1 110	30.7	22	Ethiopia
6.8	2.6	…	…	98	100	4 690	5.9	98	Fiji
9.4	1.9	8	…	98	98	38 220	…	172	Finland
8.7	2.0	12	…	98	99	36 720	…	97	France
9.2	4.1	114	89	…	…	14 090	4.8	179	Gabon
8.4	5.8	118	51	71	76	1 830	…	85	Gambia
11.5	1.8	43	100	98	99	5 770	18.0	108	Georgia
10.5	1.4	8	…	…	…	42 230	…	112	Germany
8.3	3.9	70	71	84[n]	81[n]	1 910	28.6	101	Ghana
10.0	1.5	10	97	99	100	25 460	…	120	Greece
6.9	2.2	…	…	96	99	10 350	…	121	Grenada
5.3	3.8	92	76	96	95	4 880	13.5	138	Guatemala
10.3	5.0	146	25	81	70	970	43.3	42	Guinea
12.2	5.0	…	55	73	69	1 100	…	63	Guinea-Bissau
7.9	2.6	97	85[o]	70	80	3 340	…	69	Guyana
8.8	3.2	66	49[o]	…	…	1 220	…	60	Haiti
4.5	3.1	…	85	93	95	3 880	17.9	93	Honduras
12.9	1.4	18	99	98	98	20 710	<2.0	116	Hungary
6.2	2.1	11	…	98	99	33 480	…	108	Iceland
7.9	2.5	39	63	…	…	3 910	32.7	70	India
6.3	2.4	48	93	95	99	4 730	16.2	114	Indonesia
5.2	1.9	31	85	…	…	…	<2.0	76	Iran (Islamic Republic of)
5.1	4.1	68	78	97[n]	86[n]	4 230	2.8	82	Iraq
5.9	2.0	16	…	99	99	35 670	…	107	Ireland
5.3	2.9	14	…	97	98	…	…	121	Israel
9.4	1.5	7	99	99	99	32 920	…	160	Italy
7.1	2.3	72	87	…	…	…	…	96	Jamaica
9.4	1.4	5	…	…	…	36 300	…	111	Japan
3.7	3.3	32	96	98	97	5 980	<2.0	128	Jordan
9.7	2.5	31	100	98	100	11 780	<2.0	186	Kazakhstan
8.6	4.5	106	72[o]	82[n]	83[n]	1 730	43.4	71	Kenya
8.2	3.0	…	…	…	…	3 870	…	16	Kiribati
1.9	2.6	13	94	99	98	…	…	157	Kuwait
6.7	3.1	34	99	99	98	2 230	5.0	124	Kyrgyzstan
7.0	3.1	…	…	97	95	2 690	33.9	65	Lao People's Democratic Republic
14.1	1.6	15	100	97	99	21 920	<2.0	112	Latvia
4.5	1.5	…	90	99[n]	93[n]	14 160	…	81	Lebanon
14.1	3.1	92	76[o]	80	84	2 170	…	75	Lesotho

Member State	Population[a]						Civil registration coverage (%)		Crude birth rate[a] (per 1000 population)
	Total (000s)	Median age (years)	Aged under 15 (%)	Aged over 60 (%)	Annual growth rate (%)	Living in urban areas (%)	Births[b]	Causes of death[c]	
	2012	2012	2012	2012	2002–2012	2012	2006–2012		2012
Liberia	4 190	18	43	5	3.1	49	4[i]	...	36.0
Libya	6 155	26	29	7	1.4	78	...	...	21.1
Lithuania	3 028	39	15	21	−1.2	67	>90[i]	100	11.2
Luxembourg	524	39	17	19	1.7	86	>90[i]	100	11.6
Madagascar	22 294	18	43	4	2.9	33	80	...	34.9
Malawi	15 906	17	45	5	2.9	16	...	...	40.1
Malaysia	29 240	27	27	8	1.8	73	...	55	17.6
Maldives	338	25	29	7	1.8	42	93	84	22.2
Mali	14 854	16	47	4	3.1	36	81	...	47.4
Malta	428	41	15	23	0.4	95	>90[i]	100	9.3
Marshall Islands	53	...	30	9	0.1	...	96	...	28.0[j]
Mauritania	3 796	20	40	5	2.8	42	59	...	34.5
Mauritius	1 240	34	20	13	0.3	42	...	100	11.5
Mexico	120 847	27	29	9	1.2	78	93[i]	94	18.8
Micronesia (Federated States of)	103	21	36	7	−0.3	23	...	...	23.5
Monaco	38	...	18	24	1.4	...	>90[i]	>80	7.0[j]
Mongolia	2 796	26	27	6	1.4	69	99	89	22.9
Montenegro	621	37	19	19	0.1	63	99	100	11.8
Morocco	32 521	27	28	8	1.0	57	94[i]	24	22.6
Mozambique	25 203	17	45	5	2.7	31	48	...	39.4
Myanmar	52 797	29	25	8	0.7	33	72	...	17.4
Namibia	2 259	21	37	5	1.4	39	78[i]	...	26.4
Nauru	10	...	30	9	0.0	...	83	...	27.0[j]
Nepal	27 474	22	36	8	1.3	17	42	...	21.6
Netherlands	16 714	41	17	23	0.4	84	>90[i]	100	10.8
New Zealand	4 460	37	20	19	1.2	86	>90[i]	100	14.0
Nicaragua	5 992	23	33	7	1.3	58	85	68	23.1
Niger	17 157	15	50	4	3.7	18	32	...	49.8
Nigeria	168 834	18	44	4	2.7	50	42	...	41.5
Niue	1	...	31	9	−2.7	...	...	...	...
Norway	4 994	39	19	21	1.0	80	>90[i]	100	12.5
Oman	3 314	26	24	4	3.6	74	...	87	21.3
Pakistan	179 160	22	34	6	1.8	37	27	...	25.7
Palau	21	...	30	9	0.6	...	...	...	11.0[j]
Panama	3 802	28	29	10	1.8	76	...	90	19.7
Papua New Guinea	7 167	21	38	5	2.4	13	...	...	29.3
Paraguay	6 687	24	33	8	1.8	62	76[i]	82	23.9
Peru	29 988	26	29	9	1.2	78	96[i]	67	20.0
Philippines	96 707	23	35	6	1.8	49	90	90	24.6
Poland	38 211	39	15	20	0.0	61	>90[i]	100	10.8
Portugal	10 604	42	15	24	0.2	62	>90[i]	100	8.8
Qatar	2 051	32	13	2	11.8	99	...	82	11.2
Republic of Korea	49 003	39	15	17	0.5	83	...	99	9.6
Republic of Moldova	3 514	36	17	17	−1.2	48	100	91	12.2
Romania	21 755	39	15	21	−0.2	53	...	100	10.3
Russian Federation	143 170	38	15	19	−0.2	74	>90[i]	99	11.8
Rwanda	11 458	18	44	4	2.4	19	63	...	35.8
Saint Kitts and Nevis	54	...	26	12	1.3	...	...	82	14.0[j]

Crude death rate[c] (per 1000 population)	Total fertility rate[a] (per woman)	MDG 5 Adolescent fertility rate[d] (per 1000 girls aged 15–19 years)	Literacy rate among adults aged ≥15 years[e] (%)	MDG 2 Net primary school enrolment rate[e] (%) Male	Female	Gross national income per capita[f] (PPP int. $)	MDG 1 Population living on <$1 a day[g] (%)	MDG 8 Cellular phone subscribers[h] (per 100 population)	Member State
2012	2012	2006–2011	2006–2012	2006–2012		2012	2006–2012	2012	
8.2	4.9	177	43 [o]	42	40	580	83.8	57	Liberia
4.2	2.4	…	90	…	…	…	…	156	Libya
11.5	1.5	17	100	99	98	23 560	<2.0	165	Lithuania
6.8	1.7	7	…	94	96	60 160	…	145	Luxembourg
7.1	4.5	147	64 [o]	…	…	930	81.3	39	Madagascar
9.5	5.5	157	61 [o]	90	97	730	61.6	29	Malawi
5.0	2.0	15	93	…	…	16 270	<2.0	141	Malaysia
3.7	2.3	16	98	95	94	7 560	…	166	Maldives
11.5	6.9	…	33	78	68	1 140	50.4	98	Mali
7.0	1.4	20	…	80	82	27 000	…	127	Malta
6.6	3.4 [j]	105	…	…	…	…	…	…	Marshall Islands
7.9	4.7	…	59	68	73	2 480	23.4	106	Mauritania
7.3	1.5	31	89	98	98	15 060	…	120	Mauritius
5.0	2.2	87	94	96	98	16 450	<2.0	83	Mexico
6.2	3.3	…	…	…	…	3 920	…	30	Micronesia (Federated States of)
8.6	1.5 [j]	…	…	…	…	…	…	88	Monaco
6.8	2.4	20	97	98	97	5 020	…	121	Mongolia
9.3	1.7	24	98	98	99	14 590	<2.0	181	Montenegro
6.3	2.7	…	67	98	97	5 060	2.5	120	Morocco
12.4	5.3	167	51	89	84	1 000	59.6	36	Mozambique
8.3	2.0	…	93	…	…	…	…	10	Myanmar
6.3	3.1	…	76 [o]	87	90	7 240	…	95	Namibia
3.5	3.0 [j]	…	…	…	…	…	…	68	Nauru
6.7	2.4	81	57 [o]	98 [n]	97 [n]	1 470	24.8	60	Nepal
8.4	1.8	5	…	99	98	43 510	…	118	Netherlands
6.3	2.1	29	…	99	100	…	…	110	New Zealand
4.9	2.5	…	…	93	94	3 890	11.9	86	Nicaragua
10.5	7.6	206	…	69	58	760	43.6	31	Niger
12.3	6.0	113	51 [o]	61 [n]	56 [n]	2 450	68.0	67	Nigeria
5.8	…	16	…	…	…	…	…	…	Niue
8.3	1.9	10	…	99	99	66 960	…	117	Norway
2.9	2.9	12	87	97	98	…	…	159	Oman
7.4	3.3	16	55	77 [m]	67 [m]	2 880	21.0	67	Pakistan
5.9	1.7 [j]	…	…	…	…	16 870	…	83	Palau
5.0	2.5	86	94	92	92	15 150	6.6	178	Panama
7.8	3.8	…	62	…	…	2 740	…	38	Papua New Guinea
4.8	2.9	63	94	83	82	5 720	7.2	102	Paraguay
4.4	2.4	72	90	92	91	10 090	4.9	98	Peru
5.9	3.1	53	95	88	89	4 380	18.4	107	Philippines
9.8	1.4	16	100	97	97	21 170	<2.0	140	Poland
9.1	1.3	16	95	99	100	24 770	…	116	Portugal
1.3	2.0	16	96	…	…	…	…	127	Qatar
5.4	1.3	2	…	99	99	30 970	…	109	Republic of Korea
12.2	1.5	26	99	91 [m]	90 [m]	3 630	<2.0	102	Republic of Moldova
11.7	1.4	41	98	88	87	16 860	<2.0	105	Romania
14.7	1.5	30	100	95	96	22 720	<2.0	183	Russian Federation
6.8	4.6	41	66 [o]	97	100	1 320	63.2	50	Rwanda
8.5	1.8 [j]	…	…	82	85	17 630	…	157	Saint Kitts and Nevis

Table 9

171

Member State	Population[a]						Civil registration coverage (%)		Crude birth rate[a] (per 1000 population)
	Total (000s)	Median age (years)	Aged under 15 (%)	Aged over 60 (%)	Annual growth rate (%)	Living in urban areas (%)	Births[b]	Causes of death[c]	
	2012	2012	2012	2012	2002–2012	2012	2006–2012		2012
Saint Lucia	181	30	24	12	1.2	17	...	90	15.7
Saint Vincent and the Grenadines	109	29	26	10	0.1	50	...	100	16.6
Samoa	189	21	38	7	0.7	20	48	...	26.8
San Marino	31	...	14	27	1.1	...	>90[i]	>80	9.0[i]
Sao Tome and Principe	188	19	42	5	2.6	63	75	...	34.7
Saudi Arabia	28 288	27	30	5	2.6	83	...	51	19.9
Senegal	13 726	18	44	5	2.8	43	75	...	38.1
Serbia	9 553	38	16	21	−0.6	57	99	90	9.8
Seychelles	92	32	22	10	1.1	54	...	100	17.1
Sierra Leone	5 979	19	42	4	2.9	40	78	...	37.1
Singapore	5 303	38	16	15	2.5	100	...	75	9.9
Slovakia	5 446	38	15	19	0.1	55	>90[i]	100	10.7
Slovenia	2 068	42	14	23	0.4	50	>90[i]	100	10.1
Solomon Islands	550	20	40	5	2.3	21	...	...	31.5
Somalia	10 195	16	47	4	2.6	38	3	...	44.2
South Africa	52 386	26	30	8	1.3	62	95[i]	92	21.1
South Sudan	10 838	19	42	5	4.1	18	35	...	36.5
Spain	46 755	41	15	23	1.2	78	>90[i]	100	10.6
Sri Lanka	21 098	31	25	12	0.9	15	97	82	18.1
Sudan	37 195	19	41	5	2.4	33	59	...	33.9
Suriname	535	28	28	10	1.1	70	99	100	18.0
Swaziland	1 231	20	38	5	1.3	21	50	...	30.2
Sweden	9 511	41	17	25	0.7	85	>90[i]	100	12.0
Switzerland	7 997	42	15	23	1.0	74	>90[i]	100	10.3
Syrian Arab Republic	21 890	22	35	6	2.5	56	96	92	24.4
Tajikistan	8 009	22	36	5	2.2	27	88	...	33.1
Thailand	66 785	36	18	14	0.5	34	100	85	10.5
The former Yugoslav Republic of Macedonia	2 106	37	17	18	0.1	59	100	100	10.8
Timor-Leste	1 114	16	46	5	2.1	29	55	...	35.9
Togo	6 643	19	42	4	2.6	38	78	...	36.8
Tonga	105	21	37	8	0.6	24	...	...	26.1
Trinidad and Tobago	1 337	33	21	13	0.5	14	97	86	14.7
Tunisia	10 875	30	23	10	1.1	67	99	...	17.4
Turkey	73 997	29	26	11	1.3	72	94	71	17.1
Turkmenistan	5 173	25	29	6	1.2	49	96	...	21.5
Tuvalu	10	...	31	9	0.3	...	50	...	23.0[i]
Uganda	36 346	16	49	4	3.4	16	30	...	43.7
Ukraine	45 530	40	14	21	−0.6	69	100	99	10.9
United Arab Emirates	9 206	29	14	1	10.5	85	100[i]	83	15.1
United Kingdom	62 783	40	18	23	0.5	80	>90[i]	100	12.3
United Republic of Tanzania	47 783	17	45	5	2.9	27	16	...	39.7
United States of America	317 505	37	20	19	0.9	83	>90[i]	98	13.3
Uruguay	3 395	34	22	19	0.2	93	100[i]	99	14.6
Uzbekistan	28 541	25	29	6	1.2	36	100	...	21.8
Vanuatu	247	22	37	6	2.4	25	43	...	26.9
Venezuela (Bolivarian Republic of)	29 955	27	29	9	1.7	94	81[i]	100	20.1
Viet Nam	90 796	29	23	9	1.0	32	95	...	15.9
Yemen	23 852	19	41	5	2.5	33	17[i]	...	31.5
Zambia	14 075	17	47	4	2.8	40	14	...	43.0
Zimbabwe	13 724	19	40	6	0.8	39	49	...	31.6

Crude death rate[c] (per 1000 population)	Total fertility rate[a] (per woman)	MDG 5 Adolescent fertility rate[d] (per 1000 girls aged 15–19 years)	Literacy rate among adults aged ≥15 years[e] (%)	MDG 2 Net primary school enrolment rate[e] (%) Male	Net primary school enrolment rate Female	Gross national income per capita[f] (PPP int. $)	MDG 1 Population living on <$1 (PPP int. $) a day[g] (%)	MDG 8 Cellular phone subscribers[h] (per 100 population)	Member State
2012	2012	2006–2011	2006–2012	2006–2012		2012	2006–2012	2012	
7.0	1.9	...	...	83	83	11 300	...	126	Saint Lucia
6.4	2.0	70	...	97	97	10 870	...	124	Saint Vincent and the Grenadines
5.3	4.2	29	99	95	97	4 250	...	...	Samoa
10.1	1.5 [j]	...	...	91 [m]	93 [m]	...	...	115	San Marino
6.6	4.1	110	70 [o]	98	100	1 810	...	65	Sao Tome and Principe
3.2	2.7	7	87	91 [n]	96 [n]	...	...	187	Saudi Arabia
7.2	5.0	96	50	77	82	1 880	29.6	84	Senegal
11.9	1.4	19	98	93 [m]	93 [m]	11 430	<2.0	96	Serbia
6.7	2.2	78	92 [k]	92	95	25 740	<2.0	148	Seychelles
17.1	4.8	122	43	...	...	1 340	51.7	37	Sierra Leone
4.4	1.3	4	96	...	...	60 110	...	152	Singapore
9.4	1.4	21	...	...	...	24 770	<2.0	112	Slovakia
9.0	1.5	5	100	97	98	27 240	...	109	Slovenia
5.4	4.1	...	...	93	93	2 130	...	55	Solomon Islands
13.6	6.7	...	...	...	...	...	...	23	Somalia
11.6	2.4	54	93	90 [n]	91 [n]	11 010	13.8	131	South Africa
11.6	5.0	...	...	48 [n]	34 [n]	...	...	21	South Sudan
8.5	1.5	13	98 [p]	100	100	31 670	...	108	Spain
6.5	2.3	24	91	94	94	6 030	4.1	92	Sri Lanka
7.9	4.5	...	...	54	49	2 070	19.8	74	Sudan
4.4	2.3	66	95	92	93	8 380	...	106	Suriname
11.7	3.4	89	88	84	86	4 760	40.6	65	Swaziland
9.6	1.9	6	...	100	99	43 980	...	125	Sweden
7.7	1.5	4	...	99	100	55 090	...	130	Switzerland
6.2	3.0	...	84	100	98	5 120	...	59	Syrian Arab Republic
6.0	3.8	54	100	100	97	2 180	6.6	82	Tajikistan
7.5	1.4	47	...	96	95	9 280	<2.0	127	Thailand
9.3	1.4	20	97	98	99	11 540	<2.0	106	The former Yugoslav Republic of Macedonia
6.3	6.0	54	58	92	91	6 230	...	56	Timor-Leste
9.8	4.7	88	60	98	87	900	28.2	50	Togo
6.7	3.8	16	99	...	...	5 020	...	53	Tonga
9.4	1.8	33	99	99	98	22 860	...	141	Trinidad and Tobago
5.5	2.0	6	79	100	100	9 210	<2.0	118	Tunisia
5.7	2.1	38	94	97	96	18 190	<2.0	91	Turkey
8.7	2.4	21	100	...	...	9 070	...	76	Turkmenistan
8.7	3.1 [j]	...	...	...	...	...	...	28	Tuvalu
9.7	6.0	146	73	90	92	1 120	38.0	45	Uganda
15.1	1.5	30	100	98 [m]	99 [m]	7 180	<2.0	130	Ukraine
1.1	1.8	34	...	99 [m]	97 [m]	...	...	150	United Arab Emirates
8.9	1.9	25	...	100	100	37 340	...	135	United Kingdom
8.4	5.3	128	68 [o]	98	98	1 560	67.9	57	United Republic of Tanzania
8.4	2.0	34	...	93	93	52 610	...	95	United States of America
9.1	2.1	60	98	100	99	15 310	<2.0	147	Uruguay
6.4	2.3	26	99	93	90	3 670	...	71	Uzbekistan
4.6	3.4	...	83	...	...	4 300	...	59	Vanuatu
4.8	2.4	101	96	96	93	12 920	6.6	102	Venezuela (Bolivarian Republic of)
5.7	1.8	35	93	...	...	3 620	16.9	148	Viet Nam
6.8	4.2	...	65	95	79	2 310	17.5	58	Yemen
10.4	5.7	...	61 [o]	95 [n]	96 [n]	1 590	74.5	75	Zambia
10.1	3.6	115	84 [o]	...	...	...	...	92	Zimbabwe

Table 9

	Population[a]						Civil registration coverage (%)		Crude birth rate[a] (per 1000 population)
	Total (000s)	Median age (years)	Aged under 15 (%)	Aged over 60 (%)	Annual growth rate (%)	Living in urban areas (%)	Births[b]	Causes of death[c]	
	2012	2012	2012	2012	2002–2012	2012	2006–2012		2012

Ranges of country values

Minimum	1	15	13	1	−2.7	11	3	4	7.0
Median	7 790	27	29	9	1.3	56	>90	98	20.1
Maximum	1 384 770	46	50	32	11.8	100	100	100	49.8

WHO region

African Region	892 529	19	43	5	2.6	39	...	...	37.6
Region of the Americas	956 779	32	24	14	1.1	80	...	...	16.3
South-East Asia Region	1 833 359	27	29	8	1.3	34	...	...	19.9
European Region	904 484	38	17	20	0.3	71	...	...	12.4
Eastern Mediterranean Region	612 372	23	33	6	2.1	49	...	...	25.6
Western Pacific Region	1 844 750	35	19	14	0.7	55	...	...	13.9

Income group

Low income	846 347	20	39	6	2.2	28	...	...	32.4
Lower middle income	2 501 846	25	31	8	1.5	39	...	...	23.4
Upper middle income	2 429 452	32	21	12	0.8	61	...	...	15.5
High income	1 266 627	40	17	22	0.6	80	...	...	11.7

Global

Global	7 044 272	30	26	11	1.2	53	...	...	19.6

[a] World Population Prospects: the 2012 Revision. New York: Population Division, Department of Economic and Social Affairs, United Nations Secretariat; 2013.

[b] *UNICEF Global Databases 2014.* Based on DHS, MICS, other nationally representative surveys, censuses and vital registration systems, 2005–2012. First published in: Every Child's Birth Right. Inequities and trends in birth registration. New York: UNICEF; 2013. The standard definition includes the percentage of children under 5 years of age who were registered at the moment of the survey. The numerator of this indicator includes children whose birth certificate was seen by the interviewer, or whose mother or carer said that the birth had been registered.

[c] Mortality data [online database]. Geneva: World Health Organization; 2014 (http://www.who.int/healthinfo/statistics/mortality/en/).

[d] 2013 Update for the MDG Database: Adolescent Birth Rate. New York: United Nations, Department of Economic and Social Affairs, Population Division; 2013 (http://www.un.org/en/development/desa/population/publications/dataset/fertility/data/2013_Update_MDG(5.4)_ABR.xls). WHO regional, income-group and global figures refer to 2010. If country-level data were not available for 2010, linear interpolation between the closest data points on both sides of the year was used. In other cases, the closest data point was used.

[e] Data centre. Montreal: UNESCO Institute for Statistics; February 2014 update (http://www.uis.unesco.org/Pages/DataCentre.aspx). WHO regional and income averages are estimated using different techniques based upon the type of data most recently available. For an explanation of methods see: http://www.uis.unesco.org/Education/Pages/FAQ.aspx#theme3.

[f] PPP int. $ = Purchasing Power Parity at international dollar rate. World development indicators database [online database]. Washington, DC: World Bank; 2014 (http://data.worldbank.org/, accessed 10 January 2014). The income-group aggregates

relate only to WHO Member States and therefore may differ from those reported in the World development indicators database.

[g] World development indicators database [online database]. Washington, DC: World Bank; 2014 (http://data.worldbank.org/, accessed 10 January 2014). These figures reflect the World Bank default poverty line.

[h] World telecommunication/ICT indicators database 2013 [online database]. Geneva: International Telecommunication Union; 18th Edition (http://www.itu.int/en/ITU-D/Statistics/Pages/stat/default.aspx, accessed 10 January 2014).

[i] Demographic Yearbook 2012. New York: United Nations Statistics Division, 2012 (http://unstats.un.org/unsd/Demographic/Products/dyb/dyb2012.htm, accessed 14 January 2014). Countries with the code "C" as noted in above source table are represented here as > 90.

[j] International data base (IDB) [online database]. Washington, DC: United States Census Bureau; 2014 (http://www.census.gov/population/international/data/idb/informationGateway.php, accessed 6 January 2014).

[k] Literacy rates are estimates for current decade based on survey or census data from previous decade.

[l] Data differ from the standard definition or refer to only part of a country.

[m] National estimation.

[n] Figure estimated by UNESCO Institute for Statistics (UIS).

[o] Data based on a reading test in a national household survey. A reading test typically yields lower literacy rates than the self- or household declaration used in most censuses and surveys. Care should be taken when analysing trends over time and in interpreting the results.

[p] Literacy rates refer to the population aged 16 years and over.

Crude death rate[c] (per 1000 population)	Total fertility rate[a] (per woman)	MDG 5 Adolescent fertility rate[d] (per 1000 girls aged 15–19 years)	Literacy rate among adults aged ≥15 years[e] (%)	MDG 2 Net primary school enrolment rate[e] (%)		Gross national income per capita[f] (PPP int. $)	MDG 1 Population living on <$1 (PPP int. $) a day[g] (%)	MDG 8 Cellular phone subscribers[h] (per 100 population)	
				Male	Female				
2012	2012	2006–2011	2006–2012	2006–2012		2012	2006–2012	2012	
1.1	1.3	1	25	36	32	390	<2.0	5	Minimum
7.6	2.4	38	90	95	95	7 995	7.7	101	Median
17.1	7.6	229	100	100	100	66 960	87.7	187	Maximum
10.4	5.0	114	60	81	77	2 594	51.5	61	African Region
6.7	2.1	65	94	95	96	27 457	5.1	104	Region of the Americas
7.5	2.4	48	70	85	76	4 054	29.6	75	South-East Asia Region
10.2	1.7	23	99	98	97	26 352	…	129	European Region
6.5	3.2	37	70	97	97	3 992	11.2	87	Eastern Mediterranean Region
7.0	1.8	13	95	97	97	11 575	12.4	90	Western Pacific Region
8.8	4.1	111	61	97	98	1 369	49.1	47	Low income
7.9	2.9	49	71	84	80	3 914	28.2	83	Lower middle income
6.9	1.9	32	94	91	89	10 298	8.7	92	Upper middle income
9.1	1.7	21	…	97	96	38 562	…	122	High income
7.9	2.5	49	84	92	90	12 018	21.5	89	Global

Table 9

Annex 1.
Regional and income groupings

WHO regional groupings[1]

WHO African Region: Algeria, Angola, Benin, Botswana, Burkina Faso, Burundi, Cabo Verde, Cameroon, Central African Republic, Chad, Comoros, Congo, Côte d'Ivoire, Democratic Republic of the Congo, Equatorial Guinea, Eritrea*, Ethiopia, Gabon, Gambia, Ghana, Guinea, Guinea-Bissau, Kenya, Lesotho, Liberia, Madagascar, Malawi, Mali, Mauritania, Mauritius, Mozambique, Namibia, Niger, Nigeria, Rwanda, Sao Tome and Principe, Senegal, Seychelles, Sierra Leone, South Africa, Swaziland, Togo, Uganda, United Republic of Tanzania, Zambia, Zimbabwe.

WHO Region of the Americas: Antigua and Barbuda, Argentina, Bahamas, Barbados, Belize, Bolivia (Plurinational State of), Brazil, Canada, Chile, Colombia, Costa Rica, Cuba, Dominica, Dominican Republic, Ecuador, El Salvador, Grenada, Guatemala, Guyana, Haiti, Honduras, Jamaica, Mexico, Nicaragua, Panama, Paraguay, Peru, Saint Kitts and Nevis, Saint Lucia, Saint Vincent and the Grenadines, Suriname, Trinidad and Tobago, United States of America, Uruguay, Venezuela (Bolivarian Republic of).

WHO South-East Asia Region: Bangladesh, Bhutan, Democratic People's Republic of Korea, India, Indonesia, Maldives, Myanmar, Nepal, Sri Lanka, Thailand, Timor-Leste*.

WHO European Region: Albania, Andorra*, Armenia*, Austria, Azerbaijan*, Belarus, Belgium, Bosnia and Herzegovina*, Bulgaria, Croatia*, Cyprus, Czech Republic*, Denmark, Estonia*, Finland, France, Georgia*, Germany, Greece, Hungary, Iceland, Ireland, Israel, Italy, Kazakhstan*, Kyrgyzstan*, Latvia*, Lithuania*, Luxembourg, Malta, Monaco, Montenegro*, Netherlands, Norway, Poland, Portugal, Republic of Moldova*, Romania, Russian Federation, San Marino, Serbia*, Slovakia*, Slovenia*, Spain, Sweden, Switzerland, Tajikistan*, The former Yugoslav Republic of Macedonia*, Turkey, Turkmenistan*, Ukraine, United Kingdom, Uzbekistan*.

WHO Eastern Mediterranean Region: Afghanistan, Bahrain, Djibouti, Egypt, Iran (Islamic Republic of), Iraq, Jordan, Kuwait, Lebanon, Libya, Morocco, Oman, Pakistan, Qatar, Saudi Arabia, Somalia, South Sudan*[2], Sudan, Syrian Arab Republic, Tunisia, United Arab Emirates, Yemen.

WHO Western Pacific Region: Australia, Brunei Darussalam, Cambodia, China, Cook Islands, Fiji, Japan, Kiribati, Lao People's Democratic Republic, Malaysia, Marshall Islands*, Micronesia (Federated States of)*, Mongolia, Nauru*, New Zealand, Niue*, Palau*, Papua New Guinea, Philippines, Republic of Korea, Samoa, Singapore, Solomon Islands, Tonga, Tuvalu*, Vanuatu, Viet Nam.

---

[1]. WHO regional groupings as of December 2012, which corresponds to the most recent reference year for the majority of the statistics presented in this publication. Member States indicated with an * may have data for periods prior to their official membership of WHO.

[2]. South Sudan was reassigned to the WHO African Region in May 2013. As the majority of the statistics presented in this publication relate to time periods prior to this date, data for South Sudan are included in the figures given for the WHO Eastern Mediterranean Region, unless otherwise noted.

Income groupings[1,2]

Low income: Afghanistan, Bangladesh, Benin, Burkina Faso, Burundi, Cambodia, Central African Republic, Chad, Comoros, Democratic People's Republic of Korea, Democratic Republic of the Congo, Eritrea, Ethiopia, Gambia, Guinea, Guinea-Bissau, Haiti, Kenya, Kyrgyzstan, Liberia, Madagascar, Malawi, Mali, Mozambique, Myanmar, Nepal, Niger, Rwanda, Sierra Leone, Somalia, South Sudan, Tajikistan, Togo, Uganda, United Republic of Tanzania, Zimbabwe.

Lower middle income: Armenia, Bhutan, Bolivia (Plurinational State of), Cabo Verde, Cameroon, Congo, Côte d'Ivoire, Djibouti, Egypt, El Salvador, Georgia, Ghana, Guatemala, Guyana, Honduras, India, Indonesia, Kiribati, Lao People's Democratic Republic, Lesotho, Mauritania, Micronesia (Federated States of), Mongolia, Morocco, Nicaragua, Nigeria, Pakistan, Papua New Guinea, Paraguay, Philippines, Republic of Moldova, Samoa, Sao Tome and Principe, Senegal, Solomon Islands, Sri Lanka, Sudan, Swaziland, Syrian Arab Republic, Timor-Leste, Ukraine, Uzbekistan, Vanuatu, Viet Nam, Yemen, Zambia.

Upper middle income: Albania, Algeria, Angola, Argentina, Azerbaijan, Belarus, Belize, Bosnia and Herzegovina, Botswana, Brazil, Bulgaria, China, Colombia, Cook Islands**, Costa Rica, Cuba, Dominica, Dominican Republic, Ecuador, Fiji, Gabon, Grenada, Hungary, Iran (Islamic Republic of), Iraq, Jamaica, Jordan, Kazakhstan, Lebanon, Libya, Malaysia, Maldives, Marshall Islands, Mauritius, Mexico, Montenegro, Namibia, Nauru**, Niue**, Palau, Panama, Peru, Romania, Saint Lucia, Saint Vincent and the Grenadines, Serbia, Seychelles, South Africa, Suriname, Thailand, The former Yugoslav Republic of Macedonia, Tonga, Tunisia, Turkey, Turkmenistan, Tuvalu, Venezuela (Bolivarian Republic of).

High income: Andorra, Antigua and Barbuda, Australia, Austria, Bahamas, Bahrain, Barbados, Belgium, Brunei Darussalam, Canada, Chile, Croatia, Cyprus, Czech Republic, Denmark, Equatorial Guinea, Estonia, Finland, France, Germany, Greece, Iceland, Ireland, Israel, Italy, Japan, Kuwait, Latvia, Lithuania, Luxembourg, Malta, Monaco, Netherlands, New Zealand, Norway, Oman, Poland, Portugal, Qatar, Republic of Korea, Russian Federation, Saint Kitts and Nevis, San Marino, Saudi Arabia, Singapore, Slovakia, Slovenia, Spain, Sweden, Switzerland, Trinidad and Tobago, United Arab Emirates, United Kingdom, United States of America, Uruguay.

---

[1] World Bank analytical income of economies for fiscal year 2014 (July 2013). Washington, DC: World Bank; 2013 (http://siteresources.worldbank.orgDATASTATISTICS/Resources/OGHIST.xls).

[2] Member States marked with an ** have been classified into income groups using gross domestic product.